T0074447

MEN'S HEALTH CONCERNS

SOURCEBOOK

SEVENTH EDITION

Health Reference Series

MEN'S HEALTH CONCERNS
SOURCEBOOK

SEVENTH EDITION

Provides Basic Consumer Health Information about Issues in Men's Health, Including Information about Gender-Specific Health Differences, Male-Linked Genetic Disorders, Mental Health Concerns, Reproductive and Sexual Health, Injuries due to Accidents and Violence, and Other Health Concerns of Special Significance to Men

Along with Information about the Screenings and Self-Examinations Recommended for Men; Guidelines for Nutrition, Physical Activities, Weight Control, Vaccinations, and Other Lifestyle Choices That Affect Wellness; a Glossary of Terms Related to Men's Health; and a Directory of Resources for Further Help and Information

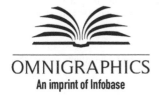

OMNIGRAPHICS
An imprint of Infobase

Bibliographic Note

Because this page cannot legibly accommodate all the copyright notices,
the Bibliographic Note portion of the Preface constitutes an extension
of the copyright notice.

* * *

OMNIGRAPHICS

An imprint of Infobase
132 W. 31st St.
New York, NY 10001
www.infobase.com
James Chambers, *Editorial Director*

* * *

Library of Congress Cataloging-in-Publication Data

Names: Chambers, James (Editor), editor.

Title: Men's health concerns sourcebook / edited by James Chambers.

Description: Seventh edition. | New York: Omnigraphics, An imprint of Infobase, [2023] | Series: Health reference series | Provides Basic Consumer Health Information about Issues in Men's Health, Including Information about Gender-Specific Health Differences, Male-Linked Genetic Disorders, Mental Health Concerns, Reproductive and Sexual Health, Accidents, Violence, and Other Health Concerns of Special Significance to Men, Along with Information about the Screenings and SelfExaminations Recommended for Men; Guidelines for Nutrition, Physical Activity, Weight Control, Vaccinations, and Other Lifestyle Choices That Affect Wellness; a Glossary of Terms Related to Men's Health; and a Directory of Resources for Further Help and Information. | Summary: "Provides basic consumer health information about health conditions of concern to men, along with tips for maintaining physical and mental wellness. Includes index, glossary of related terms, and other resources"-- Provided by publisher.

Identifiers: LCCN 2023030055 (print) | LCCN 2023030056 (ebook) | ISBN 9780780820524 (library binding) | ISBN 9780780820531 (ebook)

Subjects: LCSH: Men--Health and hygiene--Popular works.

Classification: LCC RA776.5.M457 2023 (print) | LCC RA776.5 (ebook) | DDC 613/.04234--dc23/eng/20230710

LC record available at https://lccn.loc.gov/2023030055
LC ebook record available at https://lccn.loc.gov/2023030056

Table of Contents

Part 4. Accidents, Violence, and Other Health Concerns

Part 5. Healthy Lifestyle Choices

Part 6. Additional Help and Information

Preface

ABOUT THIS BOOK

In recent years, the gap in life expectancy between men and women has started to narrow. However, men still encounter various health disparities. Men are more prone to smoking, excessive drinking, engaging in risky behaviors, and postponing essential checkups and preventative care. Men also face several disorders specific to their gender, including prostate cancer, penile and testicular disorders, low testosterone levels, and sex-related genetic disorders.

Men's Health Concerns Sourcebook, Seventh Edition discusses health issues that disproportionately affect men. It explains how men can protect themselves and maintain their health with self-examinations and screening tests. It offers detailed information about diseases that primarily impact men, their sexual and reproductive health, prostate disorders, and mental health concerns. Additionally, it provides facts about alcohol and drug use as well as injuries resulting from accidents and other health-related issues and explains how men can avoid them or lessen their impact. Lifestyle choices, nutrition, physical activities, and details about vaccinations for men are also covered. A glossary of terms related to men's health and a list of resources provide additional help and information.

HOW TO USE THIS BOOK

This book is divided into parts and chapters. Parts focus on broad areas of interest. Chapters are devoted to single topics within a part.

Part 1: Men's Health: An Overview provides fundamental information about differences in men's and women's health, screening tests, and self-examinations that are recommended for men.

Part 2: Common Medical Issues in Men discusses male-linked genetic disorders, including conditions such as color vision deficiency, hemophilia, and muscular dystrophy (MD). It also explores prevalent health risks that greatly affect men, including heart disease, cancer, diabetes, Alzheimer disease (AD), liver and kidney disease, chronic obstructive pulmonary disease (COPD), respiratory illnesses, and mental health disorders. Furthermore, it addresses men's health concerns related to conditions traditionally associated with women, such as breast cancer and osteoporosis.

Part 3: Sexual and Reproductive Health provides information about conditions that affect male reproductive organs, including prostate disorders, disorders of the scrotum and testicles, circumcision, penile concerns, and male menopause. It offers guidance on managing sexual dysfunction and male infertility. It also includes information about birth control methods, sexually transmitted diseases (STDs), and practices for safer sex.

Part 4: Accidents, Violence, and Other Health Concerns addresses prevalent injuries and accidents, often linked to fatalities in men. This includes motor vehicle accidents, falls, occupational injuries, and suicide. The part concludes with information on the consumption of alcohol, tobacco, and drugs, as well as the prevalence of body image issues that can result in eating disorders among men.

Part 5: Healthy Lifestyle Choices provides information on vaccinations recommended for men and offers guidance on managing common disease risk factors. It includes tips on weight management, nutrition, and physical activity to help men maintain a healthy lifestyle.

Part 6: Additional Help and Information includes a glossary of terms related to men's health and a directory of resources offering additional help and support for men's health concerns.

BIBLIOGRAPHIC NOTE

This volume contains documents and excerpts from publications issued by the following U.S. government agencies: Administration for Children and Families (ACF); Centers for Disease Control and Prevention (CDC); Centers for Medicare & Medicaid Services (CMS); Effective Health Care Program; *Eunice Kennedy Shriver* National Institute of Child Health and Human Development (NICHD); HIVinfo; MedlinePlus; National Cancer Institute (NCI); National Center for Posttraumatic Stress Disorder (NCPTSD); National Eye Institute (NEI); National Heart, Lung, and Blood Institute (NHLBI); National Highway Traffic Safety Administration (NHTSA); National Institute of Arthritis and Musculoskeletal and Skin

Diseases (NIAMS); National Institute of Dental and Craniofacial Research (NIDCR); National Institute of Diabetes and Digestive and Kidney Diseases (NIDDK); National Institute of Mental Health (NIMH); National Institute of Neurological Disorders and Stroke (NINDS); National Institute on Aging (NIA); National Institute on Drug Abuse (NIDA); *NIH News in Health*; Office of Disease Prevention and Health Promotion (ODPHP); Office of Population Affairs (OPA); Office of Research on Women's Health (ORWH); Substance Abuse and Mental Health Services Administration (SAMHSA); Surveillance, Epidemiology, and End Results (SEER) Program; U.S. Bureau of Labor Statistics (BLS); U.S. Department of Health and Human Services (HHS); U.S. Department of Veterans Affairs (VA); U.S. Drug Enforcement Administration (DEA); U.S. Fire Administration (USFA); U.S. Food and Drug Administration (FDA); U.S. Office of Personnel Management (OPM); and Vaccines.gov.

It also contains original material produced by Infobase and reviewed by medical consultants.

ABOUT THE *HEALTH REFERENCE SERIES*

The *Health Reference Series* is designed to provide basic medical information for patients, families, caregivers, and the general public. Each volume provides comprehensive coverage on a particular topic. This is especially important for people who may be dealing with a newly diagnosed disease or a chronic disorder in themselves or in a family member. People looking for preventive guidance, information about disease warning signs, medical statistics, and risk factors for health problems will also find answers to their questions in the *Health Reference Series*. The *Series*, however, is not intended to serve as a tool for diagnosing illness, in prescribing treatments, or as a substitute for the physician–patient relationship. All people concerned about medical symptoms or the possibility of disease are encouraged to seek professional care from an appropriate health-care provider.

A NOTE ABOUT SPELLING AND STYLE

Health Reference Series editors use *Stedman's Medical Dictionary* as an authority for questions related to the spelling of medical terms and *The Chicago Manual of Style* for questions related to grammatical structures, punctuation, and other editorial concerns. Consistent adherence is not always possible, however, because the individual volumes within the *Series* include many documents from a wide variety of different producers, and the editor's primary goal is to present material from each source as accurately as is possible. This sometimes means that information in different chapters or sections may follow other guidelines and alternate spelling authorities. For example, occasionally a copyright holder may require that eponymous terms be shown in possessive forms (Crohn's disease vs. Crohn disease) or that British spelling norms be retained (leukaemia vs. leukemia).

MEDICAL REVIEW
Infobase contracts with a team of qualified, senior medical professionals who serve as medical consultants for the *Health Reference Series*. As necessary, medical consultants review reprinted and originally written material for currency and accuracy. Medical consultation services are provided to the *Health Reference Series* editors by:

Dr. Vijayalakshmi, MBBS, DGO, MD
Dr. Senthil Selvan, MBBS, DCH, MD
Dr. K. Sivanandham, MBBS, DCH, MS (Research), PhD

HEALTH REFERENCE SERIES UPDATE POLICY
The inaugural book in the *Health Reference Series* was the first edition of *Cancer Sourcebook* published in 1989. Since then, the *Series* has been enthusiastically received by librarians and in the medical community. In order to maintain the standard of providing high-quality health information for the layperson, the editorial staff felt it was necessary to implement a policy of updating volumes when warranted.

Medical researchers have been making tremendous strides, and it is the purpose of the *Health Reference Series* to stay current with the most recent advances. Each decision to update a volume is made on an individual basis. Some of the considerations include how much new information is available and the feedback we receive from people who use the books. If there is a topic you would like to see added to the update list, or an area of medical concern you feel has not been adequately addressed, please write to: custserv@infobaselearning.com.

Part 1 | Men's Health: An Overview

Chapter 1 | **Healthy Men, Healthy Families**

Although one generally does not think of being a dad or a dad-to-be as a health issue, there is no question that it is. Just like taking the car in for an oil change or for the 25,000-mile checkup, dads also need to take themselves to the doctor's office to make sure everything is running smoothly.

However, there are still men who ask what their health has to do with their family. Plenty! Men's health issues rarely affect only the male. Many of the health issues men face are silently taking their toll on the entire family unit.

Why do our fathers, sons, brothers, and husbands continue to suffer, you ask? First, we must recognize the factors that impact men's attitudes, which lead to risky health behaviors. The reasons are manifold, including a lack of awareness, poor health education, and culturally induced behavior patterns in their work and personal lives. The end result is men's health and well-being are deteriorating steadily.

On average, men are less healthy and have a shorter life expectancy than women. They are also less likely to have health insurance, receive health screenings, or attend regular medical checkups. And, because women live longer than men, they see their fathers, brothers, sons, husbands, and partners suffer or die prematurely.

These factors have led to men suffering in higher death rates in 9 of the top 10 causes of death, which include cardiovascular disease (CVD), cancer, diabetes, and unintentional injuries. Fortunately, women and children are in a unique position to be able to help fight the obstacles men face in getting the health care they need.

It is true! Moms, wives, partners, and children can make a difference. Although most men are taught from an early age to cope quietly, their loved ones can initiate changes that will benefit the entire family. Encourage the men in your life to get regular checkups and age-appropriate screenings. Regular checkups improve health and extend life.

Research shows that children with healthy, involved fathers do better in school, are more likely to graduate high school, have more friends, have fewer psychological problems, and are less likely to smoke, abuse drugs or alcohol, engage in risky behavior, start having sex early, or become teen parents. Start working together as a family today so that you can enjoy the many Father's Days to come.

Please do your part to end the silence and remind men to stay healthy. By encouraging the men in your life to take even the smallest symptoms seriously and discuss them with their health-care providers, you will be helping them take a more active role in their own health care. And, by educating yourself about men's health issues and passing that information on to your loved ones, you may also be able to save a life and preserve a family.[1]

HOW CAN YOU TAKE CHARGE OF YOUR HEALTH?

See a doctor for regular checkups even if you feel healthy. This is important because some diseases and health conditions do not have symptoms at first. Plus, seeing a doctor will give you a chance to learn more about your health.

Here are some more things you can do to take care of your health:

- Eat healthy and get active.
- If you drink alcohol, drink only in moderation.
- Quit smoking.

---

[1] Administration for Children and Families (ACF), "Healthy Men, Healthy Families," U.S. Department of Health and Human Services (HHS), June 11, 2013. Available online. URL: www.acf.hhs.gov/archive/blog/2013/06/healthy-men-healthy-families. Accessed June 9, 2023.

- Know your family's health history.
- Get screening tests to check for health problems before you have symptoms.
- Make sure you are up-to-date on your vaccines (shots).[2]

---

[2] Office of Disease Prevention and Health Promotion (ODPHP), "Men: Take Charge of Your Health," U.S. Department of Health and Human Services (HHS), December 22, 2022. Available online. URL: https://health.gov/myhealthfinder/doctor-visits/regular-checkups/men-take-charge-your-health#the-basics-tab. Accessed June 22, 2023.

Chapter 2 | **Statistical Overview of Men's Health**

HEALTH STATUS

The percentage of men aged 18 and over in fair or poor health was 13.6 percent in 2021 (see Table 2.1).

Table 2.1. Percentage of Fair or Poor Health Status for Adults Aged 18 and Over, United States, 2019–2022

Year	Fair or Poor Health Status (%)
2019	15.3
2020	13.8
2021	13.6
2022	14.5

PHYSICAL ACTIVITY

In 2020, the percentage of men aged 18 and over who met the 2018 federal physical activity guidelines for aerobic and muscle-strengthening activity was 28.3 percent (see Figure 2.1).

Other key indicators of men's health include:

- **Alcohol use**. The percentage of men aged 18 and over who had five or more drinks in one day at least once in the past year was 30.9 percent in 2018.
- **Health insurance coverage**. The percentage of men under age 65 without health insurance coverage was 11.5 percent in 2022.

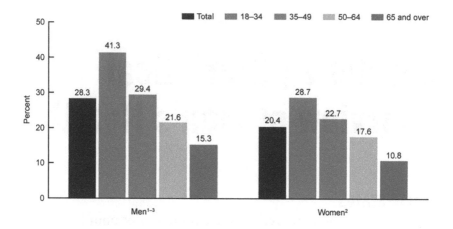

Figure 2.1. Percentage of Adults Aged 18 and Over Who Met 2018 Physical Activity Guidelines for Americans for Aerobic and Muscle-Strengthening Activities, by Sex and Age: United States, 2020

Centers for Disease Control and Prevention (CDC)

- **Hypertension**. The percentage of men aged 20 and over with hypertension (measured high blood pressure and/or taking antihypertensive medication) between 2015 and 2018 was 51.9 percent.
- **Obesity**. The percentage of men aged 20 and over with obesity between 2015 and 2018 was 40.5 percent.
- **Smoking**. The percentage of men aged 18 and over who currently smoke cigarettes was 13.1 percent in 2021 (see Table 2.2).

Table 2.2. Percentage of Current Cigarette Smoking for Adults Aged 18 and Over, United States, 2019–2022

Year	Current Cigarette Smoking (%)
2019	14
2020	12.5
2021	11.5
2022	11.6

MORTALITY

The Centers for Disease Control and Prevention (CDC) reported on men's deaths due to any underlying cause between 2018 and 2021 and noted the following data:

- number of deaths (all ages): 1,838,108
- deaths per 100,000 population: 1,118.2

Table 2.3 shows the mortality rate per 100,000 population.

Table 2.3. Mortality Data (2021)

Gender	Deaths	Population	Crude Rate per 100,000
Female	1,626,123	167,509,003	970.8
Male	1,838,108	164,384,742	1,118.20
Total	3,464,231	331,893,745	1,043.80

LEADING CAUSES OF DEATH

Among the top causes of death in men are:

- heart disease
- cancer
- COVID-19

Table 2.4 lists the leading causes of death in men in the United States.

Table 2.4. Fifteen Leading Causes of Death[1]

15 Leading Causes of Death	Deaths	Population	Crude Rate per 100,000
Diseases of heart	384,886	164,384,742	234.1
Malignant neoplasms	318,670	164,384,742	193.9
COVID-19	236,610	164,384,742	143.9
Accidents (unintentional injuries)	149,602	164,384,742	91

[1] "Men's Health," Centers for Disease Control and Prevention (CDC), May 16, 2023. Available online. URL: www.cdc.gov/nchs/fastats/mens-health.htm. Accessed June 9, 2023.

Table 2.4. Continued

15 Leading Causes of Death	Deaths	Population	Crude Rate per 100,000
Cerebrovascular diseases	70,852	164,384,742	43.1
Chronic lower respiratory diseases	67,528	164,384,742	41.1
Diabetes mellitus	58,628	164,384,742	35.7
Intentional self-harm (suicide)	38,358	164,384,742	23.3
Alzheimer disease	36,975	164,384,742	22.5
Chronic liver disease and cirrhosis	35,707	164,384,742	21.7
Nephritis, nephrotic syndrome, and nephrosis	28,589	164,384,742	17.4
Parkinson disease	23,567	164,384,742	14.3
Influenza and pneumonia	22,373	164,384,742	13.6
Assault (homicide)	21,084	164,384,742	12.8
Septicemia	20,529	164,384,742	12.5

Chapter 3 | Sex-Specific Health Differences

Chapter Contents

Section 3.1 | Why Do Men Have Shorter Life Spans than Women?

Although social and lifestyle factors are believed to play a role in adult mortality rates, evidence suggests that biological and genetic factors are also involved. Significantly, studies have found gender-related differences in life expectancy among other primates—female gorillas, chimpanzees, and orangutans consistently outlive males of their species as well. By studying the various factors that may account for increased female longevity, scientists hope that they will identify ways to help both men and women live longer, healthier lives.

BIOLOGICAL FACTORS

Biologists have put forth a number of theories to explain why women live longer than men. Some of the major genetic and biological factors they believe may contribute to increased female longevity include the following:

- **Women carry two X chromosomes, while men have one X and one Y chromosome**. This biological difference means that men are more vulnerable to genetic mutations that can cause life-threatening health conditions. While women may avoid the expression of genetic diseases by relying on a normal gene in the other X chromosome, men lack a second copy of the defective gene.
- **Women's bodies tend to be smaller in size than men's bodies**. Since larger people have more cells in their bodies, they may have a greater tendency to develop harmful cellular mutations. In addition, larger bodies use more energy, which creates wear and tear on organs and tissues and may increase the rate of long-term damage.
- **Women's immune system function declines at a slower rate than men's**. All people's immune function gradually declines with age. But blood samples of

healthy people have shown that the normal loss of
white blood cells—which help protect the body from
infection—occurs faster in men than in women. As a
result, women may enjoy protection from illness to a
more advanced age.

- **The male hormone testosterone may increase disease
  risk later in life.** Testosterone, which is secreted by
  the testicles, is the hormone primarily responsible for
  the development of male sex traits, such as deep voices
  and hairy chests. Although testosterone contributes to
  male strength and virility, it may also increase men's
  risk of developing cardiovascular disease and cancer
  later in life.

- **The female hormone estrogen may decrease disease
  risk later in life.** Estrogen, which is produced in the
  ovaries, is the hormone primarily responsible for
  female sex traits, such as breast development and
  menstruation. In contrast to testosterone, estrogen
  appears to protect against disease. Estrogen has
  antioxidant properties, meaning that it helps eliminate
  harmful chemicals that may cause cell damage. Studies
  have shown that when the ovaries are removed from
  female animals, the animals experience an increase in
  disease risk and a decrease in longevity.

- **Women develop heart disease a decade later than
  men.** Heart disease is the leading cause of death for
  both men and women in the United States. But, partly
  due to the protective effects of estrogen, which helps
  control cholesterol and prevent plaque formation in
  the arteries, women tend to develop heart disease
  10 years later than men. In fact, women's risk of heart
  disease only begins to increase after menopause when
  the production of estrogen declines. In addition,
  more than four times as many men as women smoke
  worldwide, and smoking is a major contributor to heart
  disease. Another theory to explain the delayed onset
  of cardiovascular illness in women is that women's
  heart rate tends to increase during the second half of

the menstrual cycle. Some researchers claim that this increase offers the same health benefits as moderate exercise.

LIFESTYLE FACTORS

In addition to the biological differences between men and women, studies have also suggested that sociological and lifestyle factors may contribute to women's longer life span. Some of the main factors that are believed to influence mortality rates include the following:

- **Men are more prone to risk-taking behavior.** According to the U.S. Centers for Disease Control and Prevention (CDC), unintentional injuries are the third leading cause of death for American men. For women, on the other hand, unintentional injuries rank sixth. Scientists point out that the frontal lobe of the brain develops more slowly in males than in females. Since this part of the brain is involved in calculating risks and behaving responsibly, men are more likely to exhibit dangerous or risky behavior than women of the same age. As a result, studies show that men are less likely to wear seat belts and more likely to drive aggressively and be involved in motor vehicle accidents.
- **Women have stronger social networks**. Men are often socialized to hide their emotions and keep their concerns bottled up inside. For women, however, it is more culturally acceptable to express emotions and confide in friends or family members about sources of worry or stress. Studies have shown that strong social connections can decrease a person's risk of dying by 50 percent. Men can experience the protective nature of social ties by getting married—studies have also shown that married men tend to be healthier and live longer than single men.
- **Women take better care of their health**. Another contributing factor to women's longevity is that they tend to take better care of their health. Men often

ignore or deny symptoms of illness and avoid seeking medical attention. In fact, studies have shown that men are 24 percent less likely than women to have visited a doctor within the past year.

References

Bergland, Christopher. "Why Do Women Live Longer Than Men?" *Psychology Today*, July 8, 2015. Available online. URL: www.psychologytoday.com/blog/the-athletes-way/201507/why-do-women-live-longer-men. Accessed August 7, 2023.

Innes, Emma. "Women Live Longer than Men Because Their Immune Systems Age More Slowly," MailOnline, May 15, 2013. Available online. URL: www.dailymail.co.uk/health/article-2324783/Women-live-longer-men-immune-systems-age-slowly.html. Accessed August 7, 2023.

Zeilinger, Julie. "The Real Reason Women Live Longer than Men?" *Huffington Post*, August 3, 2013. Available online. URL: www.huffingtonpost.in/entry/why-women-live-longer-than-men_n_3696114. Accessed August 7, 2023.

Section 3.2 | Influence of Gender on Health and Disease

SEX AND GENDER

Are you male or female? The answer to this seemingly simple question can have a major impact on your health. While both sexes are similar in many ways, researchers have found that sex and social factors can make a difference when it comes to your risk for disease, how well you respond to medications, and how often you seek medical care. That is why scientists are taking a closer look at the links between sex, gender, and health.

Many people use the words "sex" and "gender" interchangeably, but they are distinct concepts to scientists.

Defining Differences

Sex is biological. It is based on your genetic makeup. Males have one X and one Y chromosome in every cell of the body. Females have two X chromosomes in every cell. These cells make up all your tissues and organs, including your skin, heart, stomach, muscles, and brain.

Gender is a social or cultural concept. It refers to the roles, behaviors, and identities that society assigns to girls and boys, women and men, and gender-diverse people. Gender is determined by how we see ourselves and each other and how we act and interact with others.

There is a lot of diversity in how individuals and groups understand, experience, and express gender. Because gender influences our behaviors and relationships, it can also affect health.

Influences on Health

"Sex and gender play a role in how health and disease affect individuals. There was a time when we studied men and applied those findings to women, but we've learned that there are distinct biological differences between women and men," explains Dr. Janine Austin Clayton, who heads research on women's health at the National Institutes of Health (NIH). "Women and men have different hormones, different organs, and different cultural influences—all of which can lead to differences in health."

As scientists learn more about the biology of males and females, they are uncovering the influences of both sex and gender in many areas of health.

For instance, women and men can have different symptoms during a heart attack. For both men and women, the most common heart attack symptom is chest pain or discomfort. But women are more likely than men to have shortness of breath, nausea and vomiting, fatigue, and pain in the back, shoulders, and jaw. Knowing about such differences can lead to better diagnoses and outcomes.

Men and women also tend to have different responses to pain. The NIH-funded researchers recently learned that different cells in male and female mice drive pain processing. "Without studying both sexes, we wouldn't know if we're taking steps in the right direction toward appropriate clinical treatment for men and women," Dr. Clayton says. "Our differences also affect how we respond to medications, as well as which diseases and conditions we may be prone to and how those diseases progress in our bodies." For example, women metabolize nicotine faster than men, so nicotine replacement therapies can be less effective in women.

Attention to Addiction

Scientists are finding that addiction to nicotine and other drugs is influenced by sex as well. "When it comes to addiction, differences in sex and gender can be found across the board," says Dr. Sherry McKee, lead researcher at an NIH-funded center at Yale University that studies treatments for tobacco dependence. "There are different reasons men and women pick up a drug and keep using a drug, and in how they respond to treatment and experience relapse. Sex also influences disease risk in addiction. For example, women who smoke are more susceptible to lung and heart disease than men who smoke."

One NIH-funded research team has detected some of these differences in the brain. In a recent study, 16 people who smoke—eight men and eight women—underwent brain scans while smoking to create "movies" of how smoking affects dopamine, the chemical messenger that triggers feelings of pleasure in the brain.

These brain movies showed that smoking alters dopamine in the brain at different rates and in different locations in males and females.

Dopamine release in nicotine-dependent men occurred quickly in a brain area that reinforces the effect of nicotine and other drugs. Women also had a rapid response but in a different brain region— the part associated with habit formation. "We were able to pinpoint a different brain response between male and female smokers, a finding that could be useful in developing sex-specific treatments to help smokers quit," says lead study researcher Dr. Kelly Cosgrove, a brain-imaging expert at Yale University.

Finding better ways to help men and women quit smoking is important for everyone's health. More than 16 million Americans have diseases caused by smoking. It is the leading cause of preventable death in the United States.

Autoimmune Disorders

Scientists have found sex influences in autoimmune disorders as well. About 80 percent of those affected are women. But autoimmune conditions in men are often more severe. For instance, more women than men get multiple sclerosis (MS), a disease in which the body's immune system attacks the brain and spinal cord. But men seem more likely to get a progressive form of MS that gradually worsens and is more challenging to treat.

"Not only are women more susceptible to MS, but women also have many more considerations in the management of the disease, especially since it often begins during childbearing years," says Dr. Ellen Mowry, a specialist who studies MS at Johns Hopkins University.

"There are a lot of unanswered questions when it comes to the study of sex differences in MS and other autoimmune disorders," Dr. Mowry explains. "Researchers can learn a lot by studying women and men separately and together, considering possible risk or predictive factors that may differ based on sex or gender, and working collaboratively with other scientists to improve the likelihood of detecting these factors."[1]

ALCOHOL USE

Drinking alcohol is a common activity in most cultures around the world, for both women and men. However, while drinking in moderation may be considered generally safe, alcohol abuse poses many risks to a woman's health. For example, although men are more likely to drink alcohol than women and men often drink more and more frequently, women are more vulnerable to some of alcohol's harmful effects. These effects are based on both gender- and sex-based factors, and they include differences in metabolism.

---

[1] *NIH News in Health*, "Sex and Gender," National Institutes of Health (NIH), May 2016. Available online. URL: https://newsinhealth.nih.gov/2016/05/sex-gender. Accessed July 3, 2023.

In addition, alcohol use by women is also linked to many other physical and psychosocial health issues, such as unprotected sex, illicit drug use, and intimate partner violence (IPV). Here are some of the facts about women and alcohol use:

- Moderate, or low-risk, drinking for women is defined as no more than three drinks on any single day and no more than seven drinks per week.
- Low-to-moderate alcohol consumption in women, defined as fewer than three drinks per day, increases the risk of certain cancers, including breast cancer.
- After drinking similar amounts, women have higher blood levels of ethanol than men, and women are more susceptible to alcoholic liver disease such as hepatitis.
- A woman's moderate alcohol intake may reduce her coronary heart disease risk although details remain unclear.
- Research showed that female college student drinkers exceeded NIH-defined guidelines for weekly drinking more frequently than their male counterparts, which may have long-term consequences on drinking behavior in these women.
- The drug naltrexone is used to treat alcohol dependence, but it does not work for everyone.
- A small study showed that naltrexone worked better in women to reduce alcohol's positive subjective effects, suggesting it may be useful in therapy for alcohol dependence in women.
- Research with the model organism *Drosophila* (fruit flies) showed that female fruit flies are more prone to the sedative effects of alcohol than male flies.
- No amount of drinking during pregnancy is safe. However, 20–30 percent of women drink at some time during pregnancy, which includes the period of time before a woman knows she is pregnant.

ARRHYTHMIAS

As an electrically controlled organ, the heart beats when a wave of electricity courses through the heart muscle in a defined regular path. Any disruption of this path of conduction, called an "arrhythmia," causes the heart to beat irregularly. An arrhythmia can be very mild, even undetectable, or serious and fatal. Sex and gender differences are known to affect heart rhythms. Certain medications, including the allergy drug Seldane and the gastrointestinal drug Propulsid (both of which have been taken off the market in the United States), trigger a potentially fatal heart arrhythmia more often in women than in men.

AUTOIMMUNE DISORDERS

Thought to be one of the most complicated systems in the human body, our immune system has effects on most aspects of health and disease. It protects us from harm, such as infectious organisms, and it helps us heal through wound healing and other processes. Most of the time, our immune system does a remarkable job distinguishing outside invaders from our own cells, but sometimes, it mistakenly attacks the body's own organs, tissues, and cells. Autoimmune disorders are the result, and they appear to be on the rise.

Autoimmune disorders are a major issue in women's health because the prevalence of these conditions is much higher in women, and some are more prevalent in women who are Black, Hispanic, American Indian, Hawaiian/Pacific Islander, or Asian. More than 80 types of autoimmune conditions exist, but some examples include inflammatory bowel disease, MS, rheumatoid arthritis (RA), Sjögren syndrome, and lupus.

Estimates say that about 80 percent of those affected by autoimmune disorders are women, but a few autoimmune disorders, such as type 1 diabetes and ankylosing spondylitis, are more common in men than in women. Disease severity also differs by sex: For example, although more women get lupus and MS than men, these conditions affect males more severely.

- Researchers often study MS in mice: They get a similar condition called "experimental autoimmune encephalomyelitis" (EAE). Some of these studies are showing promise in humans, such as one small clinical trial that found a protective role for testosterone in males with MS.

21

- Certain brain regions were thinner than other brain regions in women with the painful condition irritable bowel syndrome (IBS). The changes corresponded with pain severity and did not occur in men with the disorder, suggesting that different brain mechanisms might be causing this type of pain in females and males.
- Novel transgenic mouse models can distinguish between the effects of sex hormones (such as estrogen and testosterone) and sex chromosomes (XX and XY) on disease. Scientists have learned that in mice, the female chromosome set (XX) stimulates the development of lupus.
- Gene expression in the salivary glands, which are impaired in Sjögren syndrome, differs markedly between women and men.
- Lupus flare-ups can signal preterm birth in pregnant women with a mild version of the condition.

CANCER

Cancer is often called a "disease of DNA" because tumors develop when cells divide uncontrollably, and in many cases, DNA mutations that affect the copying of DNA are to blame. Researchers today know, however, that cancers are very different from each other—almost different enough to look like a completely different health condition. In addition, as scientists learn more about the molecular roots of disease, they can classify cancers based on molecular signatures. These signatures can aid in diagnosis, treatment, and prognosis. In addition to being different from one another, the same type of cancer can be quite different in females and males. Here are a few examples:

- Some studies suggest that female cancer patients are more likely to experience inadequate pain management than male patients, but more studies are needed.
- Research comparing cell lines from women to cell lines from men reported sex differences in DNA damage to cancer-causing chemicals in tobacco smoke. For a given number of cigarettes smoked, females

appear to be at higher risk of developing lung cancer than males.

- Females are less prone to liver cancer than males (humans and mice given a liver carcinogen), possibly due to estrogen's protective effect against inflammation in the liver.

CARDIOVASCULAR RISK

For the most part, an individual has direct control over whether he or she will develop heart disease, by managing behaviors that raise or reduce the chances that heart disease will take root in their body. The NIH-funded medical research that goes back decades has defined a core set of cardiovascular risk factors that individuals can manage with the help of a doctor. The risk factors include smoking, high cholesterol and triglycerides, high blood pressure, diabetes, and being overweight or obese.

Yet, even though everyone should pay attention to these risk factors that affect heart health, the risks differ between women and men in various ways that appear subtle but can be very significant.

- In women, aspirin reduces risk of ischemic stroke, whereas in men, low-dose aspirin therapy reduces risk of heart attack.

DEPRESSION

Gender plays an important role in mental health disorders, such as depression, which is common but underdiagnosed. Epidemiological research shows that females are more likely than males to develop not only depression but also eating disorders, panic disorder, and posttraumatic stress disorder (PTSD).

INFLUENZA

Influenza, more commonly called the "flu," is a viral infection of the nose, throat, and lungs. Flu symptoms may include muscle aches, chills, cough, fever, headache, and sore throat. Research is underway to find out why the flu virus and vaccine affect men and women differently. For example, women are more likely than men to have severe flu symptoms. Here are some facts about men and women and the flu:

- Pregnant women who get the flu are more likely than women who are not pregnant to become very ill and have to go to the hospital. For this reason, doctors recommend that most pregnant women should get the flu shot.
- Women who get a half dose of the flu vaccine produce as many antibodies as men who receive a full dose.
- Men with high levels of testosterone produce fewer antibodies in response to the flu vaccine than men with low testosterone.
- The immune systems of female mice respond to the flu virus with a much stronger counterattack, known as an "inflammatory response," than those of male mice.
- When female mice are given estrogen, they have less inflammation and milder flu symptoms.

JOINTS

Sex-specific research analyses are especially important in orthopedics because of the substantial sex-based anatomical differences between females and males. Researchers are beginning to appreciate that structural differences of the knee joint and thigh muscles, differences in the ways male and female athletes move, and other sex differences help explain why women are often more susceptible to certain injuries than men. Here are some examples of sex-based factors that affect the health of joints:

- Females are two to three times more likely than males to develop patellofemoral pain syndrome, one of the most common causes of knee pain in teen and young adult athletes.
- Tears of the anterior cruciate ligament (ACL), the ligament that runs through the front of the knee, are more common in females than in males.
- Temporomandibular joint and muscle disorder–type pain is 2.25 times more prevalent in women than in men.

- Among people undergoing total hip replacement, women were 29 percent more likely than men to require repeat surgery within the first three years.
- Female college athletes have the highest risk of having a first-time noncontact ACL injury among female and male athletes in high school and college. (Noncontact injuries are caused by a person's own actions, such as landing after a jump or coming to an abrupt stop while running.)
- Women use their hamstring and quadriceps muscles differently from men when they are running and cutting from side to side during sports activities, and this puts greater stress on the knee.

LUPUS

Lupus is an autoimmune condition that causes inflammation and damage to various organs. The common symptoms include extreme fatigue, painful or swollen joints (arthritis), unexplained fever, skin rashes, hair loss, and kidney problems. Lupus develops slowly, with symptoms that come and go. The most common type, systemic lupus erythematosus (SLE), usually appears in the mid-teens, 30s, or 40s. Women are more likely to get lupus than men, and African-American, Hispanic, Asian, and American-Indian women have a higher lupus risk than White women. Here are examples of how lupus can differ in women and men:

- Although more women than men get lupus and a related disorder, systemic sclerosis, men are more likely to have more severe disease.
- In contrast, women are more likely than men to develop lupus-related urinary tract infections (UTIs), hypothyroidism, depression, esophageal reflux, asthma, and fibromyalgia.
- Among children and adults with lupus, males are at greater risk than females for kidney injury, kidney failure, and kidney-related death.
- Researchers have found a lupus-related gene (called "*IRAK1*") on the X chromosome, which may help

25

explain why women get the disease more often than men.

- Sex hormones may also have a role in making women more likely to develop lupus.

MEN'S HEALTH

As is the case with women's health, many people tend to think of men's health as it relates to the reproductive organs. However, just as in women's health, men's health is much broader. While many sex-based influences affect diseases/organs related to reproduction, such as prostate and testicular cancer, many sex-based factors influence diseases and organs unrelated to reproduction. Here are a few examples:

- Osteoporotic fractures in men over 50 are common, yet they are under-recognized and often underrated.
- SLE, or lupus, is often thought of as women's disease, yet this condition affects men, too. Moreover, males with lupus often have more severe disease than females, and they are more likely than females to experience lupus-related kidney failure.
- White male teens and young adults are 55 percent more likely to die of melanoma, the most serious type of skin cancer, than their female peers of the same age.
- Onchocerciasis, the second leading cause of infectious blindness in the world, is more common in men, who work in contaminated rivers in the developing world. Onchocerciasis is thus an example of a gender-based health disparity as it is caused by a behavior more common to males in certain societies although it is treatable with antibiotics.

OSTEOARTHRITIS

Osteoarthritis is a condition that accompanies aging, as the body's bones and joints suffer wear and tear with time and lots of use. It is painful, and there is no cure. Moreover, osteoarthritis remains the leading cause of chronic disability in the United States, and it disproportionately affects postmenopausal women. Current treatment generally involves a mix of exercise, lifestyle modification (such as weight loss), and pain relievers. Researchers are hard at work looking for new clues about how to prevent and treat osteoarthritis. It is more common among women than men in every age group, but there are subtle differences worth knowing about.

- The severity of osteoarthritis is usually significantly worse in women than it is in men.
- In women, osteoarthritis typically affects certain joints, such as the knees, hips, and/or hands.
- Before the age of 45, more men than women have osteoarthritis, but after the age of 45, the condition is more common in women.
- Black women are at a greater risk than White women for developing osteoarthritis and for experiencing complications from the condition.
- Black women and Black men with osteoarthritis are much less likely to undergo total knee replacement than White men.

PAIN

The sensation of pain is a protective response that alerts us when we are hurt or sick. Pain can be caused by injury to a specific area of the body, or it can be caused by an illness, such as the flu, that makes the whole body ache. Pain may be dull or intense; it may be constant; or it may come and go. Sometimes, the cause of the pain is unknown. Women seem to be more sensitive to pain than men. Here are some other examples of how pain is different in women and men:

- Several studies show that chronic pain is more common in women than men.
- Women experience pain from musculoskeletal, neuropathic, abdominal, and migraine-related conditions more often than men.
- Migraines are twice as common in females as in males, and the brain is affected differently in females compared with males.

- Among individuals with depression, women are more likely to report pain complaints than men.
- In imaging tests of people with IBS, brain regions that control emotions were more active in female brains, and cognitive regions were more active in male brains.
- Researchers have identified a molecular pain pathway that operates only in the spinal cords of male mice.

PRESCRIPTION PAINKILLER ABUSE

Women in America are dying from prescription drug overdoses at unprecedented rates. Most of these deaths are caused by opioids, painkillers that are chemically similar to heroin and that have similar effects in the body and can be highly addictive. Examples include OxyContin, Percocet, and Vicodin. Research has shown that males and females do not respond in similar ways to opioids. Here are some facts about sex- and gender-based differences in prescription painkiller abuse:

- Overall, men are more likely to die of a prescription painkiller overdose than women; however, since 1999, the percentage increase in deaths has been greater among women (400 percent in women compared to 265 percent in men).
- For every woman who dies of a prescription painkiller overdose, 30 go to the emergency department for painkiller misuse or abuse.
- According to the Centers for Disease Control and Prevention (CDC), the majority of people, both women and men, who misused prescription pain relievers (55%) received them free from a friend or relative; 17 percent got them using a doctor's prescription; 4 percent bought them from a drug dealer; and a small fraction (less than a 0.5%) ordered them online.
- Animal studies showed that males and females have different physiological responses to coping with opioid withdrawal, suggesting the need for gender-appropriate addiction treatment strategies.

- Studies show that overall, women and men have similar perception of pain, but that pain perception varies significantly by triggers, such as cold, hot, pressure, ischemia (RH1), or other sensation. The use of opioid drugs during pregnancy can produce drug withdrawal syndrome in newborns.

SLEEP

We spend one-third of our lives asleep: This valuable time promotes development in infants and children, cleans up waste accumulated during the body's busy waking hours, solidifies memory, and restores immune health. Sleep is regulated by the circadian clock, which in humans and many animals is controlled by the suprachiasmatic nucleus, a cluster of nerve cells in the brain. Human sleep needs vary significantly throughout life: While newborns spend 14–17 hours sleeping every day, adults need considerably less, between 7 and 9 hours. Many sex-based factors affect sleep.

- On average, women have a six-minute shorter circadian period (24 hours) than men. Although seemingly small, this difference could contribute to different sleep needs and patterns in women and men.
- Sleep deprivation raises blood pressure more strongly in women than in men.
- A study in mice showed that disrupting circadian rhythms by changing the rodents' light–dark cycle negatively affected female animals' ability to become pregnant.
- Scientists discovered sex-based differences in the sleep patterns of fruit flies, a common animal model for biomedical research. They discovered that young (but not adult) female fruit flies slept mostly at night, whereas young males slept almost as much in the middle of the day as they did at night.
- Driving performance is impaired in women but not in men the morning after taking certain sleep medications: flurazepam (30 mg, when taken at bedtime) and zolpidem (10 mg, when taken in the middle of the night).

- Hot flashes and night sweats during perimenopause and menopause affect a woman's ability to fall asleep and stay asleep.
- Obstructive sleep apnea (OSA) is more common in men than in women; however, obesity raises risk for both sexes.

SMOKING

Tobacco use is the leading cause of preventable disease and death in the United States, and worldwide, it carries a substantial health burden. Smoking is an unhealthy habit for both genders, but women and men experience different health risks, and they respond differently to techniques designed to help them quit. Here are some examples:

- Quitting smoking at any age dramatically cuts a woman's risk of death.
- Women smokers have a higher breast cancer risk.
- Women smokers who use oral contraceptives risk serious health effects, such as blood clots, heart attacks, and strokes.
- Smoking affects a woman's eyes, putting her at higher risk for vision problems, such as macular degeneration and cataracts, later in life.
- There is a strong relationship between the number of cigarettes a young woman smokes per day and the probability that she will have an ischemic stroke.
- Quitting smoking is one of the best decisions a woman can make toward a healthier tomorrow for herself and her family.
- While men are more sensitive than women to nicotine's effects on the body, women are more susceptible than men to smoking sensory triggers, such as smell and taste, as well as to social cues.
- Nicotine patches and gums do not work as well in women as they do in men.
- Quitting techniques that work better in women than in men include cognitive-behavioral therapy (CBT)

that focuses not only on quitting smoking but also on related issues, such as controlling quitting-associated weight gain and moderating mood.

STEM CELLS

Muscle-derived stem cells, which reside in skeletal muscle tissue, are one type of adult stem cell. Hematopoietic stem cells, in the bone marrow, are another type. Because stem cells are not yet specialized, they can turn into other many different types of cells, such as bone, fat, and blood.

All cells, not just stem cells, have a sex. Each cell in the body is either male or female, based on its DNA content contributed by XX (female) and XY (male) chromosomes. Other factors contribute as well, such as the source (maternal or paternal) of the X chromosome and various other biological signatures. Here are some examples of how sex affects stem cells:

- Cell sex exerts a strong effect on the regenerative capacity of muscle-derived stem cells.
- In mice, stem cells that mature to become blood cells divide faster in females than in males.
- Hormones affect the growth of stem cells in the mammary gland.

STROKE

A stroke is sort of like a heart attack in the brain. Strokes occur when blood flow to a part of the brain suddenly stops, starving brain cells of the oxygen they need to live. Clogged arteries can cause a so-called ischemic stroke, in which fat and cholesterol form plaques in artery walls, allowing less blood to flow through freely.

While some of the risk factors for stroke are the same in men and women—such as family history of stroke, high blood pressure or cholesterol, smoking, and being overweight—certain aspects of stroke are unique to women. Researchers have identified several sex/gender differences:

- While men have a higher risk of stroke than women, in general, women are usually older when they have

strokes, and they are more likely to die of strokes than men.
- Women have a poorer quality of life (QOL) after a stroke than men.
- Women with a history of preeclampsia during pregnancy are 60 percent more likely to have a nonpregnancy-related stroke later in life.
- Women who suffer from migraines with visual components, such as flashing lights, have a higher risk of having an ischemic stroke.

VIOLENCE
Men and women both experience violence, and researchers have identified ways different types of violence, such as child abuse, suicidal behavior, IPV, and elder abuse, are connected.

VISION
Vision disorders affect women disproportionately both in the United States and throughout the world. But, in addition to affecting vision, eye changes can signal the presence of other conditions, especially autoimmune diseases such as lupus and RA. Ocular manifestations of thyroid disease may be the first characteristic symptom that brings a woman to a physician's office to seek treatment. Here are some examples of how vision disorders affect women and men:
- Dry eye affects twice as many women than men over 50 years of age. Dry eye disease affects QOL—interfering with routine activities, such as reading, working on a computer, and driving a car.
- Cataracts that cloud the eye's lens are more likely to occur in women than in men. In developing countries, women are less likely than men to receive cataract surgery.
- Brain-imaging studies of people with migraines—intense headaches that are twice as common in women than men and that often affect vision—have reported sex-specific patterns.

- Adult women experience about 25 percent more uncorrected visual impairment due to refractive error—which impedes the ability to focus—compared to adult men.
- Worldwide, women account for two-thirds of all people with blindness or visual impairment, but more than three-quarters of these vision problems are preventable.[2]

Section 3.3 | Alcohol Use and Its Risks to Men's Health

Men are more likely than women to drink excessively. Excessive drinking is associated with significant risks to men's health and safety, and the risks increase with the amount of alcohol consumed. Men are also more likely than women to take other risks (such as misusing other substances, having multiple sex partners, or not wearing a seat belt) that when combined with alcohol further increase their risk of illness, injury, or death.

ADULT MEN DRINK MORE THAN WOMEN

- Almost 58 percent of adult men report drinking alcohol in the past 30 days compared with 49 percent of adult women.
- Men are more likely to binge drink than women. Approximately 21 percent of men report binge drinking, compared with 13 percent of women. Among men who binge drink, 25 percent do so at least five times a month, on average, and 25 percent consume at least nine drinks during a binge drinking occasion.
- In 2020, 13 percent of adult men had an alcohol use disorder (AUD) compared with 9 percent of adult women.

---

[2] Office of Research on Women's Health (ORWH), "How Sex/Gender Influence Health & Disease (A-Z)," National Institutes of Health (NIH), September 22, 2014. Available online. URL: https://orwh.od.nih.gov/sex-gender/sexgender-influences-health-and-disease/how-sexgender-influence-health-disease-z. Accessed July 3, 2023.

ALCOHOL IS ASSOCIATED WITH INJURY, VIOLENCE, AND OTHER HARMS

- Men have higher rates of alcohol-related hospitalizations than women.
- More than three-quarters of deaths from excessive drinking are among males, totaling more than 97,000 deaths each year in the United States.
- Among drivers in fatal motor vehicle traffic crashes, men are 50 percent more likely to have been intoxicated (i.e., a blood alcohol concentration (BAC) of 0.08% or greater) than women.
- Excessive alcohol consumption increases aggression and may increase the risk of physically assaulting another person. Alcohol is a key risk factor for sexual violence perpetration.
- Males are more than three times as likely to die by suicide than females and more likely to have been drinking prior to suicide.
- Alcohol use is one of the most important preventable risk factors for cancer. Alcohol use increases the risk of cancer of the mouth, throat, esophagus, liver, and colon, which are more common among men. Drinking alcohol also increases the risk of prostate cancer.

ALCOHOL MAY AFFECT MEN'S SEXUAL AND REPRODUCTIVE HEALTH

- Excessive alcohol use can interfere with testicular function and male hormone production, resulting in erectile dysfunction (ED) and infertility.
- Alcohol use by men also increases the chances of engaging in risky sexual activity, including unprotected sex, sex with multiple partners, or sex with a partner at risk for sexually transmitted infections (STIs).

Men can reduce the amount of alcohol they drink to reduce their risk of health problems and other harms.[3]

---

[3] "Excessive Alcohol Use Is a Risk to Men's Health," Centers for Disease Control and Prevention (CDC), October 31, 2022. Available online. URL: www.cdc.gov/alcohol/fact-sheets/mens-health.htm. Accessed June 23, 2023.

Section 3.4 | Gender Differences in Tobacco Smoking

Generally, men tend to use all tobacco products at higher rates than women. Results from neuroimaging studies suggest that smoking activates men's reward pathways more than women's. This finding is consistent with the idea that men smoke for the reinforcing effects of nicotine, whereas women smoke to regulate mood or in response to cigarette-related cues. A study of stress responses and craving among male and female smokers who were trying to quit found that during abstinence, lower levels of the stress hormone cortisol predicted relapse in men. However, high cortisol levels were predictive of relapse in women. Other work on abstinence found that smoking a cigarette with nicotine, as compared to a denicotinized cigarette, alleviated the symptoms of withdrawal and negative mood to a greater extent in men than in women. Women obtained equal relief from cigarettes with and without nicotine, suggesting that they found the drug less rewarding than men.

Cigarette craving is a major reason why smokers find it hard to quit, and this strong urge to smoke can be evoked by sensory cues and stress. Research suggests that women experience stronger craving than men in response to stress, but men may be more responsive to environmental cues. Additionally, longitudinal data from international surveys conducted in four industrialized countries indicated that men and women did not differ in their desire to quit, plans to quit, or quit attempts. However, women were 31 percent less likely to quit successfully. One reason why women may have difficulty quitting is post-cessation weight gain. This concern should be addressed in behavioral counseling and adjunct treatments for all smokers.

The overall lower cessation rate for women may reflect sex differences in response to particular medications. For example, varenicline has greater short- and immediate-term efficacy (at three and six months) among women smokers. However, women and men show similar one-year quit rates when using varenicline. In contrast, a combination of varenicline plus bupropion was less effective for cessation among women than among men.[4]

Men are more likely than women to use almost all types of illicit drugs, and illicit drug use is more likely to result in emergency department visits or overdose deaths for men than for women.

"Illicit" refers to the use of illegal drugs, including marijuana (according to federal law), and the misuse of prescription drugs. For most age groups, men have higher rates of use or dependence on illicit drugs and alcohol than women. However, women are just as likely as men to develop a substance use disorder (SUD). In addition, women may be more susceptible to craving and relapse, which are key phases of the addiction cycle.

ILLEGAL DRUGS
Marijuana (Cannabis)

Similar to other addictive drugs, fewer females than males use marijuana. For females who do use marijuana, however, the effects can be different from the effects for male users. Research indicates that marijuana impairs spatial memory in women more than it does in men, while males show a greater marijuana-induced high.

In a study specific to teenagers, male high school students who smoke marijuana reported poor family relationships and problems at school more often than female students who smoke marijuana. However, a few studies have suggested that teenage girls who use marijuana may have a higher risk of brain structural abnormalities associated with regular marijuana exposure than teenage boys.

Animal studies show that female rats are more sensitive to the rewarding, pain-relieving, and activity-altering effects of marijuana's main active ingredient, delta-9-tetrahydrocannabinol (THC). Many of these differences have been attributed to the effects of sex hormones although rodent research also points to the possibility that there are sex differences in the functioning of the

---

[4] "Are There Gender Differences in Tobacco Smoking?" National Institute on Drug Abuse (NIDA), May 2022. Available online. URL: https://nida.nih.gov/publications/research-reports/tobacco-nicotine-e-cigarettes/ are-there-gender-differences-in-tobacco-smoking. Accessed June 23, 2023.

endocannabinoid system, the system of brain signaling where THC and other cannabinoids exert their actions.

For both sexes, marijuana use disorder (see Table 3.1) is associated with an increased risk of at least one other mental health condition, such as depression or anxiety. However, men who are addicted to marijuana have higher rates of other substance use problems as well as antisocial personality disorders. By contrast, women who are addicted to marijuana have more panic attacks and anxiety disorders. Although the severity of marijuana use disorders is generally higher for men, women tend to develop these disorders more quickly after their first marijuana use. Rates of seeking treatment for marijuana use disorder are low for both sexes.

Table 3.1. Marijuana Use Disorder

Men	Women
Similarities	
• at least one other mental health disorder • low rate of seeking treatment	
Differences	
• other substance use disorders (SUDs) • antisocial personality disorder • severity of disorder	• panic attacks • anxiety disorders • disorder developing more quickly

Stimulants (Cocaine and Methamphetamine)

Research in both humans and animals suggests that women may be more vulnerable to the reinforcing (rewarding) effects of stimulants, with estrogen possibly being one factor for this increased sensitivity. In animal studies, females are quicker to start taking cocaine—and take it in larger amounts—than males. Women may also be more sensitive than men to cocaine's effects on the heart and blood vessels. In contrast, female and male cocaine users show similar deficits in learning, concentration, and academic achievement, even if women had been using it longer. Female cocaine users are also less likely than male users to exhibit abnormalities of blood flow in the brain's frontal regions. These findings suggest

37

a sex-related mechanism that may protect women from some of the detrimental effects of cocaine on the brain.

As for methamphetamine, women report using the drug because they believe it will increase energy and decrease exhaustion associated with work, home care, childcare, and family responsibilities. Weight loss is another incentive women cite for methamphetamine use—and one reported significantly more by women than by men. Women who use methamphetamine also have high rates of co-occurring depression.

Women tend to begin using methamphetamine at an earlier age than men, with female users typically being more dependent on methamphetamine compared to male users. Women are also less likely to switch to another drug when they lack access to methamphetamine. In addition, as with other substances, women tend to be more receptive than men to methamphetamine treatment.

3,4-Methylenedioxymethamphetamine (Ecstasy and Molly)

Research suggests that 3,4-Methylenedioxymethamphetamine (MDMA) produces stronger hallucinatory effects in women than in men although men show higher MDMA-induced blood pressure increases. There is some evidence that in occasional users, women are more prone than men to feeling depressed a few days after they last used MDMA. Both men and women show similar increases in aggression a few days after they stop using MDMA.

MDMA can interfere with the body's ability to eliminate water and decrease sodium levels in the blood, causing a person to drink large amounts of fluid. In rare cases, this can lead to increased water in the spaces between cells, which may eventually produce swelling of the brain and even death. Young women are more likely than men to die from this reaction, with almost all reported cases of death occurring in young females between the ages of 15 and 30. MDMA can also interfere with temperature regulation and cause acute hyperthermia, leading to neurotoxic effects and even death.

Heroin

Research suggests that women tend to use smaller amounts of heroin and for less time and are less likely than men to inject it.

Most women who inject heroin point to social pressure and sexual partner encouragement as factors. One study indicates that women are more at risk than men for overdose death during the first few years of injecting heroin, but it is unclear why this might be the case. One possibility is that women who inject heroin are more likely than their male counterparts to also use prescription drugs—a dangerous combination. Women who do not overdose within these first few years are more likely than men to survive in the long term. This could be due to differences in treatment and other environmental factors that impact heroin use.

PRESCRIPTION DRUGS

Prescription drug misuse is the use of a medication without a prescription, in a way other than as prescribed, or for the experience or feelings elicited. Prescription drug misuse can be dangerous if mixed together without a physician's guidance or mixed with other drugs or alcohol.

Prescription Opioids

Some research indicates that women are more sensitive to pain than men and more likely to have chronic pain, which could contribute to the high rates of opioid prescriptions among women of reproductive age. In addition, women may be more likely to take prescription opioids without a prescription to cope with pain, even when men and women report similar pain levels. Research also suggests that women are more likely to misuse prescription opioids to self-treat for other problems such as anxiety or tension.

A possible consequence of prescription opioid misuse is fatal overdose, which can occur because opioids suppress breathing. In 2016, 7,109 women and 9,978 men died from prescription opioid overdose (a total of 17,087), which is about 19 women per day compared to about 27 men dying from overdosing on prescription opioids. Women between the ages of 45 and 54 are more likely than women of other age groups to die from a prescription opioid overdose.

Antianxiety Medications and Sleeping Aids

Women are more likely to seek treatment for misuse of central nervous system depressants, which include sedatives sometimes prescribed to treat seizures, sleep disorders, and anxiety and to help people fall asleep prior to surgery. Women are also more likely than men to die from overdoses involving medications for mental health conditions, such as antidepressants. Antidepressants and benzodiazepines (antianxiety or sleep drugs) send more women than men to emergency departments. Because women are also more at risk than men for anxiety and insomnia, it is possible that women are being prescribed more of these types of medications; greater access can increase the risk of misuse and lead to SUD or overdose.

OTHER SUBSTANCES
Alcohol

In general, men have higher rates of alcohol use, including binge drinking. However, young adults are an exception: Girls aged 12–20 have slightly higher rates of alcohol misuse and binge drinking than their male counterparts.

Drinking over the long term is more likely to damage a woman's health than a man's, even if the woman has been drinking less alcohol or for a shorter length of time. Comparing people with alcohol use disorders, women have death rates 50–100 percent higher than men, including deaths from suicides, alcohol-related accidents, heart disease, stroke, and liver disease. In addition, there are some health risks that are unique to female drinkers. For example, heavy drinking is associated with increased risk of having unprotected sex, resulting in pregnancy or disease, and an increased risk of becoming a victim of violence and sexual assault. In addition, drinking as little as one drink per day is associated with a higher risk of breast cancer in some women, especially those who are postmenopausal or have a family history of breast cancer.

In addition, men and women metabolize alcohol differently due to differences in gastric tissue activity. In fact, after drinking comparable amounts of alcohol, women have higher blood ethanol concentrations. As a result, women become intoxicated from smaller quantities of alcohol than men.

Nicotine (Tobacco)

Research indicates that men and women differ in their smoking behaviors. For instance, women smoke fewer cigarettes per day, tend to use cigarettes with lower nicotine content, and do not inhale as deeply as men. Women may also smoke for different reasons than men, including regulation of mood and stress. It is unclear whether these differences in smoking behaviors are because women are more sensitive to nicotine, because they find the sensations associated with smoking less rewarding, or because of social factors contributing to the difference; some research also suggests women may experience more stress and anxiety as a result of nicotine withdrawal than men.

Risk of death from smoking-associated lung cancer, chronic obstructive pulmonary disease (COPD), heart disease, and stroke continues to increase among women—approaching rates for men. Some dangers associated with smoking—such as blood clots, heart attack, or stroke—increase in women using oral contraceptives.

Several factors appear to be contributing to this narrowing gender gap, including women being less likely than men to quit and more likely to relapse if they do quit.[5]

Section 3.5 | Men and COVID-19: Sex Differences in Mortality

Data suggest that more men than women have died of coronavirus disease 2019 (COVID-19) worldwide, but it is unclear why. A biopsychosocial approach has been critical for understanding the disproportionate death rate among men. Biological, psychological,

---

[5] "Sex and Gender Differences in Substance Use," National Institute on Drug Abuse (NIDA), April 2020. Available online. URL: https://nida.nih.gov/publications/research-reports/substance-use-in-women/sex-gender-differences-in-substance-use. Accessed June 23, 2023.

behavioral, and social factors may have put men at disproportionate risk of death. The Centers for Disease Control and Prevention (CDC) had proposed a stepwise approach to clinical, public health, and policy interventions to reduce COVID-19-associated morbidity and mortality among men.

In the United States, as of June 2020, 57 percent of deaths caused by COVID-19 have been men. With the exception of Massachusetts, all states in the United States have reported higher mortality among men. However, the United States has not been consistent in reporting sex-disaggregated data. In a recent analysis of 26 states, only half reported sex as a variable. Age is a significant risk factor for COVID-19 mortality, and a vast majority of the COVID-19 deaths in the United States have been among people older than 75; in addition, rates of preexisting health conditions (e.g., hypertension, obesity, diabetes) exacerbate disparities in mortality by class, race, and sex/gender.

FACTORS AFFECTING COVID-19 MORBIDITY AND MORTALITY AMONG MEN

Although epidemiological data showed a difference between men and women in the rates of mortality among those diagnosed with COVID-19, the mechanisms underlying sex differences in mortality are unclear. Because most health patterns are the result of a combination of biological, behavioral, and psychosocial factors, how sex-associated biological factors and gender-associated psychosocial and behavioral factors interact in determining health and in explaining COVID-19-associated mortality must be considered.

Biological Factors

Men and women differ in both innate and adaptive immune responses, perhaps related in part to sex-specific inflammatory responses resulting from X-chromosomal inheritance. The X chromosome contains a high density of immune-related genes; therefore, women generally mount stronger innate and adaptive immune responses than men. This differential regulation of immune responses in men and women is contributed by sex chromosome genes and sex hormones, including estrogen, progesterone, and androgens. Sex-specific disease outcomes after viral infections are attributed to the sex-dependent production of steroid hormones, different copy numbers of immune response X-linked genes, and the presence of disease susceptibility genes.

Severe acute respiratory syndrome coronavirus 2 (SARS-CoV-2) uses the SARS-CoV receptor angiotensin-converting enzyme 2 (ACE2) for entry into the host cell. The S spike of the virus attaches to the cellular ACE2 receptor (coded by the *ACE2* gene) located on the respiratory epithelial cells. The internalization of the virus is potentiated by the cellular protease transmembrane protease, serine 2 (TMPRSS2) in the host cell. The high burden of illness and high case fatality ratio in patients with COVID-19 may be driven in part by the strong affinity of the virus for ACE2, leading to virus entry and multisystem illness in pulmonary, gut, renal, cardiac, and central nervous systems.

Men have higher plasma ACE2 levels than women, and a recent study of patients with heart failure showed that plasma ACE2 concentrations were higher than normal in men and higher in men than in women, possibly reflecting higher tissue expression of the ACE2 receptor for SARS-CoV infections. This could explain why men might be more susceptible to infection with, or the consequences of, SARS-CoV-2. Unraveling which cellular factors are used by SARS-CoV-2 for entry might provide insights into viral transmission and reveal therapeutic targets. Further investigation into the association of ACE2 enzyme activity in COVID-19 and its correlation with sex is ongoing. Although biological factors clearly helped to explain the sex difference in COVID-19 mortality, psychosocial and behavioral factors also play a part.

Psychosocial and Behavioral Factors

In addition to sex differences in immune responses, hormones, and genes, there are also psychological, social, and behavioral components that influenced COVID-19 progression. Compared with women, men tend to be engaged in more high-risk behaviors that generate the potential for contracting COVID-19. Polls taken early in the first wave of COVID-19 cases in the United States showed sex differences in the perceived severity of the pandemic. Another U.S. study found that men were more likely to downplay the severity of the virus's potential to harm them, and fewer men than women had reported that they had been avoiding large public gatherings or avoiding close physical contact with others. In addition, compared with women in many countries, including the United States, men tend to have higher rates of behaviors that are linked with COVID-19 infection and mortality, including higher rates of tobacco use and alcohol consumption.

Men also had lower rates than women of handwashing, social distancing, wearing masks, and effectively and proactively seeking medical help. Many men had been socialized to mask their fear, and it is important to consider how hiding fear affected men's response to COVID-19. It is particularly important to focus on men who responded to threats such as COVID-19 with aggression and anger. Research shows that people with this response "tend to downplay risk and were resistant to risk reduction policies," which was problematic during efforts to promote social distancing and other pandemic restrictions. These socially constructed behaviors reduced the perception of susceptibility and severity, which then translated into a decrease in the practice of preventive measures, such as handwashing, and protests against pandemic-related restrictions.

Other factors that may have intersected with sex and gender were age and geography. For example, a U.S. study of associations between perceived risk and worry with age and gender found that although older men perceived their risks of COVID-19 to be higher than those of younger men, older men made the fewest behavior changes across age and gender groups. Another study highlighted the importance of considering place or geography. In a comparison of counties where populations were predominantly Black or predominantly White, the SARS-CoV-2 infection rate was three times higher, and the death rate was six times higher in counties where the population was predominantly Black.

In addition to these psychological and behavioral factors, differences in occupational risk existed between men and women. In the United States, a larger number of women than men were deemed essential workers primarily because of the large share of women employed as social workers and in health care. Nevertheless, the low-skilled or low-paid occupations that were considered essential workers (e.g., food processing, transportation, delivery, warehousing, construction, manufacturing), where men outnumber women, were associated with a greater risk of mortality.

In summary, a range of biological, psychological, and behavioral factors explained why men had higher rates of COVID-19-associated morbidity and mortality than women. Although it is critical to identify the factors associated with increased risk for men of COVID-19 mortality, it is equally important to determine how to reduce the risk of men dying of COVID-19. The factors that exacerbate men's risk were also intertwined with race, ethnicity, geography, and other proxies for factors that were markers of marginalization and social inequality.

INTERVENTION STRATEGIES TO REDUCE MEN'S COVID-19 MORTALITY RISK

To reduce virus transmission and increase screening for the virus and thereby reduce men's risk of COVID-19 mortality, the CDC proposed five strategies: health education, community engagement, and public health outreach; health promotion and preventive care; sex-disaggregated data in clinical practice and policy; rehabilitation and health-care delivery infrastructure; and health policy and legislative interventions.

Health Education, Community Engagement, and Public Health Outreach

Educational efforts to increase compliance with public health recommendations were more effective in changing the behavior of men if these efforts incorporate some of the principles from health communications research that consider how health behavior is gendered.

Although the health education of men is useful, the health education of men's partners and their families about men's health risks is also critical. One U.S. study of communication strategies examined the influence of men's partners and found that communicating with a man's loved one, combined with a reminder system implemented by providers, was associated with increases in preventive health-care screenings. As a result, a federally qualified health center in Baton Rouge, Louisiana, for example, conducted outreach to men with underlying conditions and their partners to ensure that they are aware of their susceptibility to COVID-19.

Increasing access and eliminating barriers to community-wide testing were additional ways to improve COVID-19 outcomes. Testing or screening use may be influenced by exposure to decision education and the influence of screening-related primary care practice factors. Federally qualified health centers offering primary care services were key community institutions that had increased COVID-19 testing—with no out-of-pocket costs to patients in many areas. These kinds of programs allowed men to have access to testing without cost barriers that may otherwise deter them from accessing testing. The community-wide testing also offered an opportunity for men to be tested before returning to work. These initiatives helped normalize testing and reduce the stigma of getting tested although they may not have reduced the stigma of receiving a positive test result.

Health Promotion and Preventive Care

Given the rates of cardiometabolic risk factors and underlying or preexisting conditions such as obesity or comorbid chronic diseases (e.g., diabetes, heart disease, cancer) among men, a focus on men with underlying conditions that increased their risk of COVID-19 mortality was critical. Although the greater severity of complications attributable to COVID-19 among men is not well understood, preliminary findings of a higher incidence of mortality attributable to underlying comorbid conditions suggested that clinicians tailor current treatment options with this in mind. Patients need to be reassured that although routine and elective care might be curtailed by the pandemic, new symptoms of myocardial infarction and stroke still need to be immediately addressed.

For men who were at increased risk because of a history of a chronic condition or disease, clinicians actively assessed risks; optimized antihypertensive and statin therapies where indicated; provided behavioral and pharmacotherapy for tobacco use cessation (cigarettes and vaping); educated on healthy diets rich in vegetables, legumes, grains, fruits, and nuts; and made exercise recommendations. In addition to providing information, clinicians encouraged men to participate in behavioral interventions that target psychosocial factors (e.g., self-efficacy, motivation) that can facilitate lifestyle change and maintenance of behavior changes over time. These important interventions continued during a pandemic through virtual visits and telemedicine platforms. Several professional organizations made COVID-19-specific clinical and operational guidelines in their specialties; these included patient education information on occupational risk mitigations and recognizing signs and symptoms of COVID-19 infection, hand hygiene and surface decontamination, and protecting family members.

Rehabilitation and Health-Care Delivery Infrastructure

Strategies aimed at preventing complications associated with COVID-19 were essential for a safe and effective return to personal, professional, and societal obligations. Urgent needs also existed to provide postacute care rehabilitation services for patients recovering from COVID-19 and to train a new workforce to care for these patients. Strong evidence suggested that interventions engaging community health workers improved health outcomes for patients, including men, across multiple chronic conditions. As care extenders, community health workers provided a culturally and linguistically appropriate clinical–community linkage for difficult-to-reach patients, such as men. They provided direct outreach to men with comorbidities that made them more susceptible to COVID-19 and its complications.

Health Policy and Legislative Interventions

In addition to various practice initiatives to reduce virus transmission and mortality, the potential policy efforts to address the COVID-19 epidemic in the United States were under consideration. Because men died of COVID-19 disproportionately, policymakers needed to explicitly consider gender but not conflate gender with women. To do so, local, state, and national policymakers ensured that legislation includes language that promotes data collection, disaggregation, and dissemination by race, ethnicity, and sex. Collecting and disseminating data by sex help make a vital economic case for considering men's health explicitly in the COVID-19 pandemic; however, men's health policy needed to be located in a framework that embraces gender equity and that does not treat men's and women's health as though they are competing interests or priorities. Men who were marginalized or disadvantaged because of their race, ethnicity, sexual orientation, incarceration, homelessness, or other factors were particularly vulnerable to COVID-19, and policies explored which groups of men are over-represented among essential workers, at risk because of preexisting health conditions, or most in need because of other socioeconomic factors.

PUBLIC HEALTH IMPLICATIONS

A biopsychosocial approach took into account not only the range of factors that determined risk but also the range of places where one might intervene within a population health framework that considered both biomedical and public health points of intervention to reduce mortality from COVID-19. The CDC ensured that COVID-19 screening, testing, and quarantine of all confirmed and potential cases; contact tracing; financing; and development of vaccines and clinical trials for novel therapeutic targets do not vary by sex or other socially meaningful markers of difference in our society. Moreover, they dramatically increased their investment in the prevention and control of chronic diseases such as hypertension, diabetes, cardiovascular diseases, chronic renal disorders, and mental health disorders that may help them reduce COVID-19 mortality among men.[6]

---

[6] "Preventing Chronic Disease," Centers for Disease Control and Prevention (CDC), July 16, 2020. Available online. URL: www.cdc.gov/pcd/issues/2020/20_0247.htm. Accessed June 26, 2023.

Chapter 4 | **Recommended Screening Tests for Men**

Chapter Contents

GET THE SCREENINGS YOU NEED

Screenings are tests that look for diseases before you have symptoms. Blood pressure checks and tests for high cholesterol are examples of screenings. You can get some screenings, such as blood pressure readings, in your doctor's office. Others—such as a colonoscopy, a test for colorectal cancer—need special equipment, so you may need to go to a different office. After a screening test, ask when you will see the results and who you should talk to about them.

- **Abdominal aortic aneurysm**. If you are between the ages of 65 and 75 and have ever been a smoker, talk to your doctor or nurse about being screened for abdominal aortic aneurysm (AAA). AAA is a bulging in your abdominal aorta, the largest artery in your body. An AAA may burst, which can cause dangerous bleeding and death.
- **Colorectal cancer**. Have a screening test for colorectal cancer starting at the age of 50. If you have a family history of colorectal cancer, you may need to be screened earlier. Several different tests can detect this cancer. Your doctor can help you decide which is best for you.
- **Depression**. Your emotional health is as important as your physical health. Talk to your doctor or nurse about being screened for depression especially if during the past two weeks:
  - you have felt down, sad, or hopeless
  - you have felt little interest or pleasure in doing things
- **Diabetes**. Get screened for diabetes if your blood pressure is higher than 135/80 or if you take medication for high blood pressure. Diabetes (high blood sugar) can cause problems with your heart, brain, eyes, feet, kidneys, nerves, and other body parts.

- **High blood pressure**. Starting at the age of 18, have your blood pressure checked at least every two years. High blood pressure is 140/90 or higher. It can cause strokes, heart attacks, kidney and eye problems, and heart failure.
- **High cholesterol**. If you are 35 years of age or older, have your cholesterol checked. Have your cholesterol checked starting at 20 years of age if:
  - you use tobacco
  - you are obese
  - you have diabetes or high blood pressure
  - you have a personal history of heart disease or blocked arteries
  - a man in your family had a heart attack before the age of 50 or a woman had a heart attack before the age of 60
- **Human immunodeficiency virus (HIV)**. Talk with your health-care team about HIV screening if any of the following apply to you:
  - You have had unprotected sex with multiple partners.
  - You have sex with men.
  - You use or have used injection drugs.
  - You exchange sex for money or drugs, or you have sex partners who do.
  - You have or had a sex partner who is HIV-infected or injects drugs.
  - You are being treated for a sexually transmitted disease (STD).
  - You had a blood transfusion between 1978 and 1985.
  - You have any other concerns.
- **Syphilis**. Ask your doctor or nurse whether you should be screened for syphilis.
- **Overweight and obesity**. The best way to learn if you are overweight or obese is to find your body mass index (BMI). You can find your BMI by entering your height and weight into an online BMI calculator. A BMI

between 18.5 and 25 indicates a normal weight. Persons with a BMI of 30 or higher may be obese. If you are obese, talk to your doctor or nurse about seeking intensive counseling and getting help with changing your behaviors to lose weight. Being overweight or obese can lead to diabetes and cardiovascular disease (CVD).

IT IS YOUR BODY

You know your body better than anyone else. Always tell your doctor or nurse about any changes in your health, including your vision and hearing. Ask them about being checked for any condition you are concerned about, not just the ones here. If you are wondering about diseases such as prostate cancer or skin cancer, for example, ask about them.[1]

Section 4.2 | Diabetes Screening

WHAT ARE DIABETES TESTS?

Diabetes, also known as "diabetes mellitus," is a disease that affects how your body uses glucose (blood sugar). Glucose is your body's main source of energy. A hormone called "insulin" helps move glucose from your bloodstream into your cells. If you have diabetes, your body cannot make insulin, or insulin does not work like it should. This can cause glucose levels to get too high, which can lead to serious health problems. These include heart disease, nerve damage, eye problems, and kidney disease. Diabetes tests measure glucose levels in blood or urine to see if you are at risk for or have diabetes.

---

[1] "Men: Stay Healthy at Any Age," U.S. Office of Personnel Management (OPM), August 15, 2010. Available online. URL: www.opm.gov/healthcare-insurance/special-initiatives/managing-my-own-health/healthymen.pdf. Accessed July 3, 2023.

WHAT ARE THEY USED FOR?

Diabetes tests are used to screen for and/or diagnose the following:

- **Type 1 diabetes**. If you have type 1 diabetes, your body makes little or no insulin at all. This condition happens when your immune system attacks and destroys cells that produce insulin. It can develop at any age, but it most often starts in childhood. People with type 1 diabetes must take daily doses of insulin, either by injection or a special pump.
- **Type 2 diabetes**. This is the most common form of diabetes. If you have type 2 diabetes, your body may still be able to make insulin, but the cells in your body do not respond well to insulin and cannot easily take up enough glucose from your blood. Type 2 diabetes may be caused by your genes and lifestyle factors, such as being overweight or having obesity. The condition most often occurs in adulthood but is becoming more common in children and teens.
- **Prediabetes**. This is a condition in which your blood glucose levels are higher than normal, but not high enough to be considered diabetes. But it may put you at risk for getting diabetes.

WHY DO YOU NEED A DIABETES TEST?

You may need testing if you have symptoms of diabetes, such as:

- increased thirst
- frequent urination
- increased hunger
- fatigue
- blurred vision
- unexplained weight loss
- sores that are slow to heal
- numbness or tingling in the feet

Symptoms of type 1 diabetes usually come on quickly and can be severe. Symptoms of type 2 diabetes and prediabetes often develop slowly, even over the course of years.

You may also need testing if you have certain risk factors. You may be at higher risk for diabetes if you:

- are over 45 years old (The American Diabetes Association (ADA) recommends annual diabetes screening for all adults aged 45 years and older.)
- have prediabetes
- are overweight or obese
- have a family history of diabetes
- have high blood pressure (HBP) or heart disease

WHAT HAPPENS DURING A DIABETES TEST?

There are several ways to screen for and diagnose diabetes. Most tests involve measuring glucose levels in the blood.

To get a blood sample, a health-care professional will take a blood sample from a vein in your arm, using a small needle. After the needle is inserted, a small amount of blood will be collected into a test tube or vial. You may feel a little sting when the needle goes in or out. This usually takes less than five minutes.

The different types of glucose blood tests include the following:

- **Blood glucose test, also known as "fasting blood glucose."** Before the test, you will need to fast (not eat or drink) for eight hours. This test is often used as a screening test for diabetes. It may be repeated to confirm a diagnosis.
- **Oral glucose tolerance test (OGTT).** This test also requires fasting before the test. When you arrive for your test, a blood sample will be taken. You will then drink a sugary liquid that contains glucose. About two hours later, another blood sample will be taken.
- **Random blood sugar.** This test can be taken at any time. No fasting is required.
- **Hemoglobin A1c (HbA1c).** This test measures the average amount of glucose attached to hemoglobin over the past three months. Hemoglobin is the part of your red blood cells (RBCs) that carries oxygen from your lungs to the rest of your body. No fasting is required for this test.

Glucose may also be measured in urine. Urine tests are not used to diagnose diabetes but may show if you are at risk of getting the disease. If your glucose in urine levels are higher than normal, you will probably need a blood test to confirm the diagnosis.

For a glucose in urine test, your provider may recommend an at-home test kit. The kit will include a test strip that you hold under your stream of urine. The test strip will change colors to show different levels of glucose.

WOULD YOU NEED TO DO ANYTHING TO PREPARE FOR THIS TEST?

You will need to fast (not eat or drink) for a blood glucose test and an OGTT.

You do not need any special preparations for a random blood sugar, hemoglobin A1c, or glucose in urine test.

ARE THERE ANY RISKS TO THIS TEST?

There is very little risk to having a blood test. There may be slight pain or bruising at the spot where the needle was put in, but most symptoms go away quickly.

There is no risk to having a urine test.

WHAT DO THE RESULTS MEAN?

Depending on the type of test or tests you had, your results may show one of the following:

- **Normal glucose levels**. This means you probably are not at risk for or do not have diabetes.
- **Prediabetes**. This means you have higher than normal glucose levels and may be at risk for getting diabetes.
- **Type 1 or type 2 diabetes**. If you have been diagnosed with type 1 diabetes, talk to your provider about how to best manage the condition. There is no cure for type 1 diabetes, but it may be controlled with regular glucose monitoring and taking insulin. If you have been diagnosed with prediabetes or type 2 diabetes, your condition may be managed or even reversed by taking

diabetes medicines and making lifestyle changes. These include eating a healthy diet, losing weight, and increasing exercise.

If you have other questions about your diabetes diagnosis or treatment, talk to your health-care provider.

IS THERE ANYTHING ELSE YOU NEED TO KNOW ABOUT DIABETES TESTING?

If you have been diagnosed with type 1 diabetes, you will need to monitor blood glucose levels daily, often several times a day. Your health-care provider can recommend a kit you can use at home. Most kits include a lancet, a device that pricks your finger. You will use this to collect a drop of blood for testing. There are some newer kits available that do not require pricking your finger.

People with type 2 diabetes will also have to check their blood sugar on a regular basis. If you have type 2 diabetes, talk to your provider about how often it should be checked.

People with type 2 diabetes may also need to have their insulin levels checked regularly. Insulin plays a key role in keeping glucose at the right levels. An insulin in blood test is done at a provider's office.[2]

MEDICARE COVERAGE FOR DIABETES SCREENINGS

Medicare Part B (Medical Insurance) covers blood glucose (blood sugar) laboratory test screenings (with or without a carbohydrate challenge) if your doctor determines you are at risk of developing diabetes. You may be eligible for up to two screenings each year. Part B covers these screenings if you have any of the following risk factors:

- HBP (hypertension)
- history of abnormal cholesterol and triglyceride levels (dyslipidemia)
- obesity
- history of high blood sugar

---

[2] MedlinePlus, "Diabetes Tests," National Institutes of Health (NIH), September 27, 2021. Available online. URL: https://medlineplus.gov/lab-tests/diabetes-tests. Accessed June 23, 2023.

Part B also covers these screenings if two or more of the following conditions apply to you:

- You are 65 or older.
- You are overweight.
- You have a family history of diabetes (parents or siblings).

Your Costs in Original Medicare

You pay nothing for these screenings if your doctor or other healthcare provider accepts the assignment.[3]

Section 4.3 | Blood Pressure Screening

Nearly half of all adults in the United States have high blood pressure (HBP). HBP increases your risk for serious health problems, including stroke and heart attack.

Get your blood pressure checked regularly starting at the age of 18 years—and do your best to keep track of your blood pressure numbers.

WHAT IS BLOOD PRESSURE?

Blood pressure is how hard your blood pushes against the walls of your arteries. Arteries are the tubes that carry blood away from your heart. Every time your heart beats, it pumps blood through your arteries to the rest of your body.

WHAT IS HYPERTENSION?

Hypertension is the medical term for HBP. HBP usually has no symptoms, so it is sometimes called a "silent killer." The only way to know if you have HBP is to get it checked.

---

[3] "Diabetes Screenings," Centers for Medicare & Medicaid Services (CMS), March 15, 2006. Available online. URL: www.medicare.gov/coverage/diabetes-screenings. Accessed June 23, 2023.

WHAT PUTS YOU AT HIGHER RISK FOR HIGH BLOOD PRESSURE?

Your risk for HBP goes up as you get older. You are also at increased risk for HBP if you:

- are African American
- are overweight or have obesity
- are currently pregnant or had HBP during a past pregnancy
- do not get enough physical activity
- drink too much alcohol
- smoke
- do not eat a healthy diet
- have kidney failure, diabetes, or some types of heart disease

HOW OFTEN DO YOU NEED TO GET YOUR BLOOD PRESSURE CHECKED?

- If you are aged 40 or over, or if you are at higher risk for HBP, get your blood pressure checked at least once a year.
- If you are 18–39 years old and you are not at increased risk for HBP, get your blood pressure checked at least every three to five years.

HOW IS BLOOD PRESSURE MEASURED?
What Do Blood Pressure Numbers Mean?

A blood pressure test measures how hard your heart is working to pump blood through your body.

Blood pressure is measured with two numbers. The first number (called "systolic blood pressure") is the pressure in your arteries when your heart beats. The second number (called "diastolic blood pressure") is the pressure in your arteries when your heart relaxes between beats.

Compare your blood pressure to these numbers:

- Normal blood pressure is lower than 120/80 (said as "120 over 80").
- HBP is 130/80 or higher.
- Blood pressure that is between normal and high (e.g., 125/80) is called "elevated blood pressure."

If your blood pressure is elevated, it means you are at risk of developing HBP. Talk to your doctor and make a plan to control your blood pressure.

HOW COULD YOU GET YOUR BLOOD PRESSURE CHECKED?

To test your blood pressure, a nurse or doctor will put a cuff around your upper arm. The nurse or doctor will pump the cuff with air until it feels tight, then slowly let it out. This takes just a few minutes.

You can find out what your blood pressure numbers are right after the test is over. If the test shows that your blood pressure is high, ask the doctor what to do next.

Blood pressure can go up and down, so it is a good idea to get it checked more than once.

Could You Check Your Blood Pressure by Yourself?

Yes. You can buy a home blood pressure monitor at a drugstore. Many shopping malls, pharmacies, and grocery stores also have blood pressure machines you can use in the store.

If the test shows that your blood pressure is elevated or high, talk to your doctor and make a plan to control it.

If you have HBP, your doctor might ask you to monitor your blood pressure at home to keep track of your numbers—and to see if treatments are working.

MEDICARE COVERAGE FOR BLOOD PRESSURE SCREENING

Under the Affordable Care Act (ACA), insurance plans must cover blood pressure testing. Depending on your insurance plan, you may be able to get your blood pressure checked by a doctor or nurse at no cost to you. Check with your insurance company to find out more.

Medicare also covers blood pressure testing at no cost as part of your yearly wellness visit.

If you do not have insurance, you may still be able to get free or low-cost blood pressure tests. Find a health center near you and ask about getting your blood pressure checked.[4]

Section 4.4 | Cholesterol Screening

WHAT IS CHOLESTEROL?

Cholesterol is a waxy material that is found naturally in your blood. Your body makes cholesterol and uses it to do important things, such as making hormones and digesting fatty foods.

If you have too much cholesterol in your body, it can build up inside your blood vessels and make it hard for blood to flow through them. Over time, this can lead to heart disease.

HOW COULD YOU TELL IF YOU HAVE HIGH CHOLESTEROL?

Most people who have high cholesterol do not have any signs or symptoms. That is why it is so important to get your cholesterol checked.

HOW COULD YOU GET YOUR CHOLESTEROL CHECKED?

Your doctor will check your cholesterol levels with a blood test called a "lipid profile." A nurse will take a small sample of blood from your finger or arm for this test.

There are other blood tests that can check cholesterol, but a lipid profile gives the most information.

---

[4] Office of Disease Prevention and Health Promotion (ODPHP), "Get Your Blood Pressure Checked," U.S. Department of Health and Human Services (HHS), May 22, 2023. Available online. URL: https://health.gov/myhealthfinder/doctor-visits/screening-tests/get-your-blood-pressure-checked#take-action-tab. Accessed June 9, 2023.

TYPES OF CHOLESTEROL

If you get a lipid profile test, the results will show a few numbers. A lipid profile measures:

- total cholesterol
- low-density lipoprotein (LDL; bad) cholesterol
- high-density lipoprotein (HDL; good) cholesterol
- triglycerides

Total cholesterol is a measure of all the cholesterol in your blood. It is based on the LDL, HDL, and triglycerides numbers.

LDL cholesterol is a "bad" type of cholesterol that can block your arteries—so a lower level is better for you. Having a high LDL level can increase your risk for heart disease.

HDL cholesterol is the "good" type of cholesterol that helps clear LDL cholesterol out of your arteries—so a higher level is better for you. Having a low HDL cholesterol level can increase your risk for heart disease.

Triglycerides are a type of fat in your blood that can increase your risk for heart attack and stroke.

The results of your lipid profile test may also show your non-HDL cholesterol number. Non-HDL cholesterol is LDL cholesterol and the other "bad" types of cholesterol. In other words, it is your total cholesterol minus your HDL cholesterol. Having a high non-HDL level can increase your risk for heart disease.

ARE YOU AT RISK OF DEVELOPING CHOLESTEROL?
What Can Cause Unhealthy Cholesterol Levels?

Causes of high LDL (bad) cholesterol or low HDL (good) cholesterol levels include the following:

- age
- smoking, using other tobacco products, or drinking alcohol
- not getting enough physical activity
- eating too much saturated fat or not enough fruits and vegetables
- taking certain medicines, such as medicines to lower blood pressure

- family history of high cholesterol
- familial hypercholesterolemia (a condition passed down through families that causes very high LDL cholesterol levels)
- certain other health problems, such as type 2 diabetes or obesity

What If Your Cholesterol Levels Are Not Healthy?

As your LDL cholesterol gets higher, so does your risk of heart disease. Take the following steps to lower your cholesterol and reduce your risk of heart disease:

- Eat heart-healthy foods.
- Get active.
- Stay at a healthy weight.
- If you smoke, quit.
- Drink only a moderate (limited) amount of alcohol.
- If you have other chronic conditions—such as type 2 diabetes or high blood pressure (HBP)—take steps to manage them.
- Ask your doctor about taking medicine to lower your risk of heart attack and stroke.

HOW OFTEN DO YOU NEED TO GET YOUR CHOLESTEROL CHECKED?

The general recommendation is to get your cholesterol checked every four to six years. Some people may need to get their cholesterol checked more often depending on their risk of heart disease.

For example, high cholesterol can run in families. If someone in your family has high cholesterol or takes medicine to control cholesterol, you might need to get tested more often. Talk to your doctor about what is best for you.

GET TESTED FOR CHOLESTEROL LEVELS

Find out what your cholesterol levels are. If your cholesterol is high or you are at risk for heart disease, take steps to control your cholesterol levels.

Make an Appointment to Get Your Cholesterol Checked

Call your doctor's office or health center to schedule the test. Be sure to ask for a complete lipid profile—and find out what instructions you will need to follow before the test. For example, you may need to fast (not eat or drink anything except water) for 9–12 hours before the test.

MEDICARE COVERAGE FOR CHOLESTEROL SCREENING

Under the Affordable Care Act (ACA), insurance plans must cover cholesterol testing. Depending on your insurance plan, you may be able to get your cholesterol checked at no cost to you. Check with your insurance company to find out more.

Medicare may also cover cholesterol testing at no cost. If you have Medicare, learn about Medicare coverage for cholesterol testing.

If you do not have insurance, you may still be able to get free or low-cost cholesterol testing. Find a health center near you and ask about cholesterol testing.[5]

Section 4.5 | Osteoporosis Screening

WHAT IS OSTEOPOROSIS?

Osteoporosis is a bone disease. It means your bones are weak and more likely to break. People with osteoporosis most often break bones in the hip, spine, and wrist.

There are no signs or symptoms of osteoporosis. You might not know you have the disease until you break a bone. That is why it is so important to get a bone density test to measure your bone strength.

[5] Office of Disease Prevention and Health Promotion (ODPHP), "Get Your Cholesterol Checked," U.S. Department of Health and Human Services (HHS), July 29, 2022. Available online. URL: https://health.gov/myhealthfinder/ doctor-visits/screening-tests/get-your-cholesterol-checked. Accessed June 9, 2023.

ARE YOU AT RISK OF DEVELOPING OSTEOPOROSIS?

Women are at higher risk for osteoporosis than men, and the risk increases with age.

- If you are a woman aged 65 or older, schedule a bone density test.
- If you are a woman aged 64 or younger and you have gone through menopause, ask your doctor if you need a bone density test.

Men can get osteoporosis, too. If you are a man over the age of 65 and you are concerned about your bone strength, talk with your doctor or nurse.

Other things can increase your risk for osteoporosis, including the following:

- hormone changes (especially for women who have gone through menopause)
- not getting enough calcium and vitamin D
- having certain diseases or taking certain medicines
- smoking cigarettes or drinking too much alcohol
- not getting enough physical activity
- having a low body weight
- having a parent who had osteoporosis or broke a bone

GET TESTED FOR OSTEOPOROSIS

If you have osteoporosis, you can still slow down bone loss. Finding and treating the disease early can keep you healthier and more active—and help lower your risk of breaking bones.

Ask your doctor if you are at risk for osteoporosis and if you need to schedule a bone density test.

Depending on the results of your bone density test, you may need to do the following:

- Add more calcium and vitamin D to your diet.
- Get more physical activity.
- Take medicine to slow down bone loss and lower your chances of breaking a bone.

Your doctor can tell you what steps are right for you. It does not matter how old you are—it is never too late to improve your bone health.

WHAT HAPPENS DURING A BONE DENSITY TEST?

A bone density test measures how strong your bones are. The test will tell you if you have osteoporosis (or weak bones), and it can help you understand your risk of breaking a bone in the future.

A bone density test is like an x-ray or scan of your body. The test does not hurt, and you do not need to do anything to prepare for it. It only takes about 15 minutes.[6]

Section 4.6 | Abdominal Aortic Aneurysm Screening

WHAT IS ABDOMINAL AORTIC ANEURYSM?

The aorta is your body's main artery. An artery is a blood vessel (or tube) that carries blood from your heart. The aorta carries blood from your heart to your abdomen, pelvis, and legs.

If the wall of your aorta is weak, it can start to bulge. This balloon-like bulge is called an "aneurysm." An abdominal aortic aneurysm (AAA) is an aneurysm that happens in the part of the aorta running through the abdomen.

ARE YOU AT RISK FOR ABDOMINAL AORTIC ANEURYSM?

Men over the age of 65 who have smoked at any point in their lives have the highest risk of AAA. Both men and women can have AAA, but it is more common in men.

Risk factors for AAA include the following:

- smoking, both if you smoke now or you smoked in the past

---

[6] Office of Disease Prevention and Health Promotion (ODPHP), "Get a Bone Density Test," U.S. Department of Health and Human Services (HHS), July 14, 2022. Available online. URL: https://health.gov/myhealthfinder/doctor-visits/screening-tests/get-bone-density-test. Accessed June 12, 2023.

- family history—for example, if a parent or sibling had AAA
- older age, especially age 65 years or older
- being White
- having other aneurysms, such as thoracic aortic aneurysm (similar to AAA but in the chest instead of the abdomen)
- high blood pressure (HBP) or high cholesterol
- heart disease or vascular disease (problems with blood vessels)

If you are a man aged 65–75 and have ever smoked, ask your doctor about getting screened (tested) for AAA.

Why Do You Need to Talk to the Doctor?

Aneurysms usually grow slowly without any symptoms. When aneurysms grow large enough to rupture (burst), they can cause dangerous bleeding inside the body that can lead to death. The aneurysm can also create a tear in the wall, which is a serious problem, too.

If AAA is found early, it can be treated before it bursts. That is why it is so important to talk to your doctor about your risk.

GET SCREENED FOR ABDOMINAL AORTIC ANEURYSM

To screen for AAA, your doctor may order an ultrasound. An ultrasound uses sound waves to look inside the body. It can help your doctor see if there is any swelling in your aorta. Ultrasounds can be a little bit uncomfortable, but they do not usually cause pain.

MEDICARE COVERAGE FOR ABDOMINAL AORTIC ANEURYSM SCREENING

Under the Affordable Care Act (ACA), insurance plans must cover AAA screening for men aged 65–75 who have ever smoked. Depending on your insurance plan, you may be able to get screened at no cost to you. Check with your insurance company to find out more.

Medicare may also cover AAA screening for men aged 65–75 who have ever smoked at no cost.

If you do not have insurance, you may still be able to get free or low-cost AAA screening. Find a health center near you and ask about AAA screening (https://findahealthcenter.hrsa.gov).[7]

[7] Office of Disease Prevention and Health Promotion (ODPHP), "Talk to Your Doctor about Abdominal Aortic Aneurysm," U.S. Department of Health and Human Services (HHS), March 30, 2023. Available online. URL: https://health.gov/myhealthfinder/health-conditions/heart-health/talk-your-doctor-about-abdominal-aortic-aneurysm. Accessed July 4, 2023.

Chapter 5 | Cancer Screening Tests Recommended for Men

Section 5.1 | Breast Self-Examination

Many people are not aware that men can develop breast cancer. Males do have breast tissue, however, and malignant (cancerous) cells can develop there—just as they can in any other part of the body. Although less than 1 percent of all cases of breast cancer occur in males, several factors may increase the risk of male breast cancer, including:

- inherited gene mutations, such as *BRCA1* or *BRCA2*
- a family history of breast cancer
- exposure to radiation
- high levels of estrogen
- advanced age (Most cases are detected in men between the ages of 60 and 70.)

Since early detection of male breast cancer can lead to improved treatment options and prognosis, many health-care practitioners and cancer-prevention organizations recommend that men with an increased risk of breast cancer perform monthly breast self-examinations.

Breast self-examination is a technique people can use to visually and manually check their own breast tissue for lumps or other changes. People who conduct regular self-exams become familiar with the normal appearance and feel of their breast tissue, which enables them to recognize changes and discover lumps that may require medical attention. The following are some of the changes that should be checked by a doctor:

- hard lumps or new areas of thickness, which may or may not be painful
- discharge of fluid from the nipples
- dimpling, puckering, rashes, or other changes to the skin
- changes to the size or shape of the breast

HOW TO PERFORM A BREAST SELF-EXAMINATION

Doctors recommend that men at risk of breast cancer perform a regular breast self-examination once per month. It should cover the entire surface area of each breast, from the collarbone down to the abdomen and from the armpit across to the center of the chest. Perhaps the easiest way for men to examine their breast area is in the shower. Using soap and water to create a slippery surface allows the fingers to slide easily over the breast tissue.

The main steps in performing a male breast self-examination are as follows:

- Raise your right arm and place it behind or on top of your head.
- Examine your right breast by using the pads of the three middle fingers on your left hand.
- Move your fingers in small circles, about the size of a quarter.
- Begin under the armpit and work from top to bottom along the outer part of your breast.
- After completing one vertical strip, move over one finger width and begin a new strip, working from bottom to top. Do not lift the fingers between rows.
- Check the entire breast area in an up-and-down pattern, as if mowing a lawn.
- Repeat the process by using the left hand to examine the right breast.
- Gently squeeze each nipple between your fingers to check for any fluid discharge, puckering, or retraction.
- After stepping out of the shower and drying off, visually examine your breasts in front of a mirror. They should appear symmetrical in size and shape, and the skin should not show signs of dimpling, puckering, or rashes.

Men who find a lump or notice other changes in their breast tissue during a self-examination should not become alarmed. Around 80 percent of all breast lumps are not cancerous. In addition, most lumps or inflammation detected in male breasts is due to a benign condition called "gynecomastia." This condition is commonly associated with the hormonal changes of puberty, but it may also occur as a side effect of certain medications. Still, any hard lumps or other areas of concern should be checked by a medical practitioner.

References

"Check Yourself for Male Breast Cancer," MaleCare, 2016. Available online. URL: http://malecare.org/male-breast-cancer/check-yourself-for-male-breast-cancer. Accessed August 7, 2023.

Pam, Stephan. "Male Breast Self-Examination," VeryWell, December 16, 2014. Available online. URL: www.verywell.com/male-breast-self-exam-430634. Accessed August 7, 2023.

Section 5.2 | Oral Cancer Self-Examination

WHAT IS ORAL CANCER?

Oral cancer is cancer of the mouth. It is a type of head and neck cancer. Most oral cancers are squamous cell cancers. They begin in the flat cells that cover the surfaces of your mouth, tongue, and lips. The cancer cells may spread into deeper tissue as the cancer grows.

Most oral cancers are related to tobacco use, heavy alcohol use, or a human papillomavirus (HPV) infection.

WHO IS MORE LIKELY TO DEVELOP ORAL CANCER?

Anyone can get oral cancer, but you are more likely to develop it if you:

- use tobacco or drink lots of alcohol (Your risk of developing oral cancer is even higher if you do both.)
- are male
- are over the age of 40
- have HPV
- have a history of head or neck cancer
- get frequent sun exposure (for lip cancer)

WHAT ARE THE SYMPTOMS OF ORAL CANCER?

The symptoms of oral cancer may include:

- a white or red patch in your mouth
- a lip or mouth sore that will not heal

- bleeding, pain, or numbness in the lip or mouth
- loose teeth or dentures that no longer fit well
- problems or pain with swallowing
- a lump in your neck
- ear pain
- trouble moving your mouth or jaw
- swelling of the jaw
- a sore throat or feeling that something is caught in the throat

If you have any of these symptoms for more than two weeks, see your health-care provider or dentist. Oral cancer can spread quickly, so it is important to find it early.

HOW IS ORAL CANCER DIAGNOSED?

To find out if you have oral cancer, your provider may use:
- a physical exam of the lips and mouth
- an endoscopy
- a biopsy or other procedure to collect cells from the lip or oral cavity (The cells are viewed under a microscope to find out if they are abnormal.)
- imaging tests

WHAT ARE THE TREATMENTS FOR ORAL CANCER?

The treatments for oral cancer include surgery, radiation therapy, or both. After surgery, some people also need chemotherapy to kill any cancer cells that are left.

CAN ORAL CANCER BE PREVENTED?

There are steps you can take to help prevent oral cancer:
- not smoking
- limiting alcohol use or not drinking at all
- getting regular dental exams[1]

---

[1] MedlinePlus, "Oral Cancer," National Institutes of Health (NIH), May 22, 2023. Available online. URL: https://medlineplus.gov/oralcancer.html. Accessed July 3, 2023.

HOW ORAL CANCER SELF-EXAMINATION IS DONE?

An oral cancer exam is painless and quick—it takes only a few minutes. Your regular dental checkup is an excellent opportunity to have the exam.

Here is what to expect:

- Prepare for the exam—if you have dentures (plates) or partials, you will be asked to remove them.
- Your health-care provider will inspect your face, neck, lips, and mouth to look for any signs of cancer.
- With both hands, he or she will feel the area under your jaw and the side of your neck, checking for lumps that may suggest cancer.
- He or she will then look at and feel the insides of your lips and cheeks to check for possible signs of cancer, such as red and/or white patches.
- Next, your provider will have you stick out your tongue so that it can be checked for swelling or abnormal color or texture.
- Using gauze, he or she will then gently pull your tongue to one side, then the other, to check the base of your tongue. The underside of your tongue will also be checked.
- In addition, he or she will look at the roof and floor of your mouth, as well as the back of your throat.
- Finally, your provider will put one finger on the floor of your mouth and, with the other hand under your chin, gently press down to check for lumps or sensitivity.[2]

---

[2] "The Oral Cancer Exam," National Institute of Dental and Craniofacial Research (NIDCR), September 2018. Available online. URL: www.nidcr.nih.gov/sites/default/files/2018-10/oral-cancer-exam.pdf. Accessed July 3, 2023.

Section 5.3 | **Skin Cancer Screening**

Skin cancer is the most common type of cancer. The main types of skin cancer are squamous cell carcinoma, basal cell carcinoma, and melanoma. Melanoma is much less common than the other types but much more likely to invade nearby tissue and spread to other parts of the body. Most deaths from skin cancer are caused by melanoma.[3]

WHAT IS SKIN CANCER SCREENING?

Skin cancer screening includes looking at all of your skin to check for signs of skin cancer. Signs of skin cancer can be seen with just your eyes.

Skin cancer is very common, and screening can help find it when it is easier to treat. Your health-care provider can do skin cancer screening, and you can also check your skin yourself. To do skin cancer screening, you or your provider check your skin for moles, birthmarks, or other areas that have an unusual color, size, shape, or texture. If an area of skin does not look normal, you may need tests to find out if it is cancer.

The most common types of skin cancer are basal cell and squamous cell cancers. These cancers rarely spread to other parts of the body, and treatment usually cures them.

Melanoma is a less common type of skin cancer, but it is more serious. That is because it is more likely to spread to nearby tissues and other parts of your body. It can be harder to cure and may be fatal. Melanoma is easier to cure if it is found when it is growing only in the top layer of the skin. And it is less likely to be fatal when it is treated early.

WHAT IS IT USED FOR?

Skin cancer screening is used to look for signs of skin cancer. It is not used to diagnose cancer. If a screening test finds signs of skin

---

[3] "Skin Cancer (Including Melanoma)—Patient Version," National Cancer Institute (NCI), May 15, 2023. Available online. URL: www.cancer.gov/types/skin. Accessed June 15, 2023.

cancer, you may need to have a test called a "skin biopsy" to find out whether you have cancer.

WHY DO YOU NEED SKIN CANCER SCREENING?

Some medical experts recommend checking your own skin regularly starting at the age of 18. That is because skin cancer is very common, and people of all skin colors can get it.

Skin cancer screening with your provider or with a dermatologist (a doctor who specializes in skin disorders) may be important if you:

- find a suspicious area of skin during a self-exam
- have had skin cancer in the past (In this case, it is usually recommended to have regular yearly skin cancer screening with your provider or a dermatologist.)
- have a higher-than-normal risk for getting skin cancer:
  - Your risk for all types of skin cancer is higher if you have:
    - had frequent exposure to natural sunlight or artificial sunlight, such as tanning beds
    - pale skin that burns and freckles easily
    - skin that tans a little or not at all
    - blond or red hair
    - light-colored eyes, including blue or green
  - Your risk for basal cell or squamous cell cancer is higher if you have had:
    - actinic keratosis, patches of thick, scaly skin
    - radiation therapy for cancer
    - a weakened immune system
    - exposure to arsenic
  - Your risk for melanoma is higher if you:
    - had many blistering sunburns, especially as a child or teenager
    - have a personal and/or family health history of melanoma
    - have a family health history of unusual moles, such as Gorlin syndrome or xeroderma pigmentosum
    - have several large or many small moles

Ask your provider how often to do a self-exam and whether you need to have regular skin cancer screening from a provider, too.

WHAT HAPPENS DURING SKIN CANCER SCREENING?

For a self-exam to screen for skin cancer, you will check your skin to look for:

- changes in the size, shape, or color of an existing mole or spot
- moles or other skin spots that ooze, bleed, or become scaly or crusty
- moles that are painful to the touch
- sores that have not healed within two weeks
- shiny pink, red, pearly white, or translucent bumps
- the "ABCDE" of melanoma, which stands for:
    - **Asymmetry.** Does the mole or spot have an irregular shape with two parts that look very different?
    - **Border.** Is the border of the mole ragged or irregular?
    - **Color.** Is the color uneven?
    - **Diameter.** Is the mole or spot bigger than the size of a pea or a pencil eraser?
    - **Evolving.** Has the mole or spot changed during the past few weeks or months?

To do a head-to-toe self-exam, do the following:

- Choose a well-lit room with a full-length mirror. You will also need a handheld mirror.
- Check your scalp. Part your hair and look with a hand mirror. Using a blow-dryer to move your hair as you look may also help.
- Check the back of your neck, too.
- Look at your face, ears, and front of your neck.
- Look at the front of your chest and belly. Lift breasts to check the skin underneath.
- Raise your arms and check the skin on your left and right sides, including your underarms.

- Look at the front and back of your arms.
- Check your hands, including between your fingers and fingernails (without nail polish).
- Check your back and buttocks with a hand mirror.
- Sit down to check the front and sides of your legs and use the hand mirror to check the backs of your legs and your genitals.
- Check your feet, including the bottoms, the spaces between your toes, and the nails of each toe (without nail polish).

For skin cancer screening by a provider, you will remove your clothing and put on a gown. Your provider will do a full exam that includes your scalp, behind your ears, fingers, buttocks, and feet. Your provider may use a special magnifying glass with a light to look more closely at certain moles or spots. The exam should take 10–15 minutes.

WILL YOU NEED TO DO ANYTHING TO PREPARE FOR THE TEST?
You should not wear makeup or nail polish. You will need to have your hair loose so that your scalp can be checked.

ARE THERE ANY RISKS TO THE TEST?
Skin cancer screening is not always helpful and may have risks. You may want to discuss these possible risks with your provider:
- Your screening test could find a cancer that would never cause health problems. Not all skin cancers cause symptoms or threaten your life. But, if they are found during screening, you may have cancer treatment that could cause side effects.
- Finding advanced skin cancer may not help you live longer. Advanced skin cancer is cancer that is unlikely to be cured or controlled with treatment. It may have spread to other parts of your body. Finding advanced skin cancer during screening may not change how the cancer affects you.

- Your screening test results could show that you have skin cancer, but you really do not. This is called a "false positive." If you have a false positive, you may have other tests that have risks, such as a skin biopsy. A skin biopsy may cause scarring. Thinking you have cancer may also make you feel anxious.
- Your skin cancer screening result could be normal, but you have skin cancer. This is called a "false negative." A false negative may delay your medical care for the cancer.

WHAT DO THE RESULTS MEAN?

If you find a mole or other spot on your skin that concerns you, contact your provider. If you or your provider finds a sign of skin cancer, you will probably have a skin biopsy to find out whether you have cancer.

A skin biopsy is a procedure that removes a small sample of skin for testing. The skin sample is checked under a microscope to look for cancer cells. Not all suspicious spots turn out to be skin cancer. If the biopsy shows that you do have skin cancer, your provider will talk with you about your treatment options.

IS THERE ANYTHING ELSE YOU NEED TO KNOW ABOUT SKIN CANCER SCREENING?

There are mobile phone apps that use the camera of your phone to check skin moles and spots to help find skin cancer. These apps need to be studied to see if they are accurate and useful for skin cancer screening.[4]

---

[4] MedlinePlus, "Skin Cancer Screening," National Institutes of Health (NIH), December 15, 2022. Available online. URL: https://medlineplus.gov/lab-tests/skin-cancer-screening. Accessed June 15, 2023.

Section 5.4 | **Colorectal Cancer Screening**

WHAT IS COLORECTAL CANCER?

Colorectal cancer is a cancer that develops in the colon or the rectum. The colon is the longest part of the large intestine. The rectum is the bottom part of the large intestine.

Like all cancers, colorectal cancer can spread to other parts of your body.

ARE YOU AT RISK OF DEVELOPING COLORECTAL CANCER?

The risk of developing colorectal cancer increases as you get older. That is why screening is recommended for everyone aged 45–75.

Other risk factors are as follows:

- having certain types of polyps (growths) inside the colon
- having a personal or family history of colorectal cancer
- smoking cigarettes
- being overweight or having obesity
- not getting enough physical activity
- drinking too much alcohol
- having inflammatory bowel disease (IBD), such as Crohn's disease, ulcerative colitis (UC), or other health conditions that cause chronic (long-term) problems with the small intestine and colon

WHAT ARE THE DIFFERENT KINDS OF COLORECTAL CANCER SCREENING TESTS?

There are several kinds of screening tests for colorectal cancer. The main types are:

- stool-based tests
- tests that look directly inside the colon and rectum

Stool tests are done at home. You collect a stool (poop) sample and send it to your doctor's office or a lab for testing.

Tests that look directly at your colon and rectum—such as a colonoscopy—happen in a doctor's office or hospital. For these tests, you need to take a laxative to clean out your bowels before the appointment. For a colonoscopy, you will get anesthesia before the test, and you will need someone to drive you home after the test.

Your doctor will tell you how to get ready for your test, including if you need to avoid certain foods or medicines beforehand.

Does It Hurt to Get a Colonoscopy?

Preparing for a colonoscopy can be unpleasant, but most people agree that the benefits to their health outweigh any discomfort. And getting anesthesia means you will not have any pain or feel uncomfortable during the test.

HOW DO YOU DECIDE WHICH TYPE OF COLORECTAL CANCER SCREENING TEST TO GET?

Your doctor can help you decide which type of screening test is right for you. Before you talk with your doctor about which screening to get, it can be helpful to think about your values and preferences.

TAKE CONTROL: GET SCREENED REGULARLY

If you get screened regularly, you have a good chance of preventing colorectal cancer or finding it when it can be treated more easily.

During a colonoscopy, the following procedures can occur:

- If your doctor finds polyps inside your colon, they can remove the polyps during your test—before they turn into cancer.
- If your doctor finds cancer during the test, you can take steps to get treatment right away.

If you get an unusual result on a stool test, your doctor will do a follow-up colonoscopy to look for cancer.

Get Support

If you are nervous about getting colorectal cancer screening, get support:

- Ask a family member or friend to go with you when you talk to the doctor.

- Talk with people you know who have been screened to learn what to expect.

Screening tests can help prevent colorectal cancer or find it early when it may be easier to treat.

You may need to get screened before the age of 45 if colorectal cancer runs in your family. Your doctor may also recommend that you continue to get screened if you are between the ages of 76 and 85, depending on certain risk factors and your overall health.

Talk with your doctor about your risk for colorectal cancer.

HOW OFTEN SHOULD YOU GET SCREENED FOR COLORECTAL CANCER?

How often you need to get screened will depend on:
- your risk for colorectal cancer
- which screening test you choose

MEDICARE COVERAGE FOR COLORECTAL CANCER SCREENING

Under the Affordable Care Act (ACA), health insurance plans must cover screening for colorectal cancer. Depending on your plan, you may be able to get screened at no cost to you. Check with your insurance company to find out more.

Medicare may also cover screening for colorectal cancer at no cost. If you have Medicare, find out about Medicare coverage for different colorectal cancer screening tests.

If you do not have insurance, you may still be able to get free or low-cost colorectal cancer screening.[5]

---

[5] Office of Disease Prevention and Health Promotion (ODPHP), "Get Screened for Colorectal Cancer," U.S. Department of Health and Human Services (HHS), February 9, 2023. Available online. URL: https://health.gov/myhealthfinder/doctor-visits/screening-tests/get-screened-colorectal-cancer. Accessed June 12, 2023.

Section 5.5 | Testicular Self-Examination

Although testicular cancer has a relatively low rate of occurrence, accounting for just 1 percent of malignancies in all men, it is the most common neoplasm, or abnormal growth, in adolescent males and young men under 35 years of age. Testicular cancer is easily diagnosable and can be successfully treated, with a high survival rate of more than 10 years in nearly 90 percent of patients. As with most types of cancer, the prognosis is particularly good with early detection. While significant advances have been made in developing treatments for testicular cancer in the last few decades, the benefits of early detection through self-examination have not received much attention, often resulting in delays before medical attention is sought.

IMPORTANCE OF TESTICULAR SELF-EXAMINATION

In the absence of standard or routine screening for testicular cancer, the condition is most often detected either by a doctor during a routine physical examination or by an individual during the course of a self-exam. The outlook for testicular cancer depends on whether or not the disease has metastasized to lymph nodes, tissues, and organs, and this underscores the importance of early detection by testicular self-examination (TSE). Early detection involves the diagnosis of testicular cancer through stages 1 and 2. Stage 1 refers to a "localized" tumor restricted to the primary site, the testes. Stage 2 is the term for a "regional" tumor, one that has spread to other areas. An early diagnosis resulting from a self-exam can greatly enhance treatment outcomes and also reduce the side effects commonly associated with chemotherapy, radiation, and surgery.

HOW TO PERFORM A SELF-EXAM

Self-examination is a common screening method that helps you identify any abnormalities in the size, shape, and consistency of your testes. This also helps you distinguish the epididymis—a highly coiled duct behind the testis for the temporary storage of sperm—from an abnormal lump or growth. Furthermore, it is quite normal for most men to have testicular asymmetry. Differently sized testes with one hanging lower than the other are a normal anatomical feature and should not be construed as a sign of abnormality.

The ideal time to perform a self-exam is right after a warm shower when the scrotum is relaxed and can be easily drawn back to examine the testicles.

TSE is a simple procedure that takes no more than a couple of minutes:

- Hold the penis away from the scrotum to enable close examination of the testes.
- Hold the testicles between your thumb and fingers and roll gently.
- Feel each testicle for any painless lump, usually grain- or pea-sized, in the front or sides, taking care not to confuse a lump with supporting tissues and blood vessels.
- If you detect any thickening, discomfort, or pain in the testicles or groin, contact your health-care professional immediately.

Studies show that men often delay seeking medical attention because early symptoms are typically mild, and many men tend to believe that a lump is benign or harmless and may go away on its own. Concerns about loss of sexuality, or sterility, may also get in the way of seeking professional help when an abnormality is detected.

While the majority of scrotal and testicular irregularities may not be associated with malignancy, it is important for all men—especially those who carry a high risk for testicular tumors—to perform regular self-exams. A family history of testicular cancer and previous history of malignant tumors in one or both of the testes are regarded as high-risk factors, as are conditions such as cryptorchidism, a common birth defect associated with undescended testes.

References

"How to Perform a Testicular Self-Examination," Nemours Foundation, 2012. Available online. URL: https://kidshealth. org/en/teens/tse.html. Accessed August 7, 2023.

"SEER Stat Fact Sheets: Testis Cancer," National Institutes of Health (NIH), April 2016. Available online. URL: https://seer. cancer.gov/statfacts/html/testis.html. Accessed August 7, 2023.

"Testicular Examination and Testicular Self-Examination (TSE)," *Web*MD, June 4, 2014. Available online. URL: www.webmd. com/men/testicular-exam. Accessed August 7, 2023.

Section 5.6 | Prostate Cancer Screening

Prostate cancer is a disease in which malignant cells form in the tissues of the prostate.

The prostate is a gland in the male reproductive system located just below the bladder (the organ that collects and empties urine) and in front of the rectum (the lower part of the intestine; see Figure 5.1). It is about the size of a walnut and surrounds part of the urethra (the tube that empties urine from the bladder). The prostate gland produces fluid that makes up part of semen.

As men age, the prostate may get bigger. A bigger prostate may block the flow of urine from the bladder and cause problems with sexual function. This condition is called "benign prostatic hyperplasia" (BPH), and although it is not cancer, surgery may be needed to correct it. The symptoms of benign prostatic hyperplasia or of other problems in the prostate may be similar to symptoms of prostate cancer.

WHO IS AT RISK OF DEVELOPING PROSTATE CANCER?

Prostate cancer is found mainly in older men. Although the number of men with prostate cancer is large, most men diagnosed with this disease do not die from it. Prostate cancer causes more deaths in men than any other cancer except lung cancer. Prostate cancer occurs more often in African-American men than in White men. African-American men with prostate cancer are more likely to die from the disease than White men with prostate cancer.

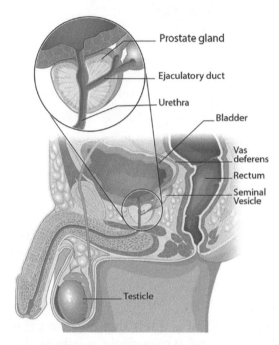

Figure 5.1. The Prostate Gland

Centers for Disease Control and Prevention (CDC)

PROSTATE CANCER SCREENING
There Is No Standard or Routine Screening Test for Prostate Cancer

Although there are no standard or routine screening tests for prostate cancer, the following tests are being used or studied to screen for it.

DIGITAL RECTAL EXAM

A digital rectal exam (DRE) is an exam of the rectum (see Figure 5.2). The doctor or nurse inserts a lubricated, gloved finger into the lower part of the rectum to feel the prostate for lumps or anything else that seems unusual.

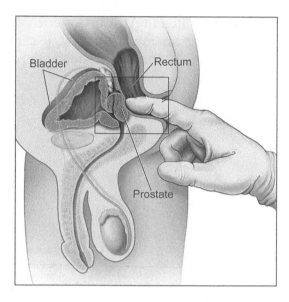

Figure 5.2. Digital Rectal Exam

National Cancer Institute (NCI)

PROSTATE-SPECIFIC ANTIGEN TEST

A prostate-specific antigen (PSA) test is a test that measures the level of PSA in the blood. PSA is a substance made mostly by the prostate that may be found in an increased amount in the blood of men who have prostate cancer. The level of PSA may also be high in men who have an infection or inflammation of the prostate or benign prostatic hyperplasia.

A PSA test or a DRE may be able to detect prostate cancer at an early stage, but it is not clear whether early detection and treatment decrease the risk of dying from prostate cancer.

Studies are being done to find ways to make PSA testing more accurate for early cancer detection.

A Prostate Cancer Gene 3 RNA Test May Be Used for Certain Patients

If a man had a high PSA level and a biopsy of the prostate did not show cancer and the PSA level remains high after the biopsy, a prostate cancer gene 3 (*PCA3*) RNA test may be done. This test measures the amount of *PCA3* RNA in the urine after a DRE. If the *PCA3* RNA level is higher than normal, another biopsy may help diagnose prostate cancer.

RISKS OF PROSTATE CANCER SCREENING
Screening Tests Have Risks

Decisions about screening tests can be difficult. Not all screening tests are helpful, and most have risks. Before having any screening test, you may want to discuss the test with your doctor. It is important to know the risks of the test and whether it has been proven to reduce the risk of dying from cancer.

The Risks of Prostate Screening
FINDING PROSTATE CANCER MAY NOT IMPROVE HEALTH OR HELP A MAN LIVE LONGER

Screening may not improve your health or help you live longer if you have cancer that has already spread to the area outside of the prostate or to other places in your body.

Some cancers never cause symptoms or become life-threatening, but if found by a screening test, the cancer may be treated. Finding these cancers is called "overdiagnosis." It is not known if treatment of these cancers would help you live longer than if no treatment were given.

Treatments for prostate cancer, such as radical prostatectomy and radiation therapy, may have long-term side effects in many men. The most common side effects are erectile dysfunction (ED) and urinary incontinence (UI).

Some studies of patients with newly diagnosed prostate cancer showed that these patients had a higher risk of death from cardiovascular (heart and blood vessel) disease or suicide. The risk was greatest in the first weeks or months after diagnosis.

FOLLOW-UP TESTS

If a PSA test is higher than normal, a biopsy of the prostate may be done. Complications from a biopsy of the prostate may include fever, pain, blood in the urine or semen, and urinary tract infection (UTI). Even if a biopsy shows that a patient does not have prostate cancer, he may worry more about developing prostate cancer in the future.

FALSE-NEGATIVE TEST RESULTS CAN OCCUR

Screening test results may appear to be normal even though prostate cancer is present. A man who receives a false-negative test result (one that shows that there is no cancer when there really is) may delay seeking medical care even if he has symptoms.

FALSE-POSITIVE TEST RESULTS CAN OCCUR

Screening test results may appear to be abnormal even though no cancer is present. A false-positive test result (one that shows there is cancer when there really is not) can cause anxiety and is usually followed by more tests (such as a biopsy), which also have risks.

Your doctor can advise you about your risk for prostate cancer and your need for screening tests.[6]

---

[6] "Prostate Cancer Screening (PDQ®)—Patient Version," National Cancer Institute (NCI), May 6, 2022. Available online. URL: www.cancer.gov/types/prostate/patient/prostate-screening-pdq#section/all. Accessed June 23, 2023.

Part 2 | Common Medical Issues in Men

Chapter 6 | **Diabetes**

Diabetes is a chronic (long-lasting) health condition that affects how your body turns food into energy.

Your body breaks down most of the food you eat into sugar (glucose) and releases it into your bloodstream. When your blood sugar goes up, it signals your pancreas to release insulin. Insulin acts like a key to let the blood sugar into your body's cells for use as energy.

With diabetes, your body does not make enough insulin or cannot use it as well as it should. When there is not enough insulin or cells stop responding to insulin, too much blood sugar stays in your bloodstream. Over time, that can cause serious health problems, such as heart disease, vision loss, and kidney disease.

TYPES OF DIABETES

There are three main types of diabetes: type 1, type 2, and prediabetes.

Type 1 Diabetes

Type 1 diabetes is thought to be caused by an autoimmune reaction (the body attacks itself by mistake). This reaction stops your body from making insulin. Approximately 5–10 percent of the people who have diabetes have type 1. Symptoms of type 1 diabetes often develop quickly. It is usually diagnosed in children, teens, and young adults. If you have type 1 diabetes, you will need to take insulin every day to survive.

Type 2 Diabetes

With type 2 diabetes, your body does not use insulin well and cannot keep blood sugar at normal levels. About 90–95 percent of people with diabetes have type 2. It develops over many years and is usually diagnosed in adults (but more and more in children, teens, and young adults). You may not notice any symptoms, so it is important to get your blood sugar tested if you are at risk.

Prediabetes

In the United States, 96 million adults—more than 1 in 3—have prediabetes. More than 8 in 10 of them do not know they have it. With prediabetes, blood sugar levels are higher than normal but not high enough for a type 2 diabetes diagnosis. Prediabetes raises your risk for type 2 diabetes, heart disease, and stroke.

RISK FACTORS FOR DIABETES
Type 1 Diabetes

Type 1 diabetes is thought to be caused by an immune reaction (the body attacks itself by mistake). Risk factors for type 1 diabetes are not as clear as for prediabetes and type 2 diabetes. Known risk factors include the following:

- **Family history**. Having a parent, brother, or sister with type 1 diabetes.
- **Age**. You can get type 1 diabetes at any age, but it usually develops in children, teens, or young adults.

In the United States, White people are more likely to develop type 1 diabetes than African-American and Hispanic or Latinx people.

Currently, no one knows how to prevent type 1 diabetes.

Type 2 Diabetes

You are at risk of type 2 diabetes if you:
- have prediabetes
- are overweight
- are 45 years or older
- have a parent, brother, or sister with type 2 diabetes
- are physically active less than three times a week

- are an African American, Hispanic or Latinx, American Indian, or Alaska Native (Some Pacific Islanders and Asian Americans are also at higher risk.)

If you have nonalcoholic fatty liver disease, you may also be at risk for type 2 diabetes.

You can prevent or delay type 2 diabetes with proven lifestyle changes. These include losing weight if you are overweight, eating a healthy diet, and getting regular physical activity.

Prediabetes
You are at risk for prediabetes if you:
- are overweight
- are 45 years or older
- have a parent, brother, or sister with type 2 diabetes
- are physically active less than three times a week
- are an African American, Hispanic or Latinx, American Indian, or Alaska Native (Some Pacific Islanders and Asian Americans are also at higher risk.)

You can prevent or reverse prediabetes with proven lifestyle changes. These include losing weight if you are overweight, eating a healthy diet, and getting regular physical activity. The National Diabetes Prevention Program led by the Centers for Disease Control and Prevention (CDC) can help you make healthy changes that have lasting results.

SYMPTOMS OF DIABETES
If you have any of the following diabetes symptoms, see your doctor about getting your blood sugar tested:
- urinate (pee) a lot, often at night
- are very thirsty
- lose weight without trying
- are very hungry

- have blurry vision
- have numb or tingling hands or feet
- feel very tired
- have very dry skin
- have sores that heal slowly
- have more infections than usual

Symptoms of Type 1 Diabetes

People who have type 1 diabetes may also have nausea, vomiting, or stomach pains. Type 1 diabetes symptoms can develop in just a few weeks or months and can be severe. Type 1 diabetes usually starts when you are a child, teen, or young adult but can happen at any age.

Symptoms of Type 2 Diabetes

Type 2 diabetes symptoms often take several years to develop. Some people do not notice any symptoms at all. Type 2 diabetes usually starts when you are an adult though more and more children and teens are developing it. Because symptoms are hard to spot, it is important to know the risk factors for type 2 diabetes. Make sure to visit your doctor if you have any of them.

DIAGNOSIS FOR DIABETES

You will need to get your blood sugar tested to find out for sure if you have type 1, type 2, or prediabetes. Testing is simple, and results are usually available quickly.

PREVENTION FOR DIABETES

Currently, no one knows how to prevent type 1 diabetes. But a few things that you can do to help include the following:

- Take medicine as prescribed.
- Get diabetes self-management education and support.
- Make and keep health-care appointments.

Diabetes

Type 2 diabetes can be prevented or delayed with healthy lifestyle changes, such as:
- losing weight
- eating healthy food
- being active

If you have prediabetes, a CDC-recognized lifestyle change program can help you take healthy steps to reverse it.[1]

---

[1] "Diabetes Basics," Centers for Disease Control and Prevention (CDC), April 24, 2023. Available online. URL: www.cdc.gov/diabetes/basics/diabetes.html. Accessed June 12, 2023.

Chapter 7 | Heart Disease

Chapter Contents

Section 7.1 | Men and Heart Disease

HOW DOES HEART DISEASE AFFECT MEN?
- Heart disease is the leading cause of death for men in the United States, killing 384,886 men in 2021—that is about one in every four male deaths.
- Heart disease is the leading cause of death for men of most racial and ethnic groups in the United States, including African Americans, American Indians or Alaska Natives, Hispanics, and Whites. For Asian-American or Pacific-Islander men, heart disease is second only to cancer.
- About 1 in 13 (7.7%) White men and 1 in 14 (7.1%) Black men have coronary heart disease (CHD). About 1 in 17 (5.9%) Hispanic men have CHD.
- Half of the men who die suddenly of CHD had no previous symptoms. Even if you have no symptoms, you may still be at risk for heart disease.

WHAT ARE THE RISKS OF HEART DISEASE?
During 2013–2016, 47 percent of men had hypertension, a major risk factor for heart disease and stroke.

Several other medical conditions and lifestyle choices can also put people at a higher risk for heart disease, including the following:
- diabetes
- overweight and obesity
- unhealthy diet
- physical inactivity
- excessive alcohol use

HOW COULD YOU REDUCE YOUR RISK OF HEART DISEASE?
To reduce your chances of getting heart disease, it is important to do the following:
- Know your blood pressure. Having uncontrolled blood pressure can result in heart disease. High blood pressure (HBP) has no symptoms, so it is important to have your blood pressure checked regularly.

- Talk to your health-care provider about whether you should be tested for diabetes. Having diabetes raises your risk of heart disease.
- Quit smoking. If you do not smoke, do not start. If you do smoke, learn ways to quit.
- Discuss checking your cholesterol and triglyceride levels with your health-care provider.
- Make healthy food habits. Having overweight or obesity raises your risk of heart disease.
- Limit alcohol intake to one drink a day.
- Lower your stress level and find healthy ways to cope with stress.

WHAT ARE THE SYMPTOMS OF HEART DISEASE?

Sometimes, heart disease may be "silent" and not diagnosed until a man experiences signs or symptoms of a heart attack, heart failure, or arrhythmia. When these events happen, symptoms may include the following:

- **Heart attack.** Chest pain or discomfort, upper back or neck pain, indigestion, heartburn, nausea or vomiting, extreme fatigue, upper body discomfort, dizziness, and shortness of breath.
- **Arrhythmia.** Fluttering feelings in the chest (palpitations).
- **Heart failure.** Shortness of breath, fatigue, or swelling of the feet, ankles, legs, abdomen, or neck veins.

Even if you have no symptoms, you may still be at risk for heart disease.

PREVENTION OF HEART DISEASE

By living a healthy lifestyle, you can help keep your blood pressure, cholesterol, and blood sugar levels normal and lower your risk for heart disease and heart attack.[1]

---

[1] "Men and Heart Disease," Centers for Disease Control and Prevention (CDC), May 15, 2023. Available online. URL: www.cdc.gov/heartdisease/men.htm. Accessed June 12, 2023.

Section 7.2 | **Heart Failure**

Heart failure, also known as "congestive heart failure," is a condition that develops when your heart does not pump enough blood for your body's needs. This can happen if your heart cannot fill up with enough blood. It can also happen when your heart is too weak to pump properly. The term "heart failure" does not mean that your heart has stopped. However, heart failure is a serious condition that needs medical care.

More than six million adults in the United States have heart failure, according to the Centers for Disease Control and Prevention (CDC).

Heart failure can develop suddenly (the acute kind) or over time as your heart gets weaker (the chronic kind). It can affect one or both sides of your heart. Left- and right-sided heart failure may have different causes. Most often, heart failure is caused by another medical condition that damages your heart. This includes coronary heart disease, heart inflammation, high blood pressure (HBP), cardiomyopathy, or an irregular heartbeat. Heart failure may not cause symptoms right away. But, eventually, you may feel tired and short of breath and notice fluid buildup in your lower body, around your stomach, or around your neck.

CAUSES AND RISK FACTORS OF HEART FAILURE

Long-term, or chronic, heart failure is often caused by other medical conditions that damage or overwork your heart. Sudden, or acute, heart failure can be caused by an injury or infection that damages your heart, a heart attack, or a blood clot in your lung.

To understand heart failure, it helps know how the heart works. The right side of your heart gets oxygen-low blood from your body. It pumps the blood to your lungs to pick up oxygen. The left side of your heart pumps oxygen-rich blood to the rest of your body.

What Causes Left-Sided Heart Failure?

Left-sided heart failure is more common than right-sided heart failure. There are two types of left-sided heart failure, each based on how well your heart pumps. This measurement is called the "ejection fraction."

- In heart failure with reduced ejection fraction (HFrEF), the left side of your heart is weak and cannot pump enough blood to the rest of your body. Chronic conditions that damage or weaken the heart muscles are the main cause of HFrEF. For example, CHD or a heart attack can prevent your heart muscle from getting enough oxygen. Other causes of this type of heart failure include faulty heart valves, an irregular heartbeat, or heart diseases that you are born with or inherit.
- In heart failure with preserved ejection fraction (HFpEF), the left side of your heart is too stiff to fully relax between heartbeats. That means it cannot fill up with enough blood to pump out to your body. HBP and other conditions that make your heart work harder are the main causes of HFpEF. Conditions that stiffen the chambers of the heart, such as obesity and diabetes, are also causes of this type of heart failure. Over time, your heart muscle thickens to adapt, which makes it stiffer.

What Causes Right-Sided Heart Failure?

Over time, left-sided heart failure can lead to right-sided heart failure.

In right-sided heart failure, your heart cannot pump enough blood to your lungs to pick up oxygen. Left-sided heart failure is the main cause of right-sided heart failure. That is because left-sided heart failure can cause blood to build up on the left side of your heart. The buildup of blood raises the pressure in the blood vessels that carry blood from your heart to your lungs. This is called "pulmonary hypertension," and it can make the right side of your heart work harder.

Congenital heart defects (CHDs) or conditions that damage the right side of your heart such as abnormal heart valves can also lead to right-side heart failure. The same is true for conditions that damage the lungs, such as chronic obstructive pulmonary disease (COPD).

What Raises Your Risk for Heart Failure?

Many things can raise your risk of heart failure. Some things you can control, such as your lifestyle habits, but many others are out of your control, including your age, race, or ethnicity. Your risk of heart failure goes up if you have more than one of the following:

- **Aging**. It can weaken and stiffen your heart. People aged 65 or older have a higher risk of heart failure. Older adults are also more likely to have other health conditions that cause heart failure.
- **Family history**. A family history of heart failure makes your risk of heart failure higher. Genetics may also play a role. Certain changes, or mutations, to genes can make your heart tissue weaker or less flexible.
- **Unhealthy lifestyle habits**. Smoking, an unhealthy diet, using cocaine or other illegal drugs, heavy alcohol use, and lack of physical activity increase your risk of heart failure.
- **Certain chronic illnesses**. Heart or blood vessel conditions, serious lung disease, or infections such as human immunodeficiency virus (HIV) or severe acute respiratory syndrome coronavirus 2 (SARS-CoV-2) raise your risk. This is also true for long-term health conditions, such as obesity, HBP, diabetes, sleep apnea, chronic kidney disease, anemia, thyroid disease, or iron overload. Cancer treatments, such as radiation and chemotherapy, can injure your heart and raise your risk as well. Atrial fibrillation (AF), a common type of irregular heart rhythm, can also cause heart failure.
- **Ethnicity**. Black and African-American people are more likely to have heart failure than people of other races, often have more serious cases of heart failure, and experience heart failure at a younger age.

Heart failure is common in both men and women although men often develop heart failure at a younger age than women. Women more commonly have HFpEF, which is when the heart does not fill with enough blood. Men are more likely to have HFrEF. Women often have worse symptoms than men.

SYMPTOMS OF HEART FAILURE

Symptoms of heart failure depend on the type of heart failure you have and how serious it is. If you have mild heart failure, you may not notice any symptoms except during hard physical work. Symptoms can depend on whether you have left- or right-sided heart failure. However, you can have symptoms of both types. Symptoms usually get worse as your heart grows weaker.

Heart failure can lead to serious and life-threatening complications.

One of the first symptoms you may notice is feeling short of breath after routine activities, such as climbing stairs. As your heart grows weaker, you may notice this while getting dressed or walking across the room. Some people have shortness of breath while lying flat.

Older adults who do not get much physical activity may not experience shortness of breath. However, they may feel tired and confused.

People who have left-sided heart failure may have the following symptoms:

- trouble breathing
- cough
- fatigue (extreme tiredness even after rest)
- general weakness
- bluish color of fingers and lips
- sleepiness and trouble concentrating
- inability to sleep lying flat

People who have right-sided heart failure may also have the following symptoms:

- nausea (feeling sick in the stomach) and loss of appetite
- pain in your abdomen (area around your stomach)
- swelling in your ankles, feet, legs, abdomen, and the veins in your neck
- needing to pee often
- weight gain

What Problems Can Heart Failure Cause?

Heart failure can cause some serious problems.

- Kidney or liver damage is caused by reduced blood flow and fluid buildup in your organs.
- Fluid may build up in or around your lungs.
- Malnutrition from nausea and swelling in your abdomen (the area around your stomach) can make it uncomfortable for you to eat.
- Reduced blood flow to your stomach can make it harder to absorb nutrients from your food.
- Other heart conditions such as an irregular heartbeat, leaking heart valves, or sudden cardiac arrest (SCA) can be caused by heart failure.
- Pulmonary hypertension may also be caused by this condition.

DIAGNOSIS OF HEART FAILURE
How Would You Find Out If You Have Heart Failure?

Your doctor will diagnose heart failure based on your medical history, a physical exam, and test results. Bring a list of your symptoms to your appointment, including how often they happen and when they started. Also, bring a list of any prescription and over-the-counter (OTC) medicines you take. Let your provider know if you have any risk factors for heart failure.

You may also be referred to a cardiologist for these tests and treatment. A cardiologist is a doctor who specializes in diagnosing and treating heart diseases.

Diagnostic Tests and Procedures
BLOOD TESTS

Your provider may order blood tests to check the levels of certain molecules, such as brain natriuretic peptide (BNP). These levels rise during heart failure. Blood tests can also show how well your liver and your kidneys are working.

TESTS TO MEASURE YOUR EJECTION FRACTION

Your provider may order an echocardiography (echo) or other imaging tests to measure your ejection fraction. Your ejection fraction is the percent of the blood in the lower left chamber of your heart (the left ventricle) that is pumped out of your heart with each heartbeat. The ejection fraction measures how well your heart pumps. This helps diagnose the type of heart failure you have and guides your treatment.

- If 40 percent or less of the blood in your left ventricle is pumped out in one beat, you have HFrEF.
- If 50 percent or more of the blood in your left ventricle is pumped out in one beat, you have HFpEF.
- If your ejection fraction is somewhere between 41 and 49 percent, you may be diagnosed with heart failure with borderline ejection fraction.

OTHER TESTS

- Other imaging tests, such as a cardiac computed tomography (CT) scan, cardiac magnetic resonance imaging (MRI), or nuclear heart scan, show how well your heart is working. You may also need cardiac catheterization with coronary angiography to look inside the arteries in your heart and see if they are blocked.
- Tests for your heart's electrical activity may also be necessary. This might include an electrocardiogram (EKG) or a Holter or event monitor that you wear for 24–48 hours or more while going about your normal activities.
- A stress test measures how much exercise your body can handle and how well it works during physical activity. Some heart problems are easier to diagnose when your heart is working hard and beating fast.

TREATMENT FOR HEART FAILURE

Heart failure has no cure. But treatment can help you live a longer, more active life with fewer symptoms. Treatment depends on the type of heart failure you have and how serious it is.

Healthy Lifestyle Changes

Your provider may recommend these heart-healthy lifestyle changes alone or as part of a cardiac rehabilitation plan:

- **Lower your sodium (salt) intake**. Salt may make fluid buildup worse.
- **Aim for a healthy weight**. Extra weight can make your heart work harder.
- **Get regular physical activity**. Ask your health-care provider about how active you should be, including during daily activities, work, leisure time, sex, and exercise. Your level of activity will depend on how serious your heart failure is. Sometimes, your provider might recommend outpatient cardiac rehabilitation services to improve your exercise level and reduce your risk factors.
- **Quit smoking**. For free help to quit smoking, you may call the Smoking Quitline of the National Cancer Institute (NCI) at 877-44U-QUIT (877-448-7848).
- **Avoid or limit alcohol**. Your provider may recommend that you limit or stop drinking alcohol. You can find resources and support at the Alcohol Treatment Navigator (https://alcoholtreatment.niaaa.nih.gov) of the National Institute on Alcohol Abuse and Alcoholism (NIAAA).
- **Manage contributing risk factors**. Controlling some of the factors that may worsen heart failure such as blood pressure, heart rhythm, and anemia will often improve heart health.
- **Manage stress**. Learning how to manage stress and cope with problems can improve your mental and physical health. Relaxation techniques, talking to a counselor, and finding a support group can all help lower stress and anxiety.
- **Get good-quality sleep**. Sleep disorders, such as sleep apnea, are common in people who have heart failure. Treating your sleep disorder helps improve your sleep and may help improve your heart failure symptoms.

Medicines
LEFT-SIDED HEART FAILURE

The following medicines are commonly used to treat heart failure with reduced ejection fraction:

- Medicines that remove extra sodium and fluid from your body, including diuretics and aldosterone antagonists (such as spironolactone), lower the amount of blood that the heart must pump. Very high doses of diuretics may cause low blood pressure, kidney disease, and worsening heart failure symptoms. Side effects of aldosterone antagonists can include kidney disease and high potassium levels.

- Medicines to relax your blood vessels make it easier for your heart to pump blood. Examples include angiotensin-converting enzyme (ACE) inhibitors and angiotensin receptor blockers (ARBs). Possible side effects include cough, low blood pressure, and short-term reduced kidney function.

- Medicines to slow your heart rate, such as beta-blockers and ivabradine, make it easier for your heart to pump blood and can help prevent long-term heart failure from getting worse. Possible side effects include a slow or irregular heart rate, HBP, and fuzzy vision or seeing bright halos.

- Newer medicines, including two new groups of medicines approved to lower blood sugar in patients with diabetes, called "sodium-glucose cotransporter-2 (SGLT-2) inhibitors" and "glucagon-like peptide (GLP) agonists," may also reduce heart failure hospitalizations. Their use in treating heart failure is currently being studied.

- Digoxin makes your heart beat stronger and pump more blood. This medicine is mostly used to treat serious heart failure when other medicines do not help improve your symptoms. Side effects may include digestive problems, confusion, and vision problems.

Currently, the main treatments for HFpEF are diuretics. Your doctor may also prescribe blood pressure medicines to help relieve your symptoms.

RIGHT-SIDED HEART FAILURE

If you have right-sided heart failure, your doctor may prescribe the following two types of medicines:

- Medicines that remove extra sodium and fluid from your body, including diuretics and aldosterone antagonists (such as spironolactone), lower the amount of blood that the heart must pump. Very high doses of diuretics may cause low blood pressure, kidney disease, and worsening heart failure symptoms. Side effects of aldosterone antagonists can include kidney disease and high potassium levels.
- Medicines to relax your blood vessels make it easier for your heart to pump blood. Examples include ACE inhibitors and ARBs. Possible side effects include cough, low blood pressure, and short-term reduced kidney function.

Procedures and Surgeries

If you have heart failure with reduced ejection fraction and it worsens, you may need one of the following medical devices:

- **Biventricular pacemaker**. Also called "cardiac resynchronization therapy," this device can help both sides of your heart contract at the same time to relieve your symptoms.
- **Mechanical heart pump**. It includes a ventricular assist device or a total artificial heart (TAH) that may be used until you have surgery or as a long-term treatment.
- **Implantable cardioverter defibrillator (ICD)**. An ICD checks your heart rate and uses electrical pulses to correct irregular heart rhythms that can cause sudden cardiac arrest.

You may also need heart surgery to repair a CHD or damage to your heart. If your heart failure is life-threatening and other treatments have not worked, you may need a heart transplant.

For people with heart failure and preserved ejection fraction, there are no currently approved devices or procedures to improve symptoms. Researchers are continuing to study possible treatments.

CAN HEART FAILURE BE PREVENTED?

Currently, heart failure is a serious condition that has no cure. However, treatments such as healthy lifestyle changes, medicines, some devices, and procedures can help many people have a higher quality of life (QOL).

You can take the following steps to lower your risk of developing heart failure. The sooner you start, the better your chances of preventing or delaying the condition.

- Choose heart-healthy foods, aim for a healthy weight, get regular physical activity, quit smoking, and manage stress to help keep your heart healthy.
- Limit or avoid alcohol and do not use illegal drugs.
- Work with your health-care provider to manage conditions that raise your risk of heart failure, such as diabetes, HBP, and obesity.[2]

Section 7.3 | Coronary Artery Disease

Coronary artery disease (CAD) is the most common type of heart disease in the United States. It is sometimes called "coronary heart disease" or "ischemic heart disease."

For some people, the first sign of CAD is a heart attack. You and your health-care team may be able to help reduce your risk for CAD.

---

[2] "Heart Failure," National Heart, Lung, and Blood Institute (NHLBI), March 24, 2022. Available online. URL: www.nhlbi.nih.gov/health/heart-failure. Accessed June 12, 2023.

WHAT CAUSES CORONARY ARTERY DISEASE?

Coronary artery disease is caused by plaque buildup in the walls of the arteries that supply blood to the heart (called "coronary arteries") and other parts of the body.

Plaque is made up of deposits of cholesterol and other substances in the artery. Plaque buildup causes the inside of the arteries to narrow over time, which can partially or totally block the blood flow (see Figure 7.1). This process is called "atherosclerosis."

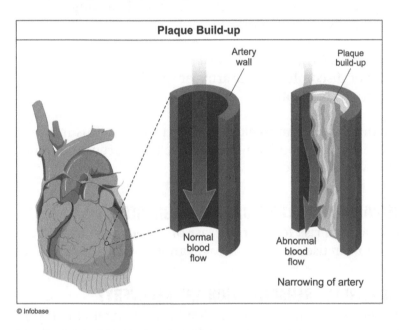

© Infobase

Figure 7.1. Plaque Buildup in Coronary Arteries

Infobase

WHAT ARE THE RISKS OF CORONARY ARTERY DISEASE?

Being overweight, physical inactivity, unhealthy eating, and smoking tobacco are risk factors for CAD. A family history of heart disease also increases your risk for CAD, especially a family history of having heart disease at an early age (50 or younger).

To find out your risk for CAD, your health-care team may measure your blood pressure, blood cholesterol, and blood sugar levels.

WHAT ARE THE SYMPTOMS OF CORONARY ARTERY DISEASE?

Angina, or chest pain and discomfort, is the most common symptom of CAD. Angina can happen when too much plaque builds up inside arteries, causing them to narrow. Narrowed arteries can cause chest pain because they can block blood flow to your heart muscle and the rest of your body.

For many people, the first clue that they have CAD is a heart attack. Symptoms of a heart attack include the following:

- chest pain or discomfort (angina)
- weakness, light-headedness, nausea (feeling sick to your stomach), or a cold sweat
- pain or discomfort in the arms or shoulder
- shortness of breath

Over time, CAD can weaken the heart muscle. This may lead to heart failure, a serious condition where the heart cannot pump blood the way it should.

HOW IS CORONARY ARTERY DISEASE DIAGNOSED?

If you are at high risk for heart disease or already have symptoms, your doctor can use several tests to diagnose CAD (see Table 7.1).

WHAT IS CARDIAC REHABILITATION AND RECOVERY?

Cardiac rehabilitation (rehab) is an important program for anyone recovering from a heart attack, heart failure, or other heart problem that requires surgery or medical care. In these people, cardiac rehab can help improve their quality of life (QOL) and can help prevent another cardiac event. Cardiac rehab is a supervised program that includes the following:

- physical activity
- education about healthy living, including healthy eating, taking medicine as prescribed, and ways to help you quit smoking
- counseling to find ways to relieve stress and improve mental health

Table 7.1. Coronary Artery Disease Tests

Test	What It Does
Electrocardiogram (ECG or EKG)	Measures the electrical activity, rate, and regularity of your heartbeat.
Echocardiogram	Uses ultrasound (special sound wave) to create a picture of the heart.
Exercise stress test	Measures your heart rate while you walk on a treadmill. This helps determine how well your heart is working when it has to pump more blood.
Chest x-ray	Uses x-rays to create a picture of the heart, lungs, and other organs in the chest.
Cardiac catheterization	Checks the inside of your arteries for blockage by inserting a thin, flexible tube through an artery in the groin, arm, or neck to reach the heart. Health-care professionals can measure blood pressure within the heart and the strength of blood flow through the heart's chambers as well as collect blood samples from the heart or inject dye into the arteries of the heart (coronary arteries).
Coronary angiogram	Monitors blockage and flow of blood through the coronary arteries. Uses x-rays to detect dye injected via cardiac catheterization.
Coronary artery calcium scan	Is a computed tomography (CT) scan that looks into the coronary arteries for calcium buildup and plaque.

A team of people may help you through cardiac rehab, including your health-care team, exercise and nutrition specialists, physical therapists, and counselors or mental health professionals.

HOW COULD YOU BE HEALTHIER IF YOU HAVE CORONARY ARTERY DISEASE?

If you have CAD, your health-care team may suggest the following steps to help lower your risk for heart attack or worsening heart disease:

- lifestyle changes, such as eating a healthier (lower sodium, lower fat) diet, increasing physical activity, reaching a healthy weight, and quitting smoking

- medicines to treat risk factors for CAD, such as high cholesterol, HBP, or an irregular heartbeat
- surgical procedures to help restore blood flow to the heart[3]

Section 7.4 | Heart Attack

A heart attack is a life-threatening medical emergency that requires immediate treatment.

A heart attack, also known as a "myocardial infarction," happens when the flow of blood that brings oxygen to a part of your heart muscle suddenly becomes blocked. Your heart cannot get enough oxygen. If blood flow is not restored quickly, the heart muscle will begin to die.

Heart attacks are very common. According to the Centers for Disease Control and Prevention (CDC), more than 800,000 people in the United States have a heart attack each year.

A heart attack is not the same as cardiac arrest, which happens when your heart suddenly and unexpectedly stops beating. A heart attack can cause sudden cardiac arrest (SCA).

CAUSES AND RISK FACTORS OF HEART ATTACK
What Causes a Heart Attack?

The most common cause of a heart attack is coronary artery disease (CAD), which is the most common type of heart disease. This is when your coronary arteries cannot carry enough oxygen-rich blood to your heart muscle. Most of the time, CAD happens when a waxy substance called "plaque" builds up inside your arteries, causing the arteries to narrow. The buildup of this plaque is called "atherosclerosis." This can happen over many years, and it can block blood flow to parts of your heart muscle. Plaques that narrow arteries slowly over time cause angina.

---

[3] "Coronary Artery Disease (CAD)," Centers for Disease Control and Prevention (CDC), July 19, 2021. Available online. URL: www.cdc.gov/heartdisease/coronary_ad.htm. Accessed June 12, 2023.

Eventually, an area of plaque can break open inside your artery. This causes a blood clot to form on the plaque's surface. If the clot becomes large enough, it can block blood flow to your heart. If the blockage is not treated quickly, a part of your heart muscle begins to die.

Other Causes of a Heart Attack

Not all heart attacks are caused by blockages from atherosclerosis. When other heart and blood vessel conditions cause a heart attack, it is called "myocardial infarction in the absence of obstructive coronary artery disease" (MINOCA). MINOCA is more common in women, younger people, and racial and ethnic minorities, including Black, Hispanic/Latinx, and Asian people.

Conditions that can cause MINOCA have different effects on the heart.

- Small plaques in your arteries may not block your blood vessels, but they can break open or their outer layer can wear away. This can cause blood clots to form on these plaques. The blood clots can then block blood flow through your coronary arteries. The formation of small plaques is more common in women, people who smoke, and people who have other blood vessel conditions.
- A sudden and serious spasm (tightening) of your coronary artery can block blood flow through your artery, even if there is not a buildup of plaque. Smoking is a risk factor for coronary spasms. If you smoke, you may be more likely to have a spasm triggered by extreme cold or very stressful situations. Drugs such as cocaine may also cause coronary spasms.
- A coronary artery embolism occurs when a blood clot travels through your bloodstream and gets stuck in your coronary artery. This can block blood flow through your artery. This is more common in people who have atrial fibrillation (AF) or conditions that raise the risk of blood clots, such as thrombocytopenia or pregnancy.

- Spontaneous coronary artery dissection (SCAD) occurs when a tear forms inside your coronary artery. A blood clot can then form at the tear, or the torn tissue itself can block your artery. SCAD can be caused by stress or extreme physical activity. This condition is more common in people who have Marfan syndrome.

Other conditions may cause symptoms similar to a heart attack. Your doctor will look at all of your test results to rule them out.

What Raises the Risk of a Heart Attack?
Certain risk factors make it more likely that you will develop CAD and have a heart attack.

RISK FACTORS YOU CAN CONTROL
The following are a few lifestyle habits that you can control:
- an unhealthy diet, including eating too many foods high in saturated fat or sodium
- lack of regular physical activity
- smoking

The following are a few medical conditions that you can control::
- high blood cholesterol
- high blood pressure (HBP) or high blood preeclampsia (HBP during pregnancy)
- high blood sugar or diabetes
- high blood triglycerides
- overweight and obesity

If you have three or more of these conditions that raise your risk for heart disease, it is called "metabolic syndrome." This greatly increases your risk of a heart attack.

RISK FACTORS YOU CANNOT CONTROL
- age (The risk of heart disease increases for men after age 45.)

- family history of early heart disease (You have a higher risk if your father or a brother was diagnosed with CAD before 55 years of age or if your mother or a sister was diagnosed with CAD before 65 years of age.)
- infections from bacteria and viruses

SYMPTOMS OF HEART ATTACK

Not all heart attacks begin with the sudden and crushing chest pain that comes when the blood flow to the heart gets blocked. Heart attack symptoms can start slowly and can be mild or more serious and sudden. Symptoms may also come and go over several hours. The symptoms of a heart attack can be different from person to person and different between men and women. If you have already had a heart attack, your symptoms may not be the same for another one.

What Are the Symptoms of a Heart Attack?

If you are having a heart attack, you may experience one or more of the following symptoms:

- chest pain, heaviness, or discomfort in the center or left side of the chest (which is the most common symptom)
- pain or discomfort in one or both arms, your back, shoulders, neck, jaw, or above your belly button
- shortness of breath when resting or doing a little bit of physical activity (which is more common in older adults)
- sweating a lot for no reason
- feeling unusually tired for no reason, sometimes for days (which is more common in women)
- nausea (feeling sick to the stomach) and vomiting
- light-headedness or sudden dizziness
- rapid or irregular heartbeat

It is also possible to have mild symptoms or even no symptoms at all and still have a heart attack.

WHEN TO CALL 911

Any time you think you might be having a heart attack, do not ignore it. Call 911 for emergency medical care, even if you are not sure that you are having a heart attack.

- Acting fast can limit damage to your heart and save your life. The 911 operator or emergency medical services (EMS) personnel can give you advice that can help prevent damage to your heart.
- An ambulance is the best and safest way to get to the hospital. Do not drive to the hospital or let someone else drive you. EMS personnel can check how you are doing and start tests and lifesaving medicines right away. People who arrive by ambulance often get faster treatment at the hospital.

Every minute matters. Never delay calling 911, taking aspirin, or doing anything else you think might help.

Knowing the difference between stable angina (chest pain in people who have CAD) and a heart attack is important.

- **Angina**. The pain from angina usually happens after physical activity and goes away in a few minutes when you rest or take medicine to treat it.
- **Heart attack**. The pain from a heart attack is more serious than the pain from angina. Heart attack pain does not go away when you rest or take medicine.

If you do not know whether your chest pain is angina or a heart attack, call 911.

DIAGNOSIS OF HEART ATTACK

Calling 911 for an ambulance and getting to the emergency room quickly if you suspect a heart attack is critical. Once at the hospital, you will likely get tests to see whether you are having a heart attack or whether you have already had one.

An electrocardiogram (EKG) is the most common initial test and may be given within minutes of your arrival at the hospital. An EKG will check whether you may be having a heart attack.

Based on the results of the EKG, your doctor may then order more tests, ask you about your medical history, and do a physical exam.

Blood Tests

During a heart attack, heart muscle cells die and release proteins into your bloodstream. Blood tests can measure the amount of these proteins in your blood. For example, you may get a troponin test to measure the amount of a protein called "troponin" in your blood. Troponin leaks when heart muscle cells die during a heart attack.

Blood tests are often repeated to check for changes over time.

Heart Imaging Tests

Imaging tests, such as a chest x-ray or computed tomography (CT), help your doctor check whether your heart is working properly. You may also need a stress test, which can help your doctor determine the amount of damage to your heart or if the cause of the heart attack is CAD.

TREATMENT OF HEART ATTACK

Your doctor or emergency medical personnel (EMS) may start treatment even before they confirm that you are having a heart attack.

Early treatment to remove the blood clot or plaque can prevent or limit damage to your heart, help your heart work better, and save your life.

Emergency Treatment
MEDICINES

- Aspirin or other medicines can prevent more blood clots from forming. In some people, aspirin may cause bleeding in the stomach.
- Nitroglycerin, or nitrates, can make it easier for your heart to pump blood and improve blood flow through your

coronary arteries. Nitroglycerin also treats chest pain. You may also be given other medicines for chest pain. Side effects of this medicine include nausea, vomiting, weakness, a slow heartbeat, and low blood pressure.

- Thrombolytic medicines, also called "clot busters," can help dissolve blood clots that are blocking your coronary arteries. These medicines may cause bleeding problems. You may be given these if you were unable to reach a hospital that can do a percutaneous coronary intervention (PCI) quickly enough.

OXYGEN THERAPY

Oxygen therapy is a treatment that delivers oxygen gas for you to breathe. You can receive oxygen therapy from tubes resting in your nose, a face mask, or a tube placed in your trachea (windpipe). You may need oxygen therapy if you have a condition that causes your blood oxygen levels to be too low.

Oxygen therapy can be given for a short or long period of time in the hospital, in another medical setting, or at home. Oxygen poses a fire risk, so you should never smoke or use flammable materials when using oxygen. You may experience side effects from this treatment, such as a dry or bloody nose, tiredness, and morning headaches. Oxygen therapy is generally safe.

Procedures

You may need one of the following procedures at the hospital or later to help restore blood flow to your heart. These procedures are often done as soon as your health-care team confirms that you are having a heart attack.

PERCUTANEOUS CORONARY INTERVENTION

PCI, also called "coronary angioplasty," is a nonsurgical procedure that improves blood flow to your heart. Doctors use PCI to open blood vessels to the heart that are narrowed or blocked by a buildup of plaque. PCI requires cardiac catheterization.

A cardiologist, a doctor who specializes in the heart, performs PCI in a hospital cardiac catheterization laboratory. Live x-rays help your doctor guide a catheter through your blood vessels into your heart, where a special contrast dye is injected to highlight any blockage. To open a blocked artery, your doctor will insert another catheter over a guidewire and inflate a balloon at the tip of that catheter. Your doctor may also put a small mesh tube called a "stent" in your artery to help keep the artery open.

You may develop a bruise and soreness where the catheters were inserted. It is common to have discomfort or bleeding where the catheters were inserted. You will recover in a special unit of the hospital for a few hours or overnight. You will get instructions on how much activity you can do and what medicines to take. You will need a ride home because of the medicines and anesthesia you received. Your doctor will check your progress during a follow-up visit. If a stent is implanted, you will have to take certain anticlotting medicines exactly as prescribed, usually for at least 6–12 months.

Serious complications during a PCI procedure or as you are recovering after one are rare, but they can happen. This might include the following:
- bleeding
- blood vessel damage
- treatable allergic reaction to the contrast dye
- need for emergency coronary artery bypass grafting (CABG) during the procedure
- arrhythmias, or irregular heartbeats
- damaged arteries
- kidney damage
- heart attack
- stroke
- blood clots

Sometimes, chest pain can occur during PCI because the balloon briefly blocks blood supply to the heart. Restenosis, when tissue regrows where the artery was treated, may occur in the months after PCI. This may cause the artery to become narrow or blocked again. The risk of complications from this procedure is higher if you are older, have chronic kidney disease (CKD), are experiencing heart failure at the time of the procedure, or have extensive heart disease and more than one blockage in your coronary arteries.

STENTING

A stent is a small mesh tube that holds open passages in the body, such as weak or narrow arteries. Stenting is a minimally invasive procedure. The most common complication after a stenting procedure is a blockage or blood clot in the stent. You may need to take certain medicines, such as aspirin and other antiplatelet medicines, for a year or longer after receiving a stent in your artery to prevent serious complications such as blood clots.

CORONARY ARTERY BYPASS GRAFTING

CABG is a procedure to improve poor blood flow to the heart. It may be needed when the arteries supplying blood to heart tissue, called "coronary arteries," are narrowed or blocked. This surgery may lower the risk of serious complications for people who have a type of heart disease called "obstructive coronary artery disease." CABG may also be used in an emergency, such as a severe heart attack.

CAN YOU PREVENT A HEART ATTACK?

You can lower your risk of a heart attack by changing behaviors that can raise your risks or treating any known CAD. Healthy lifestyle changes, including heart-healthy eating, staying active, quitting smoking, managing stress, and maintaining a healthy weight, can help prevent heart disease. Even if you already have CAD, these changes can lower your risk of a heart attack.

It is also important for you to get treatment for other health conditions that raise your risk of a heart attack. Talk to your doctor about whether taking aspirin can help you prevent blood clots that can lead to a heart attack.[4]

---

[4] "Heart Attack," National Heart, Lung, and Blood Institute (NHLBI), March 24, 2022. Available online. URL: www.nhlbi.nih.gov/health/heart-attack. Accessed June 12, 2023.

Chapter 8 | Stroke

Stroke is a leading cause of death in men. Stroke is also a leading cause of long-term disability, and men under age 44 are hospitalized for certain types of strokes at a higher rate than women in the same age-group.

About four in five strokes are preventable. That is why it is important to know your risk for stroke and take action to protect your health.

WHAT IS A STROKE?

A stroke, sometimes called a "brain attack," happens when blood flow to an area of the brain is blocked or when a blood vessel in the brain bursts. When brain cells are starved of oxygen, they die.

A stroke is a medical emergency. It is important to act fast and get treatment as soon as possible. Call 911 right away if you or someone you are with shows any signs of having a stroke.

Some treatments for stroke work only if given within the first three hours after symptoms start. A delay in treatment increases the risk of permanent brain damage or death.

WHAT PUTS MEN AT RISK FOR STROKE?

High blood pressure (HBP), also called "hypertension," is a major risk factor for stroke. Half of men (50.4%) have HBP greater than or equal to 130/80 mm Hg or are taking medicine for their blood pressure. Four out of five men with HBP do not have their blood pressure controlled.

Other risk factors for stroke include the following:
- **Smoking**. It damages blood vessels, which can cause a stroke. About one in seven men smokes. Men are also more likely to be smokers than women.

- **Overweight and obesity**. Having overweight or obesity increases stroke risk. About three in four men in the United States have overweight or obesity.
- **Diabetes**. It increases stroke risk because it can harm blood vessels in the brain. About one in seven men has diabetes.
- **Too much alcohol**. Drinking too much alcohol can raise blood pressure levels and increase the risk of stroke. It also increases levels of triglycerides, a form of fat in your blood that can harden your arteries. Men are more likely than women to drink too much alcohol.
- **Not enough physical activity**. Not getting enough physical activity can lead to other health conditions that can raise the risk of stroke.

WHY ARE AFRICAN-AMERICAN MEN AT HIGHER RISK FOR STROKE?

- More than one in two African-American men have a blood pressure greater than or equal to 130/80 mm Hg or are taking medicine to control their blood pressure.
- About one in nine African-American men has been diagnosed with diabetes, and many more have the disease but do not know it.
- Sickle cell disease (SCD), a common genetic disorder in African Americans, can lead to a stroke. About 1 in 365 African-American babies are born with SCD.
- About one in five African-American men smoke.
- About 7 in 10 African-American men have overweight or obesity.
- U.S. adults, including African Americans, consume more than the recommended amounts of salt or sodium, which raises blood pressure and increases the risk of stroke.

WHY ARE HISPANIC MEN AT RISK FOR STROKE?

- About half of Hispanic men have a blood pressure greater than or equal to 130/80 mm Hg or are taking medicine to lower blood pressure—a major risk factor for stroke.

- About one in seven Hispanic men has been diagnosed with diabetes, and many more have the disease but do not know it. Diabetes is also more common in people of Mexican and Puerto Rican ancestry than in people of Cuban or Central/South American ancestry.
- About one in seven Hispanic men smokes.
- More than four in five Hispanic men have overweight or obesity.

HOW COULD YOU PREVENT STROKE?

Most strokes can be prevented by keeping medical conditions under control and making healthy lifestyle changes:
- Know your ABCS of heart and brain health:
  - **Aspirin**. It may help reduce your risk for stroke by preventing blood clots, but you should check with your doctor before taking aspirin to make sure it is right for you.
  - **Blood pressure**. Control your blood pressure with healthy lifestyle changes. If a blood pressure medicine is prescribed, take it as directed.
  - **Cholesterol**. Manage your blood cholesterol with healthy lifestyle changes. If a cholesterol medicine is prescribed, take it as directed.
  - **Smoking**. Do not start smoking. If you do smoke, learn how to quit (www.cdc.gov/tobacco/campaign/tips/quit-smoking/index.html?s_cid=OSH_tips_D9385).
- Make lifestyle changes:
  - **Eat healthy**. Choose healthy foods, including foods with less salt, or sodium, to lower your blood pressure and foods that are rich in fiber and whole grains to manage your cholesterol. Learn more about healthy eating basics from ChooseMyPlate.gov, as well as small steps you can take to boost your healthy eating habits from the "Live to the Beat" campaign.
  - **Get regular physical activity**. Regular physical activity helps you reach and maintain a healthy weight and keeps your heart and blood vessels

healthier. Adults aged 18 and older should get at least 150 minutes (2 hours and 30 minutes) of physical activity each week and do muscle-strengthening activities on two or more days each week.

- Work with your health-care team:
  - Talk to your doctor about your chances of having a stroke, including your age and whether anyone in your family has had a stroke.
  - Get other health conditions under control, such as diabetes or heart disease.[1]

---

[1] "Men and Stroke," Centers for Disease Control and Prevention (CDC), May 4, 2023. Available online. URL: www.cdc.gov/stroke/men.htm. Accessed July 18, 2023.

Chapter 9 | **Chronic Obstructive Pulmonary Disease**

Chronic obstructive pulmonary disease (COPD) refers to a group of diseases that cause airflow blockage and breathing-related problems. It includes emphysema and chronic bronchitis.

WHO HAS CHRONIC OBSTRUCTIVE PULMONARY DISEASE?
More than 50 percent of adults with low pulmonary function were not aware that they had COPD, so the actual number may be higher.
- people aged 65–74 and 75 or younger
- American Indians/Alaska Natives and multiracial non-Hispanics
- people who were unemployed, retired, or unable to work
- people with less than a high school education
- people who were divorced, widowed, or separated
- current or former smokers
- people with a history of asthma

WHAT CAUSES CHRONIC OBSTRUCTIVE PULMONARY DISEASE?
In the United States, tobacco smoke is a key factor in the development and progression of COPD. Exposure to air pollutants in the home and workplace, genetic factors, and respiratory infections also play a role. In the developing world, indoor air quality is thought to play a larger role than it does in the United States. People should

try to avoid inhaling tobacco smoke, home and workplace air pollutants, and respiratory infections to prevent developing COPD. Early detection of COPD may change its course and progress.

WHAT ARE THE SYMPTOMS OF CHRONIC OBSTRUCTIVE PULMONARY DISEASE?

Symptoms of COPD include the following:

- frequent coughing or wheezing
- excess phlegm, mucus, or sputum production
- shortness of breath
- trouble taking a deep breath

WHAT ARE THE COMPLICATIONS OR EFFECTS OF CHRONIC OBSTRUCTIVE PULMONARY DISEASE?

Compared to adults without COPD, those with this disease are more likely to:

- have activity limitations, such as difficulty walking or climbing stairs
- be unable to work
- need special equipment, such as portable oxygen tanks
- not engage in social activities, such as eating out, going to places of worship, going to group events, or getting together with friends or neighbors
- have increased confusion or memory loss
- have more emergency room visits or overnight hospital stays
- have other chronic diseases, such as arthritis, congestive heart failure, diabetes, coronary heart disease, stroke, or asthma
- have depression or other mental or emotional conditions
- report a fair or poor health status

HOW IS CHRONIC OBSTRUCTIVE PULMONARY DISEASE DIAGNOSED?

A simple test, called "spirometry," can be used to measure pulmonary—or lung—function and detect COPD in anyone with breathing problems.

HOW IS CHRONIC OBSTRUCTIVE PULMONARY DISEASE TREATED?

Treatment of COPD requires a careful and thorough evaluation by a physician. COPD treatment can alleviate symptoms, decrease the frequency and severity of exacerbations, and increase exercise tolerance. Treatment options that your physician may consider include the following:

- **Quit smoking.** For people who smoke, the most important part of treatment is smoking cessation.
- **Avoid tobacco smoke.** Air pollutants and tobacco smoke must be avoided at home and at work.
- **Ask your doctor about pulmonary rehabilitation.** It is a personalized treatment program that teaches COPD management strategies to improve quality of life (QOL). Programs may include plans that teach people how to breathe better and conserve their energy, as well as provide advice on food and exercise.
- **Take medication.** Symptoms such as coughing or wheezing can be treated with medication.
- **Avoid lung infections.** Lung infections can cause serious problems in people with COPD. Certain vaccines, such as flu and pneumococcal vaccines, are especially important for people with COPD. Respiratory infections should be treated with antibiotics, if appropriate.
- **Use supplemental oxygen.** Some people may need to use a portable oxygen tank if their blood oxygen levels are low.[1]

---

[1] "Basics about COPD," Centers for Disease Control and Prevention (CDC), June 9, 2021. Available online. URL: www.cdc.gov/copd/basics-about.html. Accessed June 14, 2023.

Chapter 10 | Influenza and Pneumonia

Chapter Contents

Section 10.1 | Influenza

Flu is a contagious respiratory illness caused by influenza viruses that infect the nose, throat, and sometimes the lungs. It can cause mild-to-severe illness and at times can lead to death. The best way to prevent flu is by getting a flu vaccine each year.

HOW MANY PEOPLE GET SICK WITH FLU EVERY YEAR?

A 2018 Centers for Disease Control and Prevention (CDC) study published in *Clinical Infectious Diseases* (CID) looked at the percentage of the U.S. population who were sickened by flu using two different methods and compared the findings (see Table 10.1). Both methods had similar findings, which suggested that on average, about 8 percent of the U.S. population gets sick from flu each season, with a range of between 3 and 11 percent, depending on the season.

WHO IS MOST LIKELY TO GET SICK WITH FLU?

The same Clinical Infectious Diseases study found that children are most likely to get sick from the flu and that people aged 65 and older are least likely to get sick from influenza. Median incidence values (or attack rate) by age group were 9.3 percent for children between 0 and 17 years of age, 8.8 percent for adults between 18 and 64 years of age, and 3.9 percent for adults aged 65 and older. This means that children younger than 18 years of age are more than twice as likely to develop a symptomatic flu infection than adults aged 65 and older.

HOW DOES FLU SPREAD?

Most experts believe that flu viruses spread mainly by tiny droplets made when people with flu cough, sneeze, or talk. These droplets can land in the mouths or noses of people who are nearby. Less often, a person might get the flu by touching a surface or object that has the flu virus on it and then touching their own mouth, nose, or possibly their eyes.

Table 10.1. Estimates of the Incidence of Symptomatic Influenza by Season and Age Group, United States, 2010–2022

Season	Predominant Virus(es)	Season Severity	Incidence by Age Group (%)				
			0–4 years	5–17 years	18–49 years	50–64 years	<65 years
2010–2011	A/H3N2, A/H1N1pdm09	Moderate	13.7	8.42	5.5	8.2	4.5
2011–2012	A/H3N2	Low	4.7	3.7	2.6	3.2	2.3
2012–2013	A/H3N2	Moderate	17.8	12.5	8.4	12.8	9.7
2013–2014	A/H1N1pdm09	Moderate	12.7	7.4	9.6	13.7	3.8
2014–2015	A/H3N2	High	16.1	11.9	6.3	11.6	10.1
2015–2016	A/H1N1pdm09	Moderate	11	7.7	6.7	10.5	2.9
2016–2017	A/H3N2	Moderate	11.9	12	6.8	11.8	7.4
2017–2018	A/H3N2	High	17.1	13.3	9.9	18.4	10.1
2018–2019	A/H1N1pdm09, A/H3N2	Moderate	15.2	12.4	7.1	11.4	4.3
2019–2020	A/H1N1pdm09, B	Moderate/high	19.8	14.5	9.6	12.9	3.5
2020–2021*							
2021–2022	A/H3N2	Low	4.6	5.1	2.6	2.3	1
Median			13.7	11.9	6.8	11.6	4.3

* The burden estimate for the 2020–2021 season was not calculated due to the uncharacteristically low level of influenza activity that season.

PEOPLE AT HIGH RISK OF FLU

Anyone can get the flu (even healthy people), and serious problems related to the flu can happen at any age. But some people are at a high risk of developing serious flu-related complications if they get sick. This includes people aged 65 and older, people of any age with certain chronic medical conditions (such as asthma, diabetes, or heart disease), and children younger than 5 years of age.

ONSET OF FLU SYMPTOMS

The time from when a person is exposed and infected with flu to when symptoms begin is about two days, but it can range from about one to four days.

Flu symptoms usually come on suddenly. People who have flu often feel some or all of the following symptoms:

- fever* or feeling feverish/chills
- cough
- sore throat
- runny or stuffy nose
- muscle or body aches
- headaches
- fatigue (tiredness)
- rarely vomiting and diarrhea though this is more common in children than adults

It is important to note that not everyone with flu will have a fever.

PERIOD OF CONTAGIOUSNESS

You may be able to pass on the flu to someone else before you know you are sick, as well as while you are sick.

- People with flu are most contagious in the first three to four days after their illness begins.
- Some otherwise healthy adults may be able to infect others beginning one day before symptoms develop and up to five to seven days after becoming sick.
- Some people, especially young children and people with weakened immune systems, might be able to infect others with flu viruses for an even longer time.

COMPLICATIONS OF FLU

Complications of flu can include bacterial pneumonia, ear infections, sinus infections, and the worsening of chronic medical conditions, such as congestive heart failure, asthma, or diabetes.

DIAGNOSING FLU

It is very difficult to distinguish flu from other viral or bacterial respiratory illnesses based on symptoms alone. There are tests available to diagnose the flu.

TREATING FLU

There are influenza antiviral drugs that can be used to treat flu illness.

PREVENTING SEASONAL FLU

The first and most important step in preventing flu is to get a flu vaccine each year. The flu vaccine has been shown to reduce flu-related illnesses and the risk of serious flu complications that can result in hospitalization or even death. The CDC also recommends everyday preventive actions (such as staying away from people who are sick, covering coughs and sneezes, and frequent handwashing) to help slow the spread of germs that cause respiratory (nose, throat, and lungs) illnesses, such as flu.[1]

Section 10.2 | Pneumonia

Pneumonia is an infection that affects one or both lungs. It causes the air sacs, or alveoli, of the lungs to fill up with fluid or pus. Bacteria, viruses, or fungi may cause pneumonia. Symptoms can range from mild to serious and may include a cough with or without

---

[1] "Key Facts about Influenza (Flu)," Centers for Disease Control and Prevention (CDC), October 24, 2022. Available online. URL: www.cdc.gov/flu/about/keyfacts.htm. Accessed July 4, 2023.

mucus (a slimy substance), fever, chills, and trouble breathing. How serious your pneumonia is depends on your age, your overall health, and what caused your infection.

CAUSES AND RISK FACTORS OF PNEUMONIA

Most of the time your body filters germs out of the air that you breathe. Sometimes, germs, such as bacteria, viruses, or fungi, get into your lungs and cause infections.

When these germs get into your lungs, your immune system, which is your body's natural defense against germs, goes into action. Immune cells attack the germs and may cause inflammation of your air sacs, or alveoli. Inflammation can cause your air sacs to fill up with fluid and pus and cause pneumonia symptoms.

Causes of Pneumonia
BACTERIA

Bacteria are a common cause of pneumonia in adults. Many types of bacteria can cause pneumonia, but *Streptococcus pneumoniae* (also called "pneumococcus bacteria") is the most common cause in the United States.

Some bacteria cause pneumonia with different symptoms or other characteristics than the usual pneumonia. This infection is called "atypical pneumonia." For example, *Mycoplasma pneumoniae* causes a mild form of pneumonia often called "walking pneumonia."

Legionella pneumophila causes a severe type of pneumonia called "Legionnaires' disease." Bacterial pneumonia can develop on its own or after you have a cold or the flu.

VIRUSES

Viruses that infect your lungs and airways can cause pneumonia. The flu (influenza virus) and the common cold (rhinovirus) are the most common causes of viral pneumonia in adults. Respiratory syncytial virus (RSV) is the most common cause of viral pneumonia in young children.

Many other viruses can cause pneumonia, including severe acute respiratory syndrome coronavirus 2 (SARS-CoV-2), the virus that causes COVID-19.

FUNGI

Fungi, such as *Pneumocystis jirovecii*, may cause pneumonia, especially for people who have weakened immune systems. Some fungi found in the soil in the southwestern United States and in the Ohio and Mississippi River valleys can also cause pneumonia.

Risk Factors

Your risk for pneumonia may be higher because of your age, environment, lifestyle habits, and other medical conditions.

AGE

Pneumonia can affect people of all ages. However, two age groups are at higher risk of developing pneumonia and having more serious pneumonia.

Babies and children aged two or younger are at higher risk because their immune systems are still developing. This risk is higher for premature babies.

Adults aged 65 or older are also at higher risk because their immune systems generally weaken as people age. Older adults are also more likely to have other chronic (long-term) health conditions that raise the risk of pneumonia.

Babies, children, and older adults who do not get the recommended vaccines to prevent pneumonia have an even higher risk.

ENVIRONMENT OR OCCUPATION

Most people get pneumonia when they catch an infection from someone else in their community. Your chance of getting pneumonia is higher if you live or spend a lot of time in crowded places, such as military barracks, prisons, homeless shelters, or nursing homes.

Your risk is also higher if you regularly breathe in polluted air or toxic fumes.

Some germs that cause pneumonia can infect birds and other animals. You are most likely to encounter these germs if you work in a chicken- or turkey-processing center, pet shop, or veterinary clinic.

LIFESTYLE HABITS

- Smoking cigarettes can make you less able to clear mucus from your airways.
- Using drugs or alcohol can weaken your immune system. You are also more likely to accidentally breathe in saliva or vomit into your windpipe if you are sedated or unconscious from an overdose.

OTHER MEDICAL CONDITIONS

You may have an increased risk of pneumonia if you have any of the following medical conditions:

- **Brain disorders**. It includes a stroke, a head injury, dementia, or Parkinson disease (PD) that can affect your ability to cough or swallow. This can lead to food, drink, vomit, or saliva going down your windpipe instead of your esophagus and getting into your lungs.
- **Conditions that weaken your immune system**. These include pregnancy, human immunodeficiency virus (HIV)/acquired immunodeficiency syndrome (AIDS), or an organ or bone marrow transplant. Chemotherapy, which is used to treat cancer, and long-term use of steroid medicines can also weaken your immune system. They may also increase your risk of pneumonia.
- **Critical diseases that require hospitalization**. Diseases, including receiving treatment in a hospital intensive care unit (ICU), can raise your risk of hospital-acquired pneumonia. Your risk is higher if you cannot move around much or are sedated or unconscious. Using a ventilator raises the risk of a type called "ventilator-associated pneumonia."

- **Lung diseases**. These include asthma, bronchiectasis, cystic fibrosis (CF), and chronic obstructive pulmonary disease (COPD) that also increase your pneumonia risk.
- **Other serious conditions**. Conditions such as malnutrition, diabetes, heart failure, sickle cell disease (SCD), or liver or kidney disease are additional risk factors.

SYMPTOMS OF PNEUMONIA

The symptoms of pneumonia can be mild or serious. Young children, older adults, and people who have serious health conditions are at risk for developing more serious pneumonia or life-threatening complications.

The symptoms of pneumonia may include the following:
- chest pain when you breathe or cough
- chills
- cough with or without mucus
- fever
- low oxygen levels in your blood, measured with a pulse oximeter
- shortness of breath

You may also have other symptoms, including a headache, muscle pain, extreme tiredness, nausea (feeling sick to your stomach), vomiting, and diarrhea.

Older adults and people who have serious illnesses or weakened immune systems may not have the typical symptoms. They may have a lower-than-normal temperature instead of a fever. Older adults who have pneumonia may feel weak or suddenly confused.

Sometimes, babies do not have typical symptoms either. They may vomit, have a fever, cough, or appear restless or tired and without energy. Babies may also show the following signs of breathing problems:
- bluish tone to the skin and lips
- grunting

- pulling inward of the muscles between the ribs when breathing
- rapid breathing
- widening of the nostrils with each breath

DIAGNOSIS OF PNEUMONIA

Your health-care provider will diagnose pneumonia based on your medical history, a physical exam, and test results. Sometimes, pneumonia is hard to diagnose because your symptoms may be the same as a cold or flu. You may not realize that your condition is more serious until it lasts longer than these other conditions.

Medical History and Physical Exam

Your provider will ask about your symptoms and when they began. They will also ask whether you have any risk factors for pneumonia. You may also be asked about:

- exposure to sick people at home, school, or work or in a hospital
- flu or pneumonia vaccinations
- medicines you take
- past and current medical conditions and whether any have gotten worse recently
- recent travel
- exposure to birds and other animals
- smoking

During your physical exam, your provider will check your temperature and listen to your lungs with a stethoscope.

DIAGNOSTIC TESTS AND PROCEDURES

If your provider thinks you have pneumonia, he or she may do one or more of the following tests.

- **Chest x-ray**. This x-ray looks for inflammation in your lungs. A chest x-ray is often used to diagnose pneumonia.

143

- **Blood tests.** Tests such as a complete blood count (CBC) see whether your immune system is fighting an infection.
- **Pulse oximetry.** This noninvasive method measures how much oxygen is in your blood. Pneumonia can keep your lungs from getting enough oxygen into your blood. To measure the levels, a small sensor called a "pulse oximeter" is attached to your finger or ear.

If you are in the hospital, have serious symptoms, are older, or have other health problems, your provider may do other tests to diagnose pneumonia.

- **Blood gas test.** This test may be done if you are very sick. For this test, your provider measures your blood oxygen levels using a blood sample from an artery, usually in your wrist. This is called an "arterial blood gas test."
- **Sputum test.** This test, using a sample of sputum (spit) or mucus from your cough, may be used to find out what germ is causing your pneumonia.
- **Blood culture test.** This culture test can identify the germ causing your pneumonia and also show whether a bacterial infection has spread to your blood.
- **Polymerase chain reaction (PCR) test.** A PCR test quickly checks your blood or sputum sample to find the deoxyribonucleic acid (DNA) of germs that cause pneumonia.
- **Bronchoscopy.** It looks inside your airways. If your treatment is not working well, this procedure may be needed. At the same time, your doctor may also collect samples of your lung tissue and fluid from your lungs to help find the cause of your pneumonia.
- **Chest computed tomography (CT) scan.** A chest CT scan can show how much of your lungs are affected by pneumonia. It can also show whether you have complications, such as lung abscesses or pleural disorders. A CT scan shows more detail than a chest x-ray.

- **Pleural fluid culture**. It can be taken using a procedure called "thoracentesis," which is when a doctor uses a needle to take a sample of fluid from the pleural space between your lungs and chest wall. The fluid is then tested for bacteria.

TREATMENT FOR PNEUMONIA

Treatment for pneumonia depends on your risk factors and how serious your pneumonia is. Many people who have pneumonia are prescribed medicine and recover at home. You may need to be treated in the hospital or an ICU if your pneumonia is serious.

Medicines

Your health-care provider may prescribe some of the following medicines to treat your pneumonia at home or at the hospital, depending on how sick you are.

MANAGEMENT AT HOME

If your pneumonia is mild, your provider may prescribe medicines or suggest over-the-counter (OTC) medicines to treat it at home.

- **Antibiotics**. These may be prescribed for bacterial pneumonia. Most people begin to feel better after one to three days of antibiotic treatment. However, you should take antibiotics as your doctor prescribes. If you stop too soon, your pneumonia may come back.
- **Antiviral medicine**. This medicine is sometimes prescribed for viral pneumonia. However, these medicines do not work against every virus that causes pneumonia.
- **Antifungal medicines**. These medicines are prescribed for fungal pneumonia.
- **OTC medicines**. These medicines may be recommended to treat your fever and muscle pain or help you breathe easier. Talk to your provider before taking a cough or cold medicine.

MANAGEMENT AT THE HOSPITAL

If your pneumonia is serious, you may be treated in a hospital, so you can get antibiotics and fluids through an intravenous (IV) line inserted into your vein. You may also get oxygen therapy to increase the amount of oxygen in your blood. If your pneumonia is very serious, you may need to be put on a ventilator.

PROCEDURES

You may need a procedure or surgery to remove seriously infected or damaged parts of your lung. This may help you recover and may prevent your pneumonia from coming back.

PREVENTION OF PNEUMONIA

Pneumonia can be very serious and even life-threatening. You can take a few steps to try and prevent it.

Vaccines can help prevent some types of pneumonia. Good hygiene (washing your hands often), quitting smoking, and keeping your immune system strong by getting regular physical activity and eating healthy are other ways to lower your risk of getting pneumonia.

Vaccines

Vaccines can help prevent pneumonia caused by pneumococcus bacteria or the flu virus. Vaccines cannot prevent all cases of pneumonia. However, compared to people who do not get vaccinated, those who are vaccinated and still get pneumonia tend to have:

- fewer serious complications
- milder infections
- pneumonia that does not last as long

PNEUMOCOCCUS VACCINES

Two vaccines are available to prevent infections from the pneumococcus bacteria, the most common type of bacteria that causes pneumonia. Pneumococcus vaccines are especially important for people at high risk of pneumonia, including the following:

- adults aged 65 or older
- children aged two or younger

- people who have chronic (ongoing) diseases, serious long-term health problems, or weak immune systems, which may include people who have cancer, HIV, asthma, SCD, or damaged or removed spleens.
- people who smoke

FLU (INFLUENZA) VACCINE

Your yearly flu vaccine can help prevent pneumonia caused by the flu. The flu vaccine is usually given in September through October before flu season starts.

HIB VACCINE

Haemophilus influenzae type b (Hib) is a type of bacteria that can cause pneumonia and meningitis. The Hib vaccine is recommended for all children under five years old in the United States. The vaccine is often given to infants starting when they are two months old.

Other Ways to Prevent Pneumonia

You can take the following steps to help prevent pneumonia:
- **Wash your hands**. Wash your hands with soap and water or alcohol-based hand sanitizers to kill germs.
- **Do not smoke**. Smoking prevents your lungs from properly filtering out and defending your body against germs.
- **Keep your immune system strong**. Get plenty of physical activity and follow a healthy eating plan.
- **Avoid lung problems**. If you have problems swallowing, eat smaller meals of thickened food and sleep with the head of your bed raised up. These steps can help you avoid getting food, drink, or saliva into your lungs.
- **Avoid eating or drinking before your surgery**. If you have a planned surgery, your provider may recommend that you do not eat for eight hours or drink liquids for two hours before your surgery. This can help prevent

food or drink from getting into your airway while you are sedated.

- **Take antibiotics**. If your immune system is impaired or weakened, your provider may recommend you take antibiotics to prevent bacteria from growing in your lungs.[2]

[2] "Pneumonia," National Heart, Lung, and Blood Institute (NHLBI), March 24, 2022. Available online. URL: www.nhlbi.nih.gov/health/pneumonia. Accessed June 14, 2023.

Chapter 11 | **Chronic Liver Disease**

Chapter Contents

Section 11.1 | Viral Hepatitis

Viral hepatitis is an infection that causes liver inflammation and damage. Inflammation is swelling that occurs when tissues of the body become injured or infected. Inflammation can damage organs. Researchers have discovered several different viruses that cause hepatitis, including hepatitis A, B, C, D, and E.

When doctors cannot find the cause of a person's hepatitis, they may call this condition "non-A–E hepatitis" or "hepatitis X." Experts think that unknown viruses other than hepatitis A, B, C, D, and E may cause some cases of hepatitis. Researchers are working to identify these viruses.

Although non-A–E hepatitis is most often acute, it can become chronic.

HEPATITIS A
What Is Hepatitis A?
The hepatitis A virus typically spreads through contact with food or water that has been contaminated by an infected person's stool.

Hepatitis A is an acute or short-term infection, which means people usually get better without treatment after a few weeks. In rare cases, hepatitis A can be severe and lead to liver failure and the need for an emergency liver transplant to survive. Hepatitis A does not lead to long-term complications, such as cirrhosis, because the infection only lasts a short time.

You can take steps to protect yourself from hepatitis A, including getting the hepatitis A vaccine. If you have hepatitis A, you can take steps to prevent spreading hepatitis A to others.

Who Is More Likely to Get Hepatitis A?
People more likely to get hepatitis A are those who:
- travel to developing countries
- have sex with an infected person
- are men who have sex with men
- use illegal drugs, including drugs that are not injected
- experience unstable housing or homelessness

- live with or care for someone who has hepatitis A
- live with or care for a child recently adopted from a country where hepatitis A is common

HEPATITIS B
What Is Hepatitis B?
The hepatitis B virus spreads through contact with an infected person's blood, semen, or other body fluids.

You can take steps to protect yourself from hepatitis B, including getting the hepatitis B vaccine. If you have hepatitis B, you can take steps to prevent spreading hepatitis B to others.

The hepatitis B virus can cause an acute or chronic infection.

ACUTE HEPATITIS B
Acute hepatitis B is a short-term infection. Some people have symptoms, which may last several weeks. In some cases, symptoms last up to six months. Sometimes, the body is able to fight off the infection, and the virus goes away. If the body is not able to fight off the virus, the virus does not go away, and chronic hepatitis B infection occurs.

Most healthy adults and children older than five years who have hepatitis B get better and do not develop a chronic hepatitis B infection.

CHRONIC HEPATITIS B
Chronic hepatitis B is a long-lasting infection. Your chance of developing chronic hepatitis B is greater if you were infected with the virus as a young child. About 90 percent of infants infected with hepatitis B develop a chronic infection. About 25–50 percent of children infected between the ages of one and five years develop chronic infections. However, only about 5 percent of people first infected as adults develop chronic hepatitis B.

Who Is More Likely to Get Hepatitis B?
People are more likely to get hepatitis B if they are born to a mother who has hepatitis B. The virus can spread from mother to child

during birth. For this reason, people are more likely to have hepatitis B if they:

- were born in a part of the world where 2 percent or more of the population has hepatitis B infection
- were born in the United States, did not receive the hepatitis B vaccine as an infant, and have parents who were born in an area where 8 percent or more of the population had hepatitis B infection

People are also more likely to have hepatitis B if they:

- are infected with HIV because hepatitis B and HIV spread in similar ways
- have lived with or had sex with someone who has hepatitis B
- have had more than one sex partner in the past six months or have a history of sexually transmitted disease
- are men who have sex with men
- are injection drug users
- work in a profession, such as health care, in which they have contact with blood, needles, or body fluids at work
- live or work in a care facility for people with developmental disabilities
- have diabetes
- have hepatitis C
- have lived in or often travel to parts of the world where hepatitis B is common
- have been on kidney dialysis
- live or work in a prison
- had a blood transfusion or organ transplant before the mid-1980s

In the United States, hepatitis B spreads among adults mainly through contact with infected blood through the skin, such as during injection drug use, and through sexual contact.

HEPATITIS C
What Is Hepatitis C?

The hepatitis C virus spreads through contact with an infected person's blood.

Hepatitis C can cause an acute or chronic infection.

Although no vaccine for hepatitis C is available, you can take steps to protect yourself from hepatitis C. If you have hepatitis C, talk with your doctor about treatment. Medicines can cure most cases of hepatitis C.

ACUTE HEPATITIS C

Acute hepatitis C is a short-term infection. Symptoms can last up to six months. Sometimes, your body is able to fight off the infection, and the virus goes away.

CHRONIC HEPATITIS C

Chronic hepatitis C is a long-lasting infection. Chronic hepatitis C occurs when your body is not able to fight off the virus. About 75–85 percent of people with acute hepatitis C will develop chronic hepatitis C.

Early diagnosis and treatment of chronic hepatitis C can prevent liver damage. Without treatment, chronic hepatitis C can cause chronic liver disease, cirrhosis, liver failure, or liver cancer.

Who Is More Likely to Get Hepatitis C?

People more likely to get hepatitis C are those who:
- have injected drugs
- had a blood transfusion or organ transplant before July 1992
- have hemophilia and received clotting factor before 1987
- have been on kidney dialysis
- have been in contact with blood or infected needles at work
- have had tattoos or body piercings
- have worked or lived in a prison

- were born to a mother with hepatitis C
- are infected with HIV
- have had more than one sex partner in the past six months or have a history of sexually transmitted disease
- are men who have or had sex with men

In the United States, injecting drugs is the most common way that people get hepatitis C.

HEPATITIS D
What Is Hepatitis D?

The hepatitis D virus is unusual because it can only infect you when you also have a hepatitis B virus infection. In this way, hepatitis D is a double infection. You can protect yourself from hepatitis D by protecting yourself from hepatitis B by getting the hepatitis B vaccine.

Hepatitis D spreads the same way that hepatitis B spreads, through contact with an infected person's blood or other body fluids.

The hepatitis D virus can cause an acute or chronic infection or both.

ACUTE HEPATITIS D

Acute hepatitis D is a short-term infection. The symptoms of acute hepatitis D are the same as the symptoms of any type of hepatitis and are often more severe. Sometimes, your body is able to fight off the infection, and the virus goes away.

CHRONIC HEPATITIS D

Chronic hepatitis D is a long-lasting infection. Chronic hepatitis D occurs when your body is not able to fight off the virus and the virus does not go away. People who have chronic hepatitis B and D develop complications more often and more quickly than people who have chronic hepatitis B alone.

Who Is More Likely to Have Hepatitis D?

Hepatitis D infection occurs only in people who have hepatitis B. People are more likely to have hepatitis D in addition to hepatitis B if they:

- are injection drug users
- have lived with or had sex with someone who has hepatitis D
- are from an area of the world where hepatitis D is more common

HEPATITIS E
What Is Hepatitis E?

The hepatitis E virus has different types that spread in different ways.

- Some types are spread by drinking contaminated water. These types are more common in developing countries, including parts of Africa, Asia, Central America, and the Middle East.
- Other types are spread by eating undercooked pork or wild game, such as deer. These types are more common in developed countries, such as the United States, Australia, Japan, and parts of Europe and East Asia.

Hepatitis E typically causes acute or chronic infection.

ACUTE HEPATITIS E

Acute hepatitis E is a short-term infection. In most cases, people's bodies are able to recover and fight off the infection, and the virus goes away. People usually get better without treatment after several weeks.

CHRONIC HEPATITIS E

Chronic hepatitis E is a long-lasting infection that occurs when your body is not able to fight off the virus and the virus does not go away. Chronic hepatitis E is rare and occurs only in people with weakened immune systems. For example, hepatitis E may become chronic in people taking medicines that weaken their immune system after an organ transplant or in people who have HIV or AIDS.

Who Is More Likely to Get Hepatitis E?

Different types of hepatitis E are more likely to affect different groups of people. The types of hepatitis E that are more common in developing countries are more likely to affect adolescents and young adults.

In contrast, the types of hepatitis E that are more common in developed countries most often affect older men.[1]

Section 11.2 | Cirrhosis

Cirrhosis is a condition in which your liver is scarred and permanently damaged (see Figure 11.1). Scar tissue replaces healthy liver tissue and prevents your liver from working normally. Scar tissue also partly blocks the flow of blood through your liver. As cirrhosis gets worse, your liver begins to fail.

Many people are not aware that they have cirrhosis since they may not have signs or symptoms until their liver is badly damaged.

HOW COMMON IS CIRRHOSIS?

Researchers estimate that about 1 in 400 adults in the United States has cirrhosis. Cirrhosis is more common in adults aged 45–54.

About 1 in 200 adults aged 45–54 in the United States has cirrhosis. Researchers believe the actual numbers may be higher because many people with cirrhosis are not diagnosed.

---

[1] "What Is Viral Hepatitis?" National Institute of Diabetes and Digestive and Kidney Diseases (NIDDK), May 2017. Available online. URL: www.niddk.nih.gov/health-information/liver-disease/viral-hepatitis/what-is-viral-hepatitis. Accessed July 5, 2023.

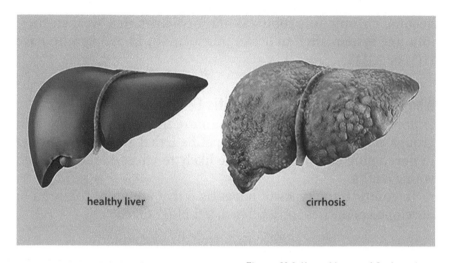

Figure 11.1. Normal Liver and Cirrhotic Liver

National Institute of Diabetes and Digestive and Kidney Diseases (NIDDK)

WHO IS MORE LIKELY TO GET CIRRHOSIS?
People are more likely to get cirrhosis if they have certain health conditions. People are also more likely to get cirrhosis if they:
- have abused alcohol for a long time
- have type 2 diabetes
- are men
- are older than age 50

WHAT ARE THE COMPLICATIONS OF CIRRHOSIS?
As the liver fails, complications may develop. In some people, complications may be the first sign of the disease. Complications of cirrhosis may include the following.

PORTAL HYPERTENSION
Portal hypertension is the most common serious complication of cirrhosis. Portal hypertension is a condition that occurs when scar tissue partly blocks and slows the normal flow of blood through your liver, which causes high blood pressure (HBP) in the portal

vein. Portal hypertension and its treatments may lead to other complications, including the following:

- enlarged veins—called "varices"—in your esophagus, stomach, or intestines, which can lead to internal bleeding if the veins burst
- swelling in your legs, ankles, or feet, called "edema"
- buildup of fluid in your abdomen—called "ascites"— which can lead to a serious infection in the space that surrounds your liver and intestines
- confusion or difficulty thinking caused by the buildup of toxins in your brain, called "hepatic encephalopathy"

INFECTIONS
Cirrhosis increases your chance of getting bacterial infections, such as urinary tract infections (UTIs) and pneumonia.

LIVER CANCER
Cirrhosis increases your chance of getting liver cancer. Most people who develop liver cancer already have cirrhosis.

LIVER FAILURE
Cirrhosis may eventually lead to liver failure. With liver failure, your liver is badly damaged and stops working. Liver failure is also called "end-stage liver disease." This may require a liver transplant.

OTHER COMPLICATIONS
Other complications of cirrhosis may include the following:

- bone diseases, such as osteoporosis
- gallstones
- problems with the bile ducts—the tubes that carry bile out of the liver
- malabsorption and malnutrition
- bruising and bleeding easily
- sensitivity to medicines
- insulin resistance and type 2 diabetes

CAUSES AND SYMPTOMS OF CIRRHOSIS
What Causes Cirrhosis?

Cirrhosis has different causes. Some people with cirrhosis have more than one cause of liver damage.

MOST COMMON CAUSES

The most common causes of cirrhosis are as follows:

- alcoholic liver disease—damage to the liver and its function due to alcohol abuse
- nonalcoholic fatty liver disease
- chronic hepatitis C
- chronic hepatitis B

LESS COMMON CAUSES

Some of the less common causes of cirrhosis include the following:

- autoimmune hepatitis
- diseases that damage, destroy, or block bile ducts, such as primary biliary cholangitis and primary sclerosing cholangitis
- inherited liver diseases—diseases passed from parents to children through genes—that affect how the liver works, such as Wilson disease, hemochromatosis, and alpha-1-antitrypsin deficiency
- long-term use of certain medicines
- chronic heart failure with liver congestion, a condition in which blood flow out of the liver is slowed

WHAT ARE THE SYMPTOMS OF CIRRHOSIS?

You may have no signs or symptoms of cirrhosis until your liver is badly damaged.

Early symptoms of cirrhosis may include the following:

- feeling tired or weak
- poor appetite
- losing weight without trying
- nausea and vomiting

- mild pain or discomfort in the upper right side of your abdomen

As liver function gets worse, you may have other symptoms, including the following:
- bruising and bleeding easily
- confusion, difficulties thinking, memory loss, personality changes, or sleep disorders
- swelling in your lower legs, ankles, or feet, called "edema"
- bloating from the buildup of fluid in your abdomen, called "ascites"
- severe itchy skin
- darkening of the color of your urine
- a yellowish tint to the whites of your eyes and skin, called "jaundice"

DIAGNOSIS OF CIRRHOSIS
How Do Doctors Diagnose Cirrhosis?
Doctors diagnose cirrhosis based on your medical history, a physical exam, and the results of tests.

MEDICAL HISTORY
Your doctor will ask about your symptoms. He or she will also ask if you have a history of health conditions that make you more likely to develop cirrhosis.

Your doctor will ask about your use of alcohol and over-the-counter (OTC) and prescription medicines.

PHYSICAL EXAM
Your doctor will examine your body, use a stethoscope to listen to sounds in your abdomen, and tap or press on specific areas of your abdomen. He or she will check to see if your liver is larger than it should be. Your doctor will also check for tenderness or pain in your abdomen.

What Tests Do Doctors Use to Diagnose Cirrhosis?
BLOOD TESTS

Your doctor may recommend the following blood tests:

- **Liver tests.** These tests can show abnormal liver enzyme levels, which may be a sign of liver damage. Your doctor may suspect cirrhosis if you have:
  - increased levels of the liver enzymes alanine transaminase (ALT), aspartate transaminase (AST), and alkaline phosphatase (ALP)
  - increased levels of bilirubin
  - decreased levels of blood proteins
- **Complete blood count (CBC).** CBC can show signs of infection and anemia that may be caused by internal bleeding.
- **Tests for viral infections.** These tests help see if you have hepatitis B or C.
- **Blood tests for autoimmune liver conditions.** These tests include the antinuclear antibody (ANA), anti-smooth muscle antibody (SMA), and anti-mitochondrial antibody (AMA) tests.

Based on the blood test results, your doctor may be able to diagnose certain causes of cirrhosis.

Your doctor can use blood tests to tell how serious your cirrhosis is.

IMAGING TESTS

Imaging tests can show the size, shape, texture, and stiffness of your liver. Measuring the stiffness of the liver can show scarring. Your doctor can use stiffness measures to see if the scarring is getting better or worse. Imaging tests can also show how much fat is in the liver. Your doctor may use one or more of the following imaging tests:

- magnetic resonance imaging (MRI)
- ultrasound
- x-rays, such as computerized tomography (CT) scans
- transient elastography, a special ultrasound that measures the stiffness of your liver and can measure liver fat

LIVER BIOPSY

Your doctor may perform a liver biopsy to see how much scarring is in your liver. A liver biopsy can diagnose cirrhosis when the results of other tests are uncertain. The biopsy may show the cause of cirrhosis. Sometimes, your doctor may find that something other than cirrhosis has caused your liver to become damaged or enlarged. Your doctor can also diagnose liver cancer based on liver biopsy results.

TREATMENT FOR CIRRHOSIS
How Do Doctors Treat Cirrhosis?

Doctors do not have specific treatments that can cure cirrhosis. However, they can treat many of the diseases that cause cirrhosis.

Some of the diseases that cause cirrhosis can be cured. Treating the underlying causes of cirrhosis may keep your cirrhosis from getting worse and help prevent liver failure. Successful treatment may slowly improve some of your liver scarring.

How Do Doctors Treat the Causes of Cirrhosis?

Doctors most often treat the causes of cirrhosis with medicines. Your doctor will recommend that you stop activities, such as drinking alcohol and taking certain medicines that may have caused cirrhosis or may make cirrhosis worse.

ALCOHOLIC LIVER DISEASE

If you have alcoholic liver disease, your doctor will recommend that you completely stop drinking alcohol. He or she may refer you for alcohol treatment.

NONALCOHOLIC FATTY LIVER DISEASE

If you have nonalcoholic fatty liver disease, your doctor may recommend losing weight. Weight loss through healthy eating and regular physical activity can reduce fat in the liver, inflammation, and scarring.

CHRONIC HEPATITIS C

If you have chronic hepatitis C, your doctor may prescribe one or more medicines that have been approved to treat hepatitis C. Studies have shown that these medicines can cure chronic hepatitis C in 80–95 percent of people with this disease.

CHRONIC HEPATITIS B

For chronic hepatitis B, your doctor may prescribe antiviral medicines that slow or stop the virus from further damaging your liver.

AUTOIMMUNE HEPATITIS

Doctors treat autoimmune hepatitis with medicines that suppress, or decrease the activity of, your immune system.

DISEASES THAT DAMAGE, DESTROY, OR BLOCK BILE DUCTS

Doctors usually treat diseases that damage, destroy, or block bile ducts with medicines such as ursodiol (Actigall and Urso). Doctors may use surgical procedures to open bile ducts that are narrowed or blocked. Diseases that damage, destroy, or block bile ducts include primary biliary cholangitis and primary sclerosing cholangitis.

INHERITED LIVER DISEASES

Treatment of inherited liver diseases depends on the disease. Treatment most often focuses on managing symptoms and complications.

LONG-TERM USE OF CERTAIN MEDICINES

The only specific treatment for most cases of cirrhosis caused by certain medicines is to stop taking the medicine that caused the problem. Talk with your doctor before you stop taking any medicines.

What Can You Do to Help Keep Your Cirrhosis from Getting Worse?

To help keep your cirrhosis from getting worse, you can do the following:

- Do not drink alcohol or use illegal drugs.
- Talk with your doctor before taking:
  - prescription medicines
  - prescription and OTC sleep aids
  - OTC medicines, including nonsteroidal anti-inflammatory drugs (NSAIDs) and acetaminophen
  - dietary supplements, including herbal supplements
- Take your medicines as directed.
- Get a vaccine for hepatitis A, hepatitis B, flu, pneumonia caused by certain bacteria, and shingles.
- Get a screening blood test for hepatitis C.
- Eat a healthy, well-balanced diet.
- Avoid raw or undercooked shellfish, fish, and meat.
- Try to keep a healthy body weight.
- Talk with your doctor about your risk of getting liver cancer and how often you should be checked.

When Do Doctors Consider a Liver Transplant for Cirrhosis?

Your doctor will consider a liver transplant when cirrhosis leads to liver failure. Doctors consider liver transplants only after they have ruled out all other treatment options. Talk with your doctor about whether a liver transplant is right for you.[2]

---

[2] "Cirrhosis," National Institute of Diabetes and Digestive and Kidney Diseases (NIDDK), March 2018. Available online. URL: www.niddk.nih.gov/health-information/liver-disease/cirrhosis. Accessed June 14, 2023.

Chapter 12 | **Kidney and Urological Disorders**

Chapter Contents

WHAT ARE KIDNEY STONES?

Kidney stones are hard, pebble-like pieces of material that form in one or both of your kidneys when high levels of certain minerals are in your urine. They rarely cause permanent damage if treated by a health-care professional.

Kidney stones vary in size and shape. They may be as small as a grain of sand or as large as a pea (see Figure 12.1). Rarely, some kidney stones are as big as golf balls. Kidney stones may be smooth or jagged and are usually yellow or brown.

A small kidney stone may pass through your urinary tract on its own, causing little or no pain. A larger kidney stone may get stuck along the way. A kidney stone that gets stuck can block your flow of urine, causing severe pain or bleeding.

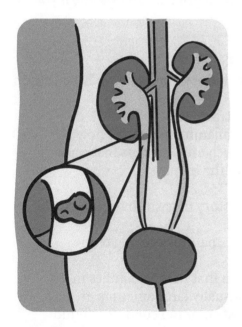

Figure 12.1. Kidney Stone

National Institute of Diabetes and Digestive and Kidney Diseases (NIDDK)

If you have symptoms of kidney stones, including severe pain or bleeding, seek care right away. A doctor, such as a urologist, can treat any pain and prevent further problems, such as a urinary tract infection (UTI).

HOW COMMON ARE KIDNEY STONES?

Kidney stones are common and are on the rise. About 11 percent of men in the United States have kidney stones at least once during their lifetime.

WHO IS MORE LIKELY TO DEVELOP KIDNEY STONES?

Men are more likely to develop kidney stones than women. If you have a family history of kidney stones, you are more likely to develop them. You are also more likely to develop kidney stones again if you have had them once.

You may also be more likely to develop a kidney stone if you do not drink enough liquids.

PEOPLE WITH CERTAIN CONDITIONS

You are more likely to develop kidney stones if you have certain conditions, including:

- a blockage of the urinary tract
- chronic, or long-lasting, inflammation of the bowel
- cystic kidney diseases, which are disorders that cause fluid-filled sacs to form in the kidneys
- cystinuria
- digestive problems or a history of gastrointestinal tract surgery
- gout, a disorder that causes painful swelling of the joints
- hypercalciuria, a condition that runs in families in which urine contains unusually large amounts of calcium, which is the most common condition found in people who form calcium stones
- hyperoxaluria, a condition in which urine contains unusually large amounts of oxalate

- hyperparathyroidism, a condition in which the parathyroid glands release too much parathyroid hormone, causing extra calcium in the blood
- hyperuricosuria, a disorder in which too much uric acid is in the urine
- obesity
- repeated or recurrent UTIs
- renal tubular acidosis, a disease that occurs when the kidneys fail to remove acids into the urine, which causes a person's blood to remain too acidic

PEOPLE WHO TAKE CERTAIN MEDICINES
You are more likely to develop kidney stones if you are taking one or more of the following medicines over a long period of time:
- diuretics, often called "water pills," which help rid your body of water
- calcium-based antacids
- indinavir, a protease inhibitor used to treat human immunodeficiency virus (HIV) infection
- topiramate, an anti-seizure medication

WHAT ARE THE COMPLICATIONS OF KIDNEY STONES?
Complications of kidney stones are rare if you seek treatment from a health-care professional before problems occur.
   If kidney stones are not treated, they can cause:
- hematuria, or blood in the urine
- severe pain
- UTIs, including kidney infections
- loss of kidney function

WHAT CAUSES KIDNEY STONES?
Kidney stones are caused by high levels of calcium, oxalate, and phosphorus in the urine. These minerals are normally found in urine and do not cause problems at low levels.
   Certain foods may increase the chances of having a kidney stone in people who are more likely to develop them.

WHAT ARE THE SYMPTOMS OF KIDNEY STONES?

Symptoms of kidney stones include:

- sharp pains in your back, side, lower abdomen, or groin
- pink, red, or brown blood in your urine, also called "hematuria"
- a constant need to urinate
- pain while urinating
- inability to urinate or can only urinate a small amount
- cloudy or bad-smelling urine

See a health-care professional right away if you have any of these symptoms. These symptoms may mean you have a kidney stone or a more serious condition.

Your pain may last for a short or long time or may come and go in waves. Along with pain, you may have:

- nausea
- vomiting

Other symptoms include:

- fever
- chills

DIAGNOSIS OF KIDNEY STONES
How Do Health-Care Professionals Diagnose Kidney Stones?

Health-care professionals use your medical history, a physical exam, and lab and imaging tests to diagnose kidney stones.

A health-care professional will ask if you have a history of health conditions that make you more likely to develop kidney stones. The health-care professional may also ask if you have a family history of kidney stones and about what you typically eat. During a physical exam, the health-care professional usually examines your body. The health-care professional will ask you about your symptoms.

What Tests Do Health-Care Professionals Use to Diagnose Kidney Stones?

Health-care professionals may use lab or imaging tests to diagnose kidney stones.

LAB TESTS

Urine tests can show whether your urine contains high levels of minerals that form kidney stones. Urine and blood tests can also help a health-care professional find out what type of kidney stones you have.

- **Urinalysis**. It involves a health-care professional testing your urine sample. You will collect a urine sample at a doctor's office or at a lab, and a health-care professional will test the sample. Urinalysis can show whether your urine has blood in it and minerals that can form kidney stones. White blood cells (WBC) and bacteria in the urine mean you may have a UTI.
- **Blood tests**. A health-care professional may take a blood sample from you and send the sample to a lab for testing. The blood test can show if you have high levels of certain minerals in your blood that can lead to kidney stones.

IMAGING TESTS

Health-care professionals use imaging tests to find kidney stones. The tests may also show problems that caused a kidney stone to form, such as a blockage in the urinary tract or a birth defect. You do not need anesthesia for these imaging tests.

- **Abdominal x-ray**. An abdominal x-ray is a picture of the abdomen that uses low levels of radiation and is recorded on film or on a computer. An x-ray technician takes an abdominal x-ray at a hospital or outpatient center, and a radiologist reads the images. During an abdominal x-ray, you will lie on a table or stand up. The x-ray technician will position the x-ray machine over or in front of your abdomen and ask you to hold your breath, so the picture would not be blurry. The x-ray technician then may ask you to change position for additional pictures. Abdominal x-rays can show the location of kidney stones in the urinary tract. Not all stones are visible on the abdominal x-ray.

- **Computed tomography (CT) scans.** CT scans use a combination of x-rays and computer technology to create images of your urinary tract. Although a CT scan without contrast medium is most commonly used to view your urinary tract, a health-care professional may give you an injection of contrast medium. A contrast medium is a dye or other substance that makes structures inside your body easier to see during imaging tests. You will lie on a table that slides into a tunnel-shaped device that takes the x-rays. CT scans can show the size and location of a kidney stone if the stone is blocking the urinary tract and conditions that may have caused the kidney stone to form.

TREATMENT OF KIDNEY STONES
How Do Health-Care Professionals Treat Kidney Stones?

Health-care professionals usually treat kidney stones based on their size, location, and type.

Small kidney stones may pass through your urinary tract without treatment. If you are able to pass a kidney stone, a health-care professional may ask you to catch the kidney stone in a special container. A health-care professional will send the kidney stone to a lab to find out what type it is. A health-care professional may advise you to drink plenty of liquids if you are able to help move a kidney stone along. The health-care professional also may prescribe pain medicine.

Larger kidney stones or kidney stones that block your urinary tract or cause great pain may need urgent treatment. If you are vomiting and dehydrated, you may need to go to the hospital and get fluids intravenously.

KIDNEY STONE REMOVAL

A urologist can remove the kidney stone or break it into small pieces with the following treatments:

- **Shock wave lithotripsy.** The doctor can use shock wave lithotripsy to blast the kidney stone into small pieces. The smaller pieces of the kidney stone then pass through your urinary tract. A doctor can give you anesthesia during this outpatient procedure.

- **Cystoscopy and ureteroscopy**. During cystoscopy, the doctor uses a cystoscope to look inside the urethra and bladder to find a stone in your urethra or bladder. During ureteroscopy, the doctor uses a ureteroscope, which is longer and thinner than a cystoscope, to see detailed images of the lining of the ureters and kidneys. The doctor inserts the cystoscope or ureteroscope through the urethra to see the rest of the urinary tract. Once the stone is found, the doctor can remove it or break it into smaller pieces. The doctor performs these procedures in the hospital with anesthesia. You can typically go home the same day.
- **Percutaneous nephrolithotomy**. The doctor uses a thin viewing tool, called a "nephroscope," to locate and remove the kidney stone. The doctor inserts the tool directly into your kidney through a small cut made in your back. For larger kidney stones, the doctor may also use a laser to break the kidney stones into smaller pieces. The doctor performs percutaneous nephrolithotomy in a hospital with anesthesia. You may have to stay in the hospital for several days after the procedure.

After these procedures, sometimes, the urologist may leave a thin flexible tube, called a "ureteral stent," in your urinary tract to help urine flow or a stone to pass. Once the kidney stone is removed, your doctor sends the kidney stone or its pieces to a lab to find out what type it is.

The health-care professional may also ask you to collect your urine for 24 hours after the kidney stone has passed or been removed. The health-care professional can then measure how much urine you produce in a day, along with mineral levels in your urine. You are more likely to form stones if you do not make enough urine each day or have a problem with high mineral levels.

To help prevent future kidney stones, you also need to know what caused your previous kidney stones. Once you know what type of kidney stone you had, a health-care professional can help you make changes to your eating, diet, and nutrition to prevent future kidney stones.

DRINKING LIQUIDS

In most cases, drinking enough liquids each day is the best way to help prevent most types of kidney stones. Drinking enough liquids keeps your urine diluted and helps flush away minerals that might form stones.

Though water is best, other liquids such as citrus drinks may also help prevent kidney stones. Some studies show that citrus drinks, such as lemonade and orange juice, protect against kidney stones because they contain citrate, which stops crystals from turning into stones.

Unless you have kidney failure, you should drink six to eight 8-ounce glasses a day. If you previously had cystine stones, you may need to drink even more. Talk with a health-care professional if you cannot drink the recommended amount due to other health problems, such as urinary incontinence (UI), urinary frequency, or kidney failure.

The amount of liquid you need to drink depends on the weather and your activity level. If you live, work, or exercise in hot weather, you may need more liquid to replace the fluid you lose through sweat. A health-care professional may ask you to collect your urine for 24 hours to determine the amount of urine you produce a day. If the amount of urine is too low, the health-care professional may advise you to increase your liquid intake.

MEDICINES

If you have had a kidney stone, a health-care professional may also prescribe medicines to prevent future kidney stones (see Table 12.1). Depending on the type of kidney stone you had and what type of medicine the health-care professional prescribes, you may have to take the medicine for a few weeks, several months, or longer.

For example, if you had struvite stones, you may have to take an oral antibiotic for one to six weeks or possibly longer.

If you have another type of stone, you may have to take a potassium citrate tablet one to three times daily. You may have to take potassium citrate for months or even longer until a health-care professional says you are no longer at risk for kidney stones.

Table 12.1. Kidney Stone and the Medicines Prescribed by the Doctors

Type of Kidney Stone	Possible Medicines Prescribed by Your Doctor
Calcium stones	• potassium citrate, which is used to raise the citrate and pH levels in urine • diuretics, often called water pills, that help rid your body of water
Uric acid stones	• allopurinol, which is used to treat high levels of uric acid in the body • potassium citrate
Struvite stones	• antibiotics, which are bacteria-fighting medications • acetohydroxamic acid, a strong antibiotic, used with another long-term antibiotic medication to prevent infection
Cystine stones	• mercaptopropionyl glycine, an antioxidant used for heart problems • potassium citrate

Talk with a health-care professional about your health history prior to taking kidney stone medicines. Some kidney stone medicines have minor to serious side effects. Side effects are more likely to occur the longer you take the medicine and the higher the dose. Tell the health-care professional about any side effects that occur when you take kidney stone medicine.

HYPERPARATHYROIDISM SURGERY

People with hyperparathyroidism, a condition that results in too much calcium in the blood, sometimes develop calcium stones. Treatment for hyperparathyroidism may include surgery to remove the abnormal parathyroid gland. Removing the parathyroid gland cures hyperparathyroidism and can prevent kidney stones. Surgery sometimes causes complications, including infection.[1]

---

[1] "Kidney Stones," National Institute of Diabetes and Digestive and Kidney Diseases (NIDDK), September 2016. Available online. URL: www.niddk.nih.gov/health-information/urologic-diseases/kidney-stones/all-content. Accessed June 27, 2023.

Section 12.2 | **Chronic Kidney Disease**

WHAT IS CHRONIC KIDNEY DISEASE?

Chronic kidney disease (CKD) means your kidneys are damaged and cannot filter blood the way they should. The disease is called "chronic" because the damage to your kidneys happens slowly over a long period of time. This damage can cause waste to build up in your body. CKD can also cause other health problems. Figure 12.2 shows the location of kidneys in the urinary tract.

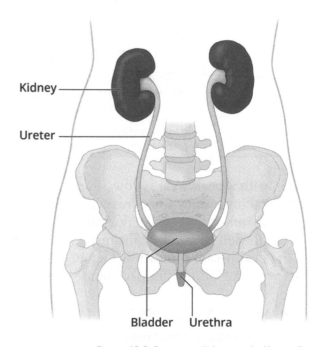

Kidney

Ureter

Bladder   Urethra

Figure 12.2. Position of Kidneys in the Urinary Tract

National Institute of Diabetes and Digestive and Kidney Diseases (NIDDK)
The kidneys are located in the middle of your back, just below your rib cage.

The kidneys' main job is to filter extra water and wastes out of your blood to make urine. To keep your body working properly, the kidneys balance the salts and minerals—such as calcium, phosphorus, sodium, and potassium—that circulate in the blood. Your kidneys also make hormones that help control blood pressure, make red blood cells (RBC), and keep your bones strong.

Kidney disease can often get worse over time and may lead to kidney failure. If your kidneys fail, you will need dialysis or a kidney transplant to maintain your health.

The sooner you know you have kidney disease, the sooner you can make changes to protect your kidneys.

HOW COMMON IS CHRONIC KIDNEY DISEASE?

Chronic kidney disease is common among adults in the United States. More than 37 million American adults may have CKD.

WHO IS MORE LIKELY TO DEVELOP CHRONIC KIDNEY DISEASE?

You are at risk for kidney disease if you have the following health problems:

- **Diabetes**. Diabetes is the leading cause of CKD. High blood glucose, also called "blood sugar," from diabetes can damage the blood vessels in your kidneys. Almost one in three people with diabetes has CKD.
- **High blood pressure**. High blood pressure is the second leading cause of CKD. Like high blood glucose, high blood pressure can also damage the blood vessels in your kidneys. Almost one in five adults with high blood pressure has CKD.
- **Heart disease**. Research shows a link between kidney disease and heart disease. People with heart disease are at higher risk for kidney disease, and people with kidney disease are at higher risk for heart disease. Researchers are working to better understand the relationship between kidney disease and heart disease.
- **Family history of kidney failure**. If your mother, father, sister, or brother has kidney failure, you are at risk for CKD. Kidney disease tends to run in families. If you have kidney disease, encourage family members to get tested.

Your chances of having kidney disease increase with age. The longer you have had diabetes, high blood pressure, or heart disease, the more likely you will have kidney disease.

African Americans, Hispanics, and American Indians tend to have a greater risk for CKD. The greater risk is mostly due to higher rates of diabetes and high blood pressure among these groups. Scientists are studying other possible reasons for this increased risk.

DOES CHRONIC KIDNEY DISEASE CAUSE OTHER HEALTH PROBLEMS?

Kidney disease can lead to other health problems, such as heart disease. If you have kidney disease, it increases your chances of having a stroke or heart attack.

HOW CAN CHRONIC KIDNEY DISEASE AFFECT YOUR DAY-TO-DAY LIFE?

Many people are afraid to learn that they have kidney disease because they think that all kidney disease leads to dialysis. However, most people with kidney disease will not need dialysis. If you have kidney disease, you can continue to live a productive life, work, spend time with friends and family, stay physically active, and do other things you enjoy. You may need to change what you eat and add healthy habits to your daily routine to help you protect your kidneys.

Will Your Kidneys Get Better?

Kidney disease is often "progressive," which means it gets worse over time. The damage to your kidneys causes scars and is permanent.

You can take steps to protect your kidneys, such as managing your blood pressure and your blood glucose, if you have diabetes.

What Happens If Your Kidneys Fail?

Kidney failure means that your kidneys have lost most of their ability to function—less than 15 percent of normal kidney function.

If you have kidney failure, you will need treatment to maintain your health.

High blood pressure can be both a cause and a result of kidney disease. High blood pressure damages your kidneys, and damaged kidneys do not work as well to help control your blood pressure.

If you have CKD, you also have a higher chance of having a sudden change in kidney function caused by illness, injury, or certain medicines. This is called "acute kidney injury" (AKI).

CAUSES OF CHRONIC KIDNEY DISEASE

Diabetes and high blood pressure are the most common causes of CKD. Your health-care provider will look at your health history and may do tests to find out why you have kidney disease. The cause of your kidney disease may affect the type of treatment you receive.

Diabetes

Too much glucose, also called "sugar," in your blood damages your kidneys' filters. Over time, your kidneys can become so damaged that they no longer do a good job filtering wastes and extra fluid from your blood.

Often, the first sign of kidney disease from diabetes is a protein in your urine. When the filters are damaged, a protein called "albumin," which you need to stay healthy, passes out of your blood and into your urine. A healthy kidney does not let albumin pass from the blood into the urine.

Diabetic kidney disease is the medical term for kidney disease caused by diabetes.

High Blood Pressure

High blood pressure can damage blood vessels in the kidneys, so they do not work as well. If the blood vessels in your kidneys are damaged, your kidneys may not work as well to remove wastes and extra fluid from your body. Extra fluid in the blood vessels may then raise blood pressure even more, creating a dangerous cycle.

Other Causes of Kidney Disease

Other causes of kidney disease include:

- a genetic disorder that causes many cysts to grow in the kidneys, polycystic kidney disease (PKD)
- an infection
- a drug that is toxic to the kidneys
- a disease that affects the entire body, such as diabetes or lupus (Lupus nephritis is the medical name for kidney disease caused by lupus.)
- immunoglobulin A (IgA) glomerulonephritis
- disorders in which the body's immune system attacks its own cells and organs, such as anti-glomerular basement membrane (GBM; Goodpasture) disease
- heavy metal poisoning, such as lead poisoning
- rare genetic conditions, such as Alport syndrome
- hemolytic uremic syndrome in children
- IgA vasculitis
- renal artery stenosis

WHAT ARE THE SYMPTOMS OF CHRONIC KIDNEY DISEASE?
Early Chronic Kidney Disease May Not Have Any Symptoms

You may wonder how you can have CKD and feel fine. Our kidneys have a greater capacity to do their job than is needed to keep us healthy. For example, you can donate one kidney and remain healthy. You can also have kidney damage without any symptoms because, despite the damage, your kidneys are still doing enough work to keep you feeling well. For many people, the only way to know if you have kidney disease is to get your kidneys checked with blood and urine tests.

As kidney disease gets worse, a person may have swelling, called "edema." Edema happens when the kidneys cannot get rid of extra fluid and salt. Edema can occur in the legs, feet, or ankles, and less often in the hands or face.

Symptoms of Advanced Chronic Kidney Disease

- chest pain
- dry skin

- itching or numbness
- feeling tired
- headaches
- increased or decreased urination
- loss of appetite
- muscle cramps
- nausea
- shortness of breath
- sleep problems
- trouble concentrating
- vomiting
- weight loss

People with CKD can also develop anemia, bone disease, and malnutrition.

DIAGNOSIS OF CHRONIC KIDNEY DISEASE
What Tests Do Doctors Use to Diagnose and Monitor Kidney Disease?

To check for kidney disease, health-care providers use the following:
- **A blood test that checks how well your kidneys are filtering your blood**. This test is called "glomerular filtration rate" (GFR).
- **A urine test to check for albumin**. Albumin is a protein that can pass into the urine when the kidneys are damaged.

If you have kidney disease, your health-care provider will use the same two tests to help monitor your kidney disease and make sure your treatment plan is working.

BLOOD TEST FOR GLOMERULAR FILTRATION RATE

Your health-care provider will use a blood test to check your kidney function. The results of the test mean the following:
- A GFR of 60 or more is in the normal range. Ask your health-care provider when your GFR should be checked again.

- A GFR of less than 60 may mean you have kidney disease. Talk with your health-care provider about how to keep your kidney health at this level.
- A GFR of 15 or less is called "kidney failure." Most people below this level need dialysis or a kidney transplant. Talk with your health-care provider about your treatment options.

You cannot raise your GFR, but you can try to keep it from going lower.

Creatinine is a waste product from the normal breakdown of muscles in your body. Your kidneys remove creatinine from your blood. Providers use the amount of creatinine in your blood to estimate your GFR. As kidney disease gets worse, the level of creatinine goes up.

URINE TEST FOR ALBUMIN

If you are at risk for kidney disease, your provider may check your urine for albumin.

Albumin is a protein found in your blood. A healthy kidney does not let albumin pass into the urine. A damaged kidney lets some albumin pass into the urine. The less albumin in your urine, the better. Having albumin in the urine is called "albuminuria."

A health-care provider can check for albumin in your urine in two ways:

- **Dipstick test for albumin**. A provider uses a urine sample to look for albumin in your urine. You collect the urine sample in a container in a health-care provider's office or lab. For the test, a provider places a strip of chemically treated paper, called a "dipstick," into the urine. The dipstick changes color if albumin is present in the urine.
- **Urine albumin-to-creatinine ratio (UACR)**. This test measures and compares the amount of albumin with the amount of creatinine in your urine sample. Providers use your UACR to estimate how much

albumin would pass into your urine over 24 hours. A urine albumin result of:
- 30 mg/g or less is normal
- more than 30 mg/g may be a sign of kidney disease

If you have albumin in your urine, your provider may want you to repeat the urine test one or two more times to confirm the results. Talk with your provider about what your specific numbers mean for you.

If you have kidney disease, measuring the albumin in your urine helps your provider know which treatment is best for you. A urine albumin level that stays the same or goes down may mean that treatments are working.

How Do You Know If Your Kidney Disease Is Getting Worse?

You can keep track of your test results over time. You can tell that your treatments are working if your:
- GFR stays the same
- urine albumin stays the same or goes down

Your health-care provider will work with you to manage your kidney disease.

PREVENTION OF CHRONIC KIDNEY DISEASE

You can protect your kidneys by preventing or managing health conditions that cause kidney damage, such as diabetes and high blood pressure.

During your next medical visit, you may want to ask your health-care provider about your kidney health. Early kidney disease may not have any symptoms, so getting tested may be the only way to know your kidneys are healthy. Your health-care provider will help decide how often you should be tested.

See a provider right away if you develop a urinary tract infection (UTI), which can cause kidney damage if left untreated.[2]

---

[2] "Chronic Kidney Disease (CKD)," National Institute of Diabetes and Digestive and Kidney Diseases (NIDDK), October 2016. Available online. URL: www.niddk.nih.gov/health-information/kidney-disease/chronic-kidney-disease-ckd/all-content. Accessed June 27, 2023.

Section 12.3 | **Urinary Incontinence in Older Adults**

Urinary incontinence means a person leaks urine by accident. While it can happen to anyone, urinary incontinence, also known as "overactive bladder," is more common in older people. Bladder control issues can be embarrassing and cause people to avoid their normal activities. However, incontinence can often be stopped or controlled.

What happens in the body to cause bladder control problems? Located in the lower abdomen, the bladder is a hollow organ that is part of the urinary system, which also includes the kidneys, ureters, and urethra. During urination, muscles in the bladder tighten to move urine into the tube-shaped urethra. At the same time, the muscles around the urethra relax and let the urine pass out of the body. When the muscles in and around the bladder do not work the way they should, urine can leak, resulting in urinary incontinence.

Incontinence can happen for many reasons, including urinary tract infections, vaginal infection or irritation, or constipation. Some medications can cause bladder control problems that last a short time. When incontinence lasts longer, it may be due to:

- weak bladder or pelvic floor muscles
- overactive bladder muscles
- damage to nerves that control the bladder from diseases such as multiple sclerosis (MS), diabetes, or Parkinson disease (PD)
- diseases such as arthritis that may make it difficult to get to the bathroom in time
- pelvic organ prolapse, which is when pelvic organs (such as the bladder, rectum, or uterus) shift out of their normal place into the vagina or anus. When pelvic organs are out of place, the bladder and urethra are not able to work normally, which may cause urine to leak.

Most incontinence in men is related to the prostate gland. Male incontinence may be caused by:

- prostatitis, a painful inflammation of the prostate gland
- injury or damage to nerves or muscles from surgery

- an enlarged prostate gland, which can lead to benign prostate hyperplasia, a condition in which the prostate grows as men age

TYPES OF URINARY INCONTINENCE

The following are the different types of incontinence:
- **Stress incontinence.** This occurs when urine leaks as pressure is put on the bladder, such as during exercise, coughing, sneezing, laughing, or lifting heavy objects. It is the most common type of bladder control problem in younger and middle-aged women. It may also begin later, around the time of menopause.
- **Urge incontinence.** This incontinence happens when people have a sudden need to urinate and can not hold their urine long enough to get to the toilet. It may be a problem for people who have diabetes, Alzheimer disease, Parkinson disease, multiple sclerosis, or stroke.
- **Overflow incontinence.** This incontinence happens when small amounts of urine leak from a bladder that is always full. A man can have trouble emptying his bladder if an enlarged prostate is blocking the urethra. Diabetes and spinal cord injuries can also cause this type of incontinence.
- **Functional incontinence.** This occurs in many older people who have normal bladder control. They just have a problem getting to the toilet because of arthritis or other disorders that make it hard to move quickly.

TREATING AND MANAGING URINARY INCONTINENCE

Today, there are more treatments and ways to manage urinary incontinence than ever before. The choice of treatment depends on the type of bladder control problem you have, how serious it is, and what best fits your lifestyle. As a general rule, the simplest and safest treatments should be tried first.

A combination of treatments may help you get better control of your bladder. Your doctor may suggest you try the following.

Bladder Control Training
- **Pelvic muscle exercises (also known as "Kegel exercises").** These exercises strengthen the muscles that support the bladder, which can help you hold urine in your bladder and avoid leaks.
- **Urgency suppression.** It helps control strong urges to urinate, so you can make it to the toilet on time. For example, you can try distracting yourself to help keep your mind off needing to urinate, taking long relaxing breaths, holding still, and squeezing the pelvic floor muscles.
- **Timed voiding.** It is used to help control your bladder by scheduling time to urinate. For example, you can set a plan to urinate every hour. As time goes on, you can slowly extend the time between toilet breaks.

Medical Treatments
- **Medications.** Medications that come in a pill, liquid, or patch may be prescribed to help with bladder control problems. However, some medications for overactive bladder have been associated with a higher risk of cognitive decline in adults over age 65. Talk with your doctor about what medications, if any, would work best for you.
- **Bulking agents.** These agents can be used to help close the bladder opening. Doctors can inject a bulking gel or paste that thickens the area around the urethra. This can reduce stress incontinence but may need to be repeated.
- **Medical devices.** Devices such as a catheter that drains urine from your bladder, a urethral insert that helps prevent leakage, and a vaginal pessary ring that provides pressure to lessen leakage may also be used to manage urinary incontinence.

- **Biofeedback.** This is a process that uses sensors to make you aware of signals from your body. This may help you regain control over the muscles in your bladder and urethra.
- **Electrical nerve stimulation.** This therapy sends mild electric currents to the nerves around the bladder that help control urination and your bladder's reflexes.
- **Surgery.** It can sometimes improve or cure incontinence if it is caused by a change in the position of the bladder or blockage due to an enlarged prostate.

Behavioral and Lifestyle Changes

Changing your lifestyle may help with bladder problems. Losing weight, quitting smoking, saying "no" to alcohol, choosing water instead of other drinks, and limiting drinks before bedtime can help with some bladder problems. Preventing constipation and avoiding lifting heavy objects may also help with incontinence. Even after treatment, some people still leak urine from time to time. There are bladder control products and other solutions, including disposable briefs or underwear, furniture pads, and urine deodorizing pills that may help.[3]

---

[3] National Institute on Aging (NIA), "Urinary Incontinence in Older Adults," National Institutes of Health (NIH), January 24, 2022. Available online. URL: www.nia.nih.gov/health/urinary-incontinence-older-adults. Accessed June 27, 2023.

Chapter 13 | Neurological Issues in Men

Section 13.1 | Alzheimer Disease

Alzheimer disease (AD) is the most common type of dementia. It is a progressive disease beginning with mild memory loss and possibly leading to loss of the ability to carry on a conversation and respond to the environment. Alzheimer disease involves parts of the brain that control thought, memory, and language. It can seriously affect a person's ability to carry out daily activities.

WHAT IS THE BURDEN OF ALZHEIMER DISEASE IN THE UNITED STATES?

- Alzheimer disease is one of the top 10 leading causes of death in the United States.
- The sixth leading cause of death among U.S. adults.
- The fifth leading cause of death among adults aged 65 or older.

In 2020, an estimated 5.8 million Americans aged 65 or older had AD. This number is projected to nearly triple to 14 million people by 2060.

In 2010, the costs of treating AD were projected to fall between $159 and $215 billion. By 2040, these costs are projected to jump to between $379 and more than $500 billion annually.

Death rates for AD are increasing, unlike heart disease and cancer death rates that are on the decline. Dementia, including AD, has been shown to be underreported in death certificates, and therefore, the proportion of older people who die from Alzheimer may be considerably higher.

RISK FACTORS OF ALZHEIMER DISEASE

Scientists do not yet fully understand what causes AD. There likely is not a single cause but rather several factors that can affect each person differently.

- **Age**. This is the best-known risk factor for AD.
- **Family history**. Researchers believe that genetics may play a role in developing AD. However, genes do not

equal destiny. A healthy lifestyle may help reduce your risk of developing AD. Studies indicate that adequate physical activity, a nutritious diet, limited alcohol consumption, and not smoking may help people.
- **Changes in the brain**. These changes can begin years before the first symptoms appear.

WHAT IS KNOWN ABOUT REDUCING YOUR RISK OF ALZHEIMER DISEASE?

The science of risk reduction is quickly evolving, and major break-throughs are within reach. For example, there is growing evidence that people who adopt healthy lifestyle habits—such as regular exercise and blood pressure management—can lower their risk of dementia. There is growing scientific evidence that healthy behaviors, which have been shown to prevent cancer, diabetes, and heart disease, may also reduce the risk for subjective cognitive decline.

WHAT ARE THE WARNING SIGNS OF ALZHEIMER DISEASE?

Alzheimer disease is not a normal part of aging. Memory problems are typically one of the first warning signs of AD and related dementias.

In addition to memory problems, someone with symptoms of AD may experience one or more of the following:
- memory loss that disrupts daily life, such as getting lost in a familiar place or repeating questions
- trouble handling money and paying bills
- difficulty completing familiar tasks at home, at work, or at leisure
- decreased or poor judgment
- misplacing things and being unable to retrace steps to find them
- changes in mood, personality, or behavior

Even if you or someone you know has several or even most of these signs, it does not mean it is AD.

WHAT TO DO IF YOU SUSPECT ALZHEIMER DISEASE

Getting checked by your health-care provider can help determine if the symptoms you are experiencing are related to AD or a more treatable condition such as a vitamin deficiency or a side effect from medication. Early and accurate diagnosis also provides opportunities for you and your family to consider financial planning, develop advance directives, enroll in clinical trials, and anticipate care needs.

HOW IS ALZHEIMER DISEASE TREATED?

Medical management can improve the quality of life (QOL) for individuals living with AD and for their caregivers. There is currently no known cure for AD. Treatment addresses several areas:
- helping people maintain brain health
- managing behavioral symptoms
- slowing or delaying symptoms of the disease

SUPPORT FOR FAMILY AND FRIENDS

Currently, many people living with AD are cared for at home by family members. Caregiving can have positive aspects for the caregiver as well as the person being cared for. It may bring personal fulfillment to the caregiver, such as satisfaction from helping a family member or friend, and lead to the development of new skills and improved family relationships.

Although most people willingly provide care to their loved ones and friends, caring for a person with AD at home can be a difficult task and may become overwhelming at times. Each day brings new challenges as the caregiver copes with changing levels of ability and new patterns of behavior. As the disease gets worse, people living with AD often need more intensive care.[1]

---

[1] "Alzheimer's Disease and Related Dementias," Centers for Disease Control and Prevention (CDC), October 26, 2020. Available online. URL: www.cdc.gov/aging/aginginfo/alzheimers.htm. Accessed July 5, 2023.

Section 13.2 | **Parkinson Disease**

Parkinson disease (PD) is a brain disorder that causes unintended or uncontrollable movements, such as shaking, stiffness, and difficulty with balance and coordination.

Symptoms usually begin gradually and worsen over time. As the disease progresses, people may have difficulty walking and talking. They may also have mental and behavioral changes, sleep problems, depression, memory difficulties, and fatigue.

While virtually anyone could be at risk of developing PD, some research studies suggest this disease affects more men than women. It is unclear why, but studies are underway to understand factors that may increase a person's risk. One clear risk is age: Although most people with PD first develop the disease after age 60, about 5–10 percent experience onset before the age of 50. Early-onset forms of PD are often, but not always, inherited, and some forms have been linked to specific alterations in genes.

WHAT CAUSES PARKINSON DISEASE?

The most prominent signs and symptoms of PD occur when nerve cells in the basal ganglia, an area of the brain that controls movement, become impaired and/or die. Normally, these nerve cells, or neurons, produce an important brain chemical known as "dopamine." When the neurons die or become impaired, they produce less dopamine, which causes the movement problems associated with the disease.

Scientists still do not know what causes the neurons to die.

People with PD also lose the nerve endings that produce norepinephrine, the main chemical messenger of the sympathetic nervous system, which controls many functions of the body, such as heart rate and blood pressure. The loss of norepinephrine might help explain some of the non-movement features of PD, such as fatigue, irregular blood pressure, decreased movement of food through the digestive tract, and sudden drop in blood pressure when a person stands up from a sitting or lying position.

Many brain cells of people with PD contain Lewy bodies, unusual clumps of the protein alpha-synuclein. Scientists are trying to better understand the normal and abnormal functions of alpha-synuclein and its relationship to genetic variants that impact PD and Lewy body dementia (LBD).

Some cases of PD appear to be hereditary, and a few cases can be traced to specific genetic variants. While genetics is thought to play a role in PD, in most cases, the disease does not seem to run in families. Many researchers now believe that PD results from a combination of genetic and environmental factors, such as exposure to toxins.

SYMPTOMS OF PARKINSON DISEASE

Parkinson disease has the following four main symptoms:
- tremor in hands, arms, legs, jaw, or head
- muscle stiffness, where muscle remains contracted for a long time
- slowness of movement
- impaired balance and coordination, sometimes leading to falls

Other symptoms may include the following:
- depression and other emotional changes
- difficulty swallowing, chewing, and speaking
- urinary problems or constipation
- skin problems

The symptoms of PD and the rate of progression differ among individuals. Early symptoms of this disease are subtle and occur gradually. For example, people may feel mild tremors or have difficulty getting out of a chair. They may notice that they speak too softly or that their handwriting is slow and looks cramped or small. Friends or family members may be the first to notice changes in someone with early PD. They may see that the person's face lacks expression and animation or that the person does not move an arm or leg normally.

People with PD often develop a Parkinsonian gait that includes a tendency to lean forward; take small, quick steps; and reduce swinging their arms. They may also have trouble initiating or continuing movement.

Symptoms often begin on one side of the body or even in one limb on one side of the body. As the disease progresses, it eventually affects both sides. However, the symptoms may still be more severe on one side than on the other.

Many people with PD note that prior to experiencing stiffness and tremor, they had sleep problems, constipation, loss of smell, and restless legs. While some of these symptoms may also occur with normal aging, talk with your doctor if these symptoms worsen or begin to interfere with daily living.

Changes in Cognition and Parkinson Disease

Some people with PD may experience changes in their cognitive function, including problems with memory, attention, and the ability to plan and accomplish tasks. Stress, depression, and some medications may also contribute to these changes in cognition.

Over time, as the disease progresses, some people may develop dementia and be diagnosed with Parkinson dementia, a type of LBD. People with Parkinson dementia may have severe memory and thinking problems that affect daily living.

Talk with your doctor if you or your loved one is diagnosed with PD and is experiencing problems with thinking or memory.

DIAGNOSIS OF PARKINSON DISEASE

There are currently no blood or laboratory tests to diagnose nongenetic cases of PD. Doctors usually diagnose the disease by taking a person's medical history and performing a neurological examination. If symptoms improve after starting to take medication, it is another indicator that the person has PD.

A number of disorders can cause symptoms similar to those of PD. People with Parkinson-like symptoms that result from other causes, such as multiple system atrophy and dementia with Lewy bodies, are sometimes said to have Parkinsonism. While these disorders initially may be misdiagnosed as PD, certain medical tests, as well as responses to drug treatment, may help better evaluate the cause. Many other diseases have similar features but require different treatments, so it is important to get an accurate diagnosis as soon as possible.

TREATMENTS FOR PARKINSON DISEASE

Although there is no cure for PD, medicines, surgical treatment, and other therapies can often relieve some symptoms.

Medicines for Parkinson Disease

Medicines can help treat the symptoms of PD by:
- increasing the level of dopamine in the brain
- having an effect on other brain chemicals, such as neurotransmitters, which transfer information between brain cells
- helping control non-movement symptoms

The main therapy for PD is levodopa. Nerve cells use levodopa to make dopamine to replenish the brain's dwindling supply. Usually, people take levodopa along with another medication called "carbidopa." Carbidopa prevents or reduces some of the side effects of levodopa therapy—such as nausea, vomiting, low blood pressure, and restlessness—and reduces the amount of levodopa needed to improve symptoms.

People living with PD should never stop taking levodopa without telling their doctor. Suddenly stopping the drug may have serious side effects, such as being unable to move or having difficulty breathing.

The doctor may prescribe other medicines to treat PD symptoms, including the following:
- dopamine agonists to stimulate the production of dopamine in the brain
- enzyme inhibitors (e.g., monoamine oxidase (MAO-B) inhibitors, catechol-O-methyltransferase (COMT) inhibitors) to increase the amount of dopamine by slowing down the enzymes that break down dopamine in the brain

- amantadine to help reduce involuntary movements
- anticholinergic drugs to reduce tremors and muscle rigidity

Deep Brain Stimulation

For people with PD who do not respond well to medications, the doctor may recommend deep brain stimulation. During a surgical procedure, a doctor implants electrodes into part of the brain and connects them to a small electrical device implanted in the chest. The device and electrodes painlessly stimulate specific areas in the brain that control movement in a way that may help stop many of the movement-related symptoms of PD, such as tremor, slowness of movement, and rigidity.

Other Therapies

Other therapies that may help manage PD symptoms include the following:

- physical, occupational, and speech therapies, which may help with gait and voice disorders, tremors and rigidity, and decline in mental functions
- a healthy diet to support overall wellness
- exercises to strengthen muscles and improve balance, flexibility, and coordination
- massage therapy to reduce tension
- yoga and tai chi to increase stretching and flexibility

SUPPORT FOR PEOPLE LIVING WITH PARKINSON DISEASE

While the progression of PD is usually slow, eventually, a person's daily routines may be affected. Activities such as working, taking care of a home, and participating in social activities with friends may become challenging. Experiencing these changes can be difficult, but support groups can help people cope. These groups can provide information, advice, and connections to resources for those living with PD, their families, and caregivers.[2]

[2] National Institute on Aging (NIA), "Parkinson's Disease: Causes, Symptoms, and Treatments," National Institutes of Health (NIH), April 14, 2022. Available online. URL: www.nia.nih.gov/health/parkinsons-disease. Accessed June 23, 2023.

Chapter 14 | Male-Linked Genetic Disorders

Chapter Contents

WHAT IS COLOR BLINDNESS?

If you have color blindness, it means you see colors differently than most people. Most of the time, color blindness makes it hard to tell the difference between certain colors.

Usually, color blindness runs in families. There is no cure, but special glasses and contact lenses can help. Most people who are color blind are able to adjust and do not have problems with everyday activities.

WHAT ARE THE TYPES OF COLOR BLINDNESS?

The most common type of color blindness makes it hard to tell the difference between red and green. Another type makes it hard to tell the difference between blue and yellow. People who are completely color blind do not see color at all, but that is not very common.

WHAT CAUSES COLOR BLINDNESS?

The most common kinds of color blindness are genetic, meaning they are passed down from parents.

Color blindness can also happen because of damage to your eye or your brain. And color vision may get worse as you get older—often because of cataracts (cloudy areas in the lens of the eye).

ARE YOU AT RISK OF COLOR BLINDNESS?

Men have a much higher risk than women for color blindness. You are also more likely to have color blindness if you:
- have a family history of color blindness
- have certain eye diseases, such as glaucoma or age-related macular degeneration (AMD)
- have certain health problems, such as diabetes, Alzheimer disease (AD), or multiple sclerosis (MS)
- take certain medicines
- are White

If you think you may have color blindness, talk with your doctor about getting checked.

WHAT ARE THE SYMPTOMS OF COLOR BLINDNESS?

The main symptom of color blindness is not seeing colors the way most people do. If you are color blind, you may have trouble seeing:

- the difference between colors
- how bright colors are
- different shades of colors

Symptoms of color blindness are often so mild that you may not notice them. And, since we get used to the way we see colors, many people with color blindness do not know they have it.

People with very serious cases of color blindness might have other symptoms, too—such as quick side-to-side eye movements (nystagmus) or sensitivity to light.

HOW COULD YOU FIND OUT IF YOU HAVE COLOR BLINDNESS?

Your eye doctor can usually use a simple test to tell you if you are color blind.

During the test, your eye doctor will show you a circle made of many different colored dots. The circle has a shape inside it that is made out of dots—such as a number, a letter, or a squiggly line. This shape is easy to see if you do not have color blindness, but people who are color blind have a hard time seeing it.

WHAT IS THE TREATMENT FOR COLOR BLINDNESS?

There is no cure for color blindness that is passed down in families, but most people find ways to adjust to it. Children with color blindness may need help with some classroom activities, and adults with color blindness may not be able to do certain jobs, such as being a pilot or graphic designer. Keep in mind that most of the time, color blindness does not cause serious problems.

If your color blindness is happening because of another health problem, your doctor will treat the condition that is causing the problem. If you are taking a medicine that causes color blindness, your doctor may adjust how much you take or suggest you switch to a different medicine.

If color blindness is causing problems with everyday tasks, there are devices and technology that can help, including the following:

- **Glasses and contacts.** Special contact lenses and glasses may help people who are color blind tell the difference between colors.
- **Visual aids.** You can use visual aids, apps, and other technology to help you live with color blindness. For example, you can use an app to take a photo with your phone or tablet and then tap on part of the photo to find out the color of that area.

Talk over your options with your eye doctor. Remember the following tips:

- Ask your doctor about visual aids and technology that can help you with everyday tasks.
- Encourage family members to get checked for color blindness since it can run in families.[1]

Section 14.2 | Fragile X Syndrome

Fragile X syndrome (FXS) and its associated conditions are caused by changes (mutations) in the *FMR1* gene found on the X chromosome. This mutation affects how the body makes a protein called "fragile X mental retardation protein" (FMRP). The mutation causes the body to make only a little bit or none of the protein, which can cause the symptoms of FXS.

In a gene, the information for making a protein has two parts: the introduction and the instructions for making the protein itself. Researchers call the introduction the promoter because of how it helps start the process of building the protein.

---

[1] "Color Blindness," National Eye Institute (NEI), July 3, 2019. Available online. URL: www.nei.nih.gov/learn-about-eye-health/eye-conditions-and-diseases/color-blindness. Accessed June 15, 2023.

The promoter part of the *FMR1* gene includes many repeats—repeated instances of a specific DNA sequence called the "CGG sequence." The *FMR1* gene usually has between 6 and 40 repeats in the promoter; the average is 30 repeats.

People with between 55 and 200 repeats have a premutation of the gene. The premutation may cause the gene to not work properly, but it does not cause intellectual and developmental disability (IDD). The premutation is linked to the disorders fragile X-associated primary ovarian insufficiency (FXPOI) and fragile X-associated tremor/ataxia syndrome (FXTAS). However, not all people with the premutation show symptoms of FXPOI or FXTAS.

People with 200 or more repeats in the promoter part of the gene have a full mutation, meaning the gene might not work at all. People with a full mutation often have FXS.

The number of repeats, also called the "size of the mutation," affects the type of symptoms and how serious the symptoms of FXS will be.

INHERITING FRAGILE X SYNDROME

Fragile X syndrome is inherited, which means it is passed down from parents to children. Anyone with the *FMR1* gene mutation can pass it to their children. However, a person who inherits the gene mutation may not develop FXS. Males will pass it down to all of their daughters and not their sons. In some cases, an *FMR1* premutation can change to a full mutation when it is passed from parent to child.

WHAT CAUSES FRAGILE X SYNDROME?

Fragile X results from a change or mutation in the *FMR1* gene, which is found on the X chromosome. The gene normally makes a protein, called "FMRP" that is important for creating and maintaining connections between cells in the brain and nervous system. The mutation causes the body to make only a little bit or none of the protein, which often causes the symptoms of FXS.

Not everyone with the mutated *FMR1* gene has symptoms of FXS because the body may still be able to make FMRP. A few things affect how much FMRP the body can make:

- **The size of the mutation**. Some people have a smaller mutation (a lower number of repeats) in their *FMR1* gene, while others have big mutations (a large number of repeats) in the gene. If the mutation is small, the body may be able to make some of the protein. Having the protein available makes the symptoms milder.
- **The number of cells that have the mutation**. Because not every cell in the body is exactly the same, some cells might have the *FMR1* mutation while others do not. This situation is called "mosaicism." If the mutation is in most of the body's cells, the person will probably have symptoms of FXS. If the mutation is in only some of the cells, the person might not have any symptoms at all or only mild symptoms.
- **Being female**. Females have two X chromosomes (XX), while males have only one. In females, if the *FMR1* gene on one X chromosome has the mutation, the *FMR1* gene on the other X chromosome might not have the mutation. Even if one of the female's genes has a very large mutation, the body can usually make at least some FMRP, leading to milder symptoms.

WHAT ARE THE SYMPTOMS OF FRAGILE X SYNDROME?

People with FXS do not all have the same signs and symptoms, but they do have some things in common. Symptoms are often milder in females than in males.

- **Intelligence and learning**. Many people with FXS have problems with intellectual functioning.
  - These problems can range from mild, such as learning disorders or problems with mathematics, to severe, such as an intellectual or developmental disability.
  - The syndrome may affect the ability to think, reason, and learn.

- Because many people with FXS also have attention disorders, hyperactivity, anxiety, and language-processing problems, a person with FXS may have more capabilities than his or her intelligence quotient (IQ) score suggests.
- **Physical**. Most infants and younger children with FXS do not have any specific physical features of this syndrome. When these children start to go through puberty, however, many will begin to develop certain features that are typical of those with FXS.
  - These features include a narrow face, large head, large ears, flexible joints, flat feet, and a prominent forehead.
  - These physical signs become more obvious with age.
- **Behavioral, social, and emotional**. Most children with FXS have some behavioral challenges.
  - They may be afraid or anxious in new situations.
  - They may have troublemaking eye contact with other people.
  - Boys, especially, may have trouble paying attention or be aggressive.
- **Speech and language**. Most boys with FXS have some problems with speech and language.
  - They may have trouble speaking clearly, may stutter, or may leave out parts of words. They may also have problems understanding other people's social cues, such as tone of voice or specific types of body language.
  - Some children with FXS begin talking later than typically developing children. Most will talk eventually, but a few might stay nonverbal throughout their lives.
- **Sensory**. Many children with FXS are bothered by certain sensations, such as bright light, loud noises, or the way certain clothing feels on their bodies.
  - These sensory issues might cause them to act out or display behavior problems.

HOW DO HEALTH-CARE PROVIDERS DIAGNOSE FRAGILE X SYNDROME?

Health-care providers often use a blood sample to diagnose FXS. The health-care provider will take a sample of blood and will send it to a laboratory, which will determine what form of the *FMR1* gene is present.

Diagnosis of Children

Many parents first notice symptoms of delayed development in their infants or toddlers. These symptoms may include delays in speech and language skills, social and emotional difficulties, and being sensitive to certain sensations. Children may also be delayed in or have problems with motor skills, such as learning to walk.

A health-care provider can perform developmental screening to determine the nature of delays in a child. If a health-care provider suspects the child has FXS, he/she can refer parents to a clinical geneticist, who can perform a genetic test for FXS.

WHAT ARE THE TREATMENTS FOR FRAGILE X SYNDROME?

There is no single treatment for FXS, but there are treatments that help minimize the symptoms of the condition. Individuals with FXS who receive appropriate education, therapy services, and medications have the best chance of using all of their individual capabilities and skills. Even those with an intellectual or developmental disability can learn to master many self-help skills.

Early intervention is important. Because a young child's brain is still forming, early intervention gives children the best start possible and the greatest chance of developing a full range of skills. The sooner a child with FXS gets treatment, the more opportunity there is for learning.[2]

---

[2] "Fragile X Syndrome," *Eunice Kennedy Shriver* National Institute of Child Health and Human Development (NICHD), May 8, 2021. Available online. URL: www.nichd.nih.gov/health/topics/fragilex. Accessed July 14, 2023.

Section 14.3 | **Hemophilia**

Hemophilia is usually an inherited bleeding disorder in which the blood does not clot properly. This can lead to spontaneous bleeding as well as bleeding following injuries or surgery. Blood contains many proteins called "clotting factors" that can help stop bleeding. People with hemophilia have low levels of either factor VIII or factor IX. The severity of hemophilia that a person has is determined by the amount of the factor in the blood. The lower the amount of the factor, the more likely it is that bleeding will occur, which can lead to serious health problems.

In rare cases, a person can develop hemophilia later in life. The majority of cases involve middle-aged or elderly people. This condition often resolves with appropriate treatment.

TYPES OF HEMOPHILIA

There are several different types of hemophilia. The following two are the most common:

- **Hemophilia A (classic hemophilia).** This type is caused by a lack or decrease of clotting factor VIII.
- **Hemophilia B (Christmas disease).** This type is caused by a lack or decrease of clotting factor IX.

WHO IS AFFECTED BY HEMOPHILIA?

Hemophilia occurs in about 1 in every 5,000 male births. Hemophilia A is about four times as common as hemophilia B, and about half of those affected have the severe form. Hemophilia affects people of all racial and ethnic groups.

CAUSES OF HEMOPHILIA

Hemophilia is caused by a mutation or change in one of the genes that provides instructions for making the clotting factor proteins needed to form a blood clot. This change or mutation can prevent the clotting protein from working properly or cause it to be missing altogether. These genes are located on the X chromosome. Males have one X and one Y chromosome (XY), and females have two X chromosomes (XX). Males inherit the X chromosome from their mothers and the Y chromosome from their fathers. Females inherit one X chromosome from each parent.

The X chromosome contains many genes that are not present on the Y chromosome. This means that males only have one copy of most of the genes on the X chromosome, whereas females have two copies. Thus, males can have a disease such as hemophilia if they inherit an affected X chromosome that has a mutation in either the factor VIII or factor IX gene. Females can also have hemophilia, but this is much rarer. In such cases, both X chromosomes are affected, or one is affected, and the other is missing or inactive. In these females, bleeding symptoms may be similar to males with hemophilia.

Even though hemophilia runs in families, some families have no prior history of family members with hemophilia. Sometimes, there are carrier females in the family but no affected boys, just by chance. However, about one-third of the time, the baby with hemophilia is the first one in the family to be affected by a mutation in the gene for the clotting factor.

Hemophilia can result in:
- bleeding within joints that can lead to chronic joint disease and pain
- bleeding in the head and sometimes in the brain that can cause long-term problems, such as seizures and paralysis
- death that can occur if the bleeding cannot be stopped or if it occurs in a vital organ such as the brain

SIGNS AND SYMPTOMS OF HEMOPHILIA
Common signs of hemophilia include the following:
- bleeding into the joints (This can cause swelling and pain or tightness in the joints; it often affects the knees, elbows, and ankles.)
- bleeding into the skin (bruising of muscle and soft tissue causing a buildup of blood in the area called a "hematoma.")

- bleeding of the mouth and gums and bleeding that is hard to stop after losing a tooth
- bleeding after circumcision (surgery performed on male babies to remove the hood of skin, called the "foreskin," covering the head of the penis)
- bleeding after having shots, such as vaccinations
- bleeding in the head of an infant after a difficult delivery
- blood in the urine or stool
- frequent and hard-to-stop nosebleeds

DIAGNOSIS OF HEMOPHILIA

Many people who have or have had family members with hemophilia will ask that their baby boys get tested soon after birth.

About one-third of babies who are diagnosed with hemophilia have a new mutation not present in other family members. In these cases, a doctor might check for hemophilia if a newborn is showing certain signs of hemophilia.

To make a diagnosis, doctors would perform certain blood tests to show if the blood is clotting properly. If it does not, then they would do clotting factor tests, also called "factor assays," to diagnose the cause of the bleeding disorder. These blood tests would show the type of hemophilia and the severity.

TREATMENT FOR HEMOPHILIA

The best way to treat hemophilia is to replace the missing blood clotting factor so that the blood can clot properly. This is done by infusing (administering through a vein) commercially prepared factor concentrates. People with hemophilia can learn how to perform these infusions themselves so that they can stop bleeding episodes and, by performing the infusions on a regular basis (called "prophylaxis"), can even prevent most bleeding episodes.

Good-quality medical care from doctors and nurses who know a lot about the disorder can help prevent some serious problems.

Often the best choice for care is to visit a comprehensive hemophilia treatment center (HTC). An HTC not only provides care to address all issues related to the disorder but also provides health education that helps people with hemophilia stay healthy.

INHIBITORS

About 15–20 percent of people with hemophilia develop an antibody (called an "inhibitor") that stops the clotting factors from being able to clot the blood and stop bleeding. Treatment of bleeding episodes becomes extremely difficult, and the cost of care for a person with an inhibitor can skyrocket because more clotting factor or a different type of clotting factor is needed. People with inhibitors often experience more joint disease and other problems from bleeding that result in a reduced quality of life (QOL).[3]

Section 14.4 | Klinefelter Syndrome

The term "Klinefelter syndrome" (KS) describes a set of features that can occur in a male who is born with an extra X chromosome in his cells. It is named after Dr. Henry Klinefelter, who identified the condition in the 1940s.

Usually, every cell in a male's body, except sperm and red blood cells (RBCs), contains 46 chromosomes. The 45th and 46th chromosomes—the X and Y chromosomes—are sometimes called "sex chromosomes" because they determine a person's sex. Normally, males have one X and one Y chromosome, making them XY. Males with KS have an extra X chromosome, making them XXY.

KS is sometimes called "47,XXY" (47 refers to total chromosomes) or the "XXY condition." Those with KS are sometimes called "XXY males."

Some males with KS may have both XY cells and XXY cells in their bodies. This is called "mosaic." Mosaic males may have fewer

---

[3] "Hemophilia," Centers for Disease Control and Prevention (CDC), August 1, 2022. Available online. URL: www.cdc.gov/ncbddd/hemophilia/facts.html. Accessed June 15, 2023.

symptoms of KS depending on the number of XY cells they have in their bodies and where these cells are located. For example, males who have normal XY cells in their testes may be fertile.

In very rare cases, males might have two or more extra X chromosomes in their cells, for instance, XXXY or XXXXY, or an extra Y, such as XXYY. This is called "poly-X Klinefelter syndrome," and it causes more severe symptoms.

WHAT CAUSES KLINEFELTER SYNDROME?

The extra chromosome results from a random error that occurs when a sperm or egg is formed; this error causes an extra X cell to be included each time the cell divides to form new cells. In very rare cases, more than one extra X or an extra Y is included.

HOW MANY PEOPLE ARE AFFECTED BY OR AT RISK FOR KLINEFELTER SYNDROME?

Researchers estimate that 1 in about 500 newborn males has an extra X chromosome, making KS among the most common chromosomal disorders seen in all newborns. The likelihood of a third or fourth X is much rarer (see Table 14.1).

Table 14.1. Prevalence of Klinefelter Syndrome Variants

Number of Extra X Chromosomes	One (XXY)	Two (XXXY)	Three (XXXXY)
Number of Newborn Males with the Condition	1 in 500	1 in 50,000	1 in 85,000– 100,000

Scientists are not sure what factors increase the risk of KS. The error that produces the extra chromosome occurs at random, meaning that the error is not hereditary or passed down from parent to child. Research suggests that older mothers might be slightly more likely to have a son with KS. However, the extra X chromosome in KS comes from the father about one-half of the time.

WHAT ARE THE COMMON SYMPTOMS OF KLINEFELTER SYNDROME?

Because XXY males do not really appear different from other males and because they may not have any or have mild symptoms, XXY males often do not know they have KS.

In other cases, males with KS may have mild or severe symptoms. Whether or not a male with KS has visible symptoms depends on many factors, including how much testosterone his body makes, if he is mosaic (with both XY and XXY cells), and his age when the condition is diagnosed and treated.

KS symptoms fall into the following main categories:
- physical symptoms
- language and learning symptoms
- social and behavioral symptoms
- symptoms of poly-X KS

Physical Symptoms

Many physical symptoms of KS result from low testosterone levels in the body. The degree of symptoms differs based on the amount of testosterone needed for a specific age or developmental stage and the amount of testosterone the body makes or has available.

During the first few years of life, when the need for testosterone is low, most XXY males do not show any obvious differences from typical male infants and young boys. Some may have slightly weaker muscles, meaning that they might sit up, crawl, and walk slightly later than average. For example, on average, baby boys with KS do not start walking until 18 months of age.

After five years of age, when compared to typically developing boys, boys with KS may be slightly:
- taller
- fatter around the belly
- clumsier
- slower in developing motor skills, coordination, speed, and muscle strength

215

Puberty for boys with KS usually starts normally. But, because their bodies make less testosterone than non-KS boys, their pubertal development may be disrupted or slow. In addition to being tall, KS boys may have:

- smaller testes and penis
- breast growth (about one-third of teens with KS have breast growth)
- less facial and body hair
- reduced muscle tone
- narrower shoulders and wider hips
- weaker bones, greater risk of bone fractures
- decreased sexual interest
- lower energy
- reduced sperm production

An adult male with KS may have the following features:

- infertility (Nearly all men with KS are unable to father a biologically related child without help from a fertility specialist.)
- small testes, with the possibility of testes shrinking slightly after the teen years
- lower testosterone levels, which lead to less muscle, hair, and sexual interest and function
- breasts or breast growth, called "gynecomastia" (In some cases, breast growth can be permanent, and about 10 percent of XXY males need breast-reduction surgery.)

Language and Learning Symptoms

Most males with KS have normal intelligence quotients (IQs) and successfully complete education at all levels. (IQ is a frequently used intelligence measure, but it does not include emotional, creative, or other types of intelligence.) Between 25 and 85 percent of all males with KS have some kind of learning or language-related problem, which makes it more likely that they will need some extra help in school. Without this help or intervention, KS males might fall behind their classmates as schoolwork becomes harder.

KS males may experience some of the following learning and language-related challenges:

- **A delay in learning to talk**. Infants with KS tend to make only a few different vocal sounds. As they grow older, they may have difficulty saying words clearly. It might be hard for them to distinguish differences between similar sounds.
- **Trouble using language to express their thoughts and needs**. Boys with KS might have problems putting their thoughts, ideas, and emotions into words. Some may find it hard to learn and remember some words, such as the names of common objects.
- **Trouble processing what they hear**. Although most boys with KS can understand what is being said to them, they might take longer to process multiple or complex sentences. In some cases, they might fidget or "tune out" because they take longer to process the information. It might also be difficult for KS males to concentrate in noisy settings. They might also be less able to understand a speaker's feelings from just speech alone.
- **Reading difficulties**. Many boys with KS have difficulty understanding what they read (called "poor reading comprehension"). They might also read more slowly than other boys.

By adulthood, most males with KS learn to speak and converse normally although they may have a harder time doing work that involves extensive reading and writing.

Social and Behavioral Symptoms

Many of the social and behavioral symptoms in KS may result from language and learning difficulties. For instance, boys with KS who have language difficulties might hold back socially and could use help building social relationships.

Boys with KS, when compared to typically developing boys, tend to be:

- quieter
- less assertive or self-confident

- more anxious or restless
- less physically active
- more helpful and eager to please
- more obedient or more ready to follow directions

In the teenage years, boys with KS may feel their differences more strongly. As a result, these teen boys are at higher risk of depression, substance abuse, and behavioral disorders. Some teens might withdraw, feel sad, or act out their frustration and anger.

As adults, most men with KS have lives similar to those of men without KS. They successfully complete high school, college, and other levels of education. They have successful and meaningful careers and professions. They have friends and families.

Contrary to research findings published several decades ago, males with KS are no more likely to have serious psychiatric disorders or to get into trouble with the law.

Symptoms of Poly-X Klinefelter Syndrome

Males with poly-X KS have more than one extra X chromosome, so their symptoms might be more pronounced than in males with KS. In childhood, they may also have seizures, crossed eyes, constipation, and recurrent ear infections. Poly-KS males might also show slight differences in other physical features.

Some common additional symptoms for several poly-X KS are as follows.

48,XXYY

- long legs
- little body hair
- lower IQ, an average of 60–80 (Normal IQ is 90–110.)
- leg ulcers and other vascular disease symptoms
- extreme shyness but also sometimes aggression and impulsiveness

48,XXXY (OR TETRASOMY)

- eyes set further apart
- flat nose bridge

- arm bones connected to each other in an unusual way
- short
- fifth (smallest) fingers curve inward (clinodactyly)
- lower IQ, an average of 40–60
- immature behavior

49,XXXXY (OR PENTASOMY)

- low IQ, usually between 20 and 60
- small head
- short
- upward-slanted eyes
- heart defects, such as when the chambers do not form properly
- high feet arches
- shy but friendly
- difficulty with changing routines

HOW DO HEALTH-CARE PROVIDERS DIAGNOSE KLINEFELTER SYNDROME?

The only way to confirm the presence of an extra chromosome is by a karyotype test. A health-care provider will take a small blood or skin sample and send it to a laboratory, where a technician inspects the cells under a microscope to find the extra chromosome. A karyotype test shows the same results at any time in a person's life.

Tests for chromosome disorders, including KS, may be done before birth. To obtain tissue or liquid for this test, a pregnant woman undergoes chorionic villus sampling (CVS) or amniocentesis. These types of prenatal testing carry a small risk for miscarriage and are not routinely conducted unless the woman has a family history of chromosomal disorders, has other medical problems, or is above 35 years of age.

Factors That Influence When Klinefelter Syndrome Is Diagnosed

Because symptoms can be mild, some males with KS are never diagnosed.

Several factors affect whether and when a diagnosis occurs:

- Few newborns and boys are tested for or diagnosed with KS.
  - Although newborns in the United States are screened for some conditions, they are not screened for XXY or other sex chromosome differences.
  - In childhood, symptoms can be subtle and overlooked easily. Only about 1 in 10 males with KS is diagnosed before puberty.
  - Sometimes, visiting a health-care provider will not produce a diagnosis. Some symptoms, such as delayed early speech, might be treated successfully without further testing for KS.
- Most XXY diagnoses occur at puberty or in adulthood.
  - Puberty brings a surge in diagnoses as some males (or their parents) become concerned about slow testes growth or breast development and consult a health-care provider.
  - Many men are diagnosed for the first time in fertility clinics. Among men seeking help for infertility, about 15 percent have KS.

WHAT ARE THE TREATMENTS FOR KLINEFELTER SYNDROME?

It is important to remember that because symptoms can be mild, many males with KS are never diagnosed or treated.

The earlier in life that KS symptoms are recognized and treated, the more likely it is that the symptoms can be reduced or eliminated. It is especially helpful to begin treatment by early puberty. Puberty is a time of rapid physical and psychological change, and treatment can successfully limit symptoms. However, treatment can bring benefits at any age.

The type of treatment needed depends on the type of symptoms being treated.

Treating Physical Symptoms
TREATMENT FOR LOW TESTOSTERONE

About one-half of XXY males' chromosomes have low testosterone levels. These levels can be raised by taking supplemental testosterone. Testosterone treatment can:

- improve muscle mass
- deepen the voice
- promote the growth of facial and body hair
- help the reproductive organs mature
- build and maintain bone strength and help prevent osteoporosis in later years
- produce a more masculine appearance, which can also help relieve anxiety and depression
- increase focus and attention

There are various ways to take testosterone:

- injections or shots, every two to three weeks
- pills
- through the skin, also called "transdermal" (Current methods include wearing a testosterone patch or rubbing testosterone gel on the skin.)

Males taking testosterone treatment should work closely with an endocrinologist, a doctor who specializes in hormones and their functions, to ensure the best outcome from testosterone therapy.

Not all males with XXY condition benefit from testosterone therapy.

For males whose testosterone level is low to normal, the benefits of taking testosterone are less clear than for those whose testosterone is very low. Side effects, although generally mild, can include acne, skin rashes from patches or gels, breathing problems (especially during sleep), and a higher risk of an enlarged prostate gland or prostate cancer in older age. In addition, testosterone supplementation will not increase testicular size, decrease breast growth, or correct infertility.

Although the majority of boys with KS grow up to live as males, some develop atypical gender identities. For these males, supplemental testosterone may not be suitable. Gender identity should be discussed with health-care specialists before starting treatment.

TREATMENT FOR ENLARGED BREASTS

No approved drug treatment exists for this condition of overdeveloped breast tissue, termed "gynecomastia." Some health-care providers recommend surgery—called "mastectomy"—to remove or reduce the breasts of XXY males.

When adult men have breasts, they are at higher risk for breast cancer than other men and need to be checked for this condition regularly. The mastectomy lowers the risk of cancer and can reduce the social stress associated with XXY males having enlarged breasts.

Because it is a surgical procedure, mastectomy carries a variety of risks. XXY males who are thinking about mastectomy should discuss all the risks and benefits with their health-care provider.

TREATMENT FOR INFERTILITY

Between 95 and 99 percent of XXY men are infertile because they do not produce enough sperm to fertilize an egg naturally. But sperm are found in more than 50 percent of men with KS.

Advances in assistive reproductive technology (ART) have made it possible for some men with KS to conceive. One type of ART called "testicular sperm extraction" (TESE) with intracytoplasmic sperm injection (ICSI) has shown success for XXY males. For this procedure, a surgeon removes sperm from the testes and places one sperm into an egg.

Like all ART, TESE-ICSI carries both risks and benefits. For instance, it is possible that the resulting child might have the XXY condition. In addition, the procedure is expensive and often is not covered by health insurance plans. Importantly, there is no guarantee the procedure will work.

Studies suggest that collecting sperm from adolescent XXY males and freezing the sperm until later might result in more pregnancies during subsequent fertility treatments. This is because, although XXY males may make some healthy sperm during puberty, this becomes more difficult as they leave adolescence and enter adulthood.

Treating Language and Learning Symptoms

Some, but not all, children with KS have language development and learning delays. They might be slow to learn to talk, read, and write, and they might have difficulty processing what they hear. But various interventions, such as speech therapy and educational assistance, can help reduce and even eliminate these difficulties. The earlier treatment begins, the better the outcomes.

Parents might need to bring these types of problems to the teacher's attention. Because these boys can be quiet and cooperative in the classroom, teachers may not notice the need for help.

Boys and men with KS can benefit by visiting therapists who are experts in areas, such as coordination, social skills, and coping. XXY males might benefit from any or all of the following:

- **Physical therapists**. They design activities and exercises to build motor skills and strength and to improve muscle control, posture, and balance.
- **Occupational therapists**. They help build skills needed for daily functioning, such as social and play skills, interaction and conversation skills, and job or career skills that match interests and abilities.
- **Behavioral therapists**. They help with specific social skills, such as asking other kids to play and starting conversations. They can also teach productive ways of handling frustration, shyness, anger, and other emotions that can arise from feeling "different."
- **Mental health therapists or counselors**. They help males with KS find ways to cope with feelings of sadness, depression, self-doubt, and low self-esteem. They can also help with substance abuse problems. These professionals can also help families deal with the emotions of having a son with KS.
- **Family therapists**. They provide counseling to a man with KS and his spouse, partner, or family. They can help identify relationship problems and help patients

develop communication skills and understand other people's needs.

Parents of XXY males have also mentioned that taking part in physical activities at low-key levels, such as karate, swimming, tennis, and golf, was helpful in improving motor skills, coordination, and confidence.

With regard to education, some boys with KS will qualify to receive state-sponsored special needs services to address their developmental and learning symptoms. But, because these symptoms may be mild, many XXY males will not be eligible for these services. Families can contact a local school district official or special education coordinator to learn more about whether XXY males can receive the following free services:

- **The Early Intervention Program for Infants and Toddlers with Disabilities**. This program is required by two national laws: the Individuals with Disabilities and Education Improvement Act (IDEIA) and the Individuals with Disabilities Education Act (IDEA). Every state operates special programs for children from birth to age three, helping them develop in areas such as behavior, development, communication, and social play.
- **Individualized education plan (IEP) for school**. IEP is created and administered by a team of people, starting with parents and including teachers and school psychologists. The team works together to design an IEP with specific academic, communication, motor, learning, functional, and socialization goals, based on the child's educational needs and specific symptoms.

Treating Social and Behavioral Symptoms

Many of the professionals and methods for treating learning and language symptoms of the XXY condition are similar to or the same as the ones used to address social and behavioral symptoms.

For instance, boys with KS may need help with social skills and interacting in groups. Occupational or behavioral therapists might be able to assist with these skills. Some school districts and health centers might also offer these types of skill-building programs or classes.

In adolescence, symptoms, such as lack of body hair, could make XXY males uncomfortable in school or other social settings, and this discomfort can lead to depression, substance abuse, and behavioral problems or "acting out." They might also have questions about their masculinity or gender identity. In these instances, consulting a psychologist, counselor, or psychiatrist may be helpful.

Contrary to research results released decades ago, research shows that XXY males are no more likely than other males to have serious psychiatric disorders or to get into trouble with the law.

IS THERE A CURE FOR KLINEFELTER SYNDROME?

Currently, there is no way to remove chromosomes from cells to "cure" the XXY condition.

But many symptoms can be successfully treated, minimizing the impact the condition has on length and quality of life (QOL). Most adult XXY men have full independence and have friends, families, and normal social relationships. They live about as long as other men, on average.[4]

Section 14.5 | Muscular Dystrophy

Muscular dystrophy (MD) are a group of muscle diseases caused by mutations in a person's genes. Over time, muscle weakness decreases mobility, making everyday tasks difficult. There are many kinds of muscular dystrophy, each affecting specific muscle groups, with signs and symptoms appearing at different ages, and varying in severity. Muscular dystrophy can run in families, or a person

---

[4] "Klinefelter Syndrome (KS): Condition Information," *Eunice Kennedy Shriver* National Institute of Child Health and Human Development (NICHD), December 1, 2016. Available online. URL: www.nichd.nih.gov/health/topics/klinefelter/conditioninfo/Default. Accessed July 17, 2023.

can be the first in their family to have a muscular dystrophy. There may be several different genetic types within each kind of muscular dystrophy, and people with the same kind of muscular dystrophy may experience different symptoms.

Muscular dystrophies are rare, with little data on how many people are affected. The Centers for Disease Control and Prevention (CDC) is working to estimate the number of people with each major kind of muscular dystrophy in the United States.

KINDS OF MUSCULAR DYSTROPHIES
Duchenne/Becker Muscular Dystrophy
Duchenne muscular dystrophy (DMD) and Becker muscular dystrophy (BMD) can have the same symptoms and are caused by mutations in the same gene. BMD symptoms can begin later in life and be less severe than DMD. However, because these two kinds are very similar, they are often studied and referred to together (Duchenne/Becker muscular dystrophy (DBMD)).

HOW MANY PEOPLE ARE AFFECTED?
About 14 in 100,000 males aged 5–24 are affected.

WHO ARE MORE LIKELY TO BE AFFECTED: MALES OR FEMALES?
Males are more likely to be affected by muscular dystrophy.

WHEN DOES MUSCLE WEAKNESS TYPICALLY BEGIN?
DMD symptoms usually begin before five years of age. In BMD, symptoms usually appear later, even into adulthood.

WHICH PARTS OF THE BODY SHOW WEAKNESS FIRST?
Initially, the upper legs and upper arms begin to show weakness.

WHAT OTHER PARTS OF THE BODY CAN BE AFFECTED?
The heart, lungs, throat, stomach, intestines, and spine can also be affected.

Myotonic Muscular Dystrophy
HOW MANY PEOPLE ARE AFFECTED?
About 8 in 100,000 people of all ages are affected.

WHO ARE MORE LIKELY TO BE AFFECTED: MALES OR FEMALES?
Males and females are equally likely to be affected by myotonic muscular dystrophy.

WHEN DOES MUSCLE WEAKNESS TYPICALLY BEGIN?
Muscle weakness typically begins between the ages of 10 and 30 but ranges from birth to 70 years of age.

WHICH PARTS OF THE BODY SHOW WEAKNESS FIRST?
Initially, the face, neck, arms, hands, hips, and lower legs begin to show weakness.

WHAT OTHER PARTS OF THE BODY CAN BE AFFECTED?
The heart, lungs, stomach, intestines, brain, eyes, and hormone-producing organs can also be affected.

Limb-Girdle Muscular Dystrophy
HOW MANY PEOPLE ARE AFFECTED?
About 2 in 100,000 people of all ages are affected.

WHO ARE MORE LIKELY TO BE AFFECTED: MALES OR FEMALES?
Males and females are equally likely to be affected by limb-girdle muscular dystrophy (LGMD).

WHEN DOES MUSCLE WEAKNESS TYPICALLY BEGIN?
Muscle weakness typically begins during childhood or adulthood, depending on the type of LGMD.

WHICH PARTS OF THE BODY SHOW WEAKNESS FIRST?
Initially, the upper arms and upper legs show weakness.

WHAT OTHER PARTS OF THE BODY CAN BE AFFECTED?
The heart, spine, hips, calves, and trunk can also be affected.

Facioscapulohumeral Muscular Dystrophy
HOW MANY PEOPLE ARE AFFECTED?
About 4 in 100,000 people of all ages are affected.

WHO ARE MORE LIKELY TO BE AFFECTED: MALES OR FEMALES?
Males and females are equally likely to be affected by facioscapulohumeral muscular dystrophy.

WHEN DOES MUSCLE WEAKNESS TYPICALLY BEGIN?
Muscle weakness typically begins in young adulthood.

WHICH PARTS OF THE BODY SHOW WEAKNESS FIRST?
Initially, the face, shoulders, and upper arms show weakness.

WHAT OTHER PARTS OF THE BODY CAN BE AFFECTED?
The eyes, ears, and lower legs can also be affected.

Congenital Muscular Dystrophy
HOW MANY PEOPLE ARE AFFECTED?
About 1 in 100,000 people of all ages are affected.

WHO ARE MORE LIKELY TO BE AFFECTED: MALES OR FEMALES?
Males and females are equally likely to be affected by congenital muscular dystrophy.

WHEN DOES MUSCLE WEAKNESS TYPICALLY BEGIN?
Muscle weakness typically begins at birth or in early infancy.

WHICH PARTS OF THE BODY SHOW WEAKNESS FIRST?
Initially, the neck, upper arms, upper legs, and lungs show weakness.

WHAT OTHER PARTS OF THE BODY CAN BE AFFECTED?
The brain, heart, and spine can also be affected.

Distal Muscular Dystrophy
HOW MANY PEOPLE ARE AFFECTED?
Less than 1 in 100,000 people are affected.

WHO ARE MORE LIKELY TO BE AFFECTED: MALES OR FEMALES?
Males and females are equally likely to be affected by distal muscular dystrophy.

WHEN DOES MUSCLE WEAKNESS TYPICALLY BEGIN?
Muscle weakness typically begins in adulthood.

WHICH PARTS OF THE BODY SHOW WEAKNESS FIRST?
Initially, the feet, hands, lower legs, and lower arms show weakness.

WHAT OTHER PARTS OF THE BODY CAN BE AFFECTED?
The heart, arms, and legs can also be affected.

Oculopharyngeal Muscular Dystrophy
HOW MANY PEOPLE ARE AFFECTED?
Less than 1 in 100,000 people is affected.

WHO ARE MORE LIKELY TO BE AFFECTED: MALES OR FEMALES?
Males and females are equally likely to be affected by oculopharyngeal muscular dystrophy.

WHEN DOES MUSCLE WEAKNESS TYPICALLY BEGIN?
Muscle weakness typically begins after 40 years of age.

WHICH PARTS OF THE BODY SHOW WEAKNESS FIRST?
Initially, the eyes and throat show weakness.

WHAT OTHER PARTS OF THE BODY CAN BE AFFECTED?
The shoulders, upper legs, and hips can also be affected.

Emery-Dreifuss Muscular Dystrophy
HOW MANY PEOPLE ARE AFFECTED?
Less than 1 in 100,000 people of all ages is affected.

WHO ARE MORE LIKELY TO BE AFFECTED: MALES OR FEMALES?
Males are more likely to be affected by Emery-Dreifuss muscular dystrophy.

WHEN DOES MUSCLE WEAKNESS TYPICALLY BEGIN?
Muscle weakness typically begins in childhood.

WHICH PARTS OF THE BODY SHOW WEAKNESS FIRST?
Initially, the arms, legs, heart, and joints show weakness.

WHAT OTHER PARTS OF THE BODY CAN BE AFFECTED?
The throat, shoulders, and hips can also be affected.[5]

HOW IS MUSCULAR DYSTROPHY DIAGNOSED AND TREATED?
Diagnosing Muscular Dystrophy
Doctors review an individual's medical history and a complete family history to determine if the muscle disease is secondary to a disease affecting other tissues or organs or is an inherited condition. It is also important to rule out any muscle weakness resulting from prior surgery, exposure to toxins, or current medications that may affect the person's functional status.

Thorough clinical and neurological exams can help doctors do the following:

- Rule out disorders of the central and/or peripheral nervous systems.

[5] "Muscular Dystrophy," Centers for Disease Control and Prevention (CDC), November 21, 2022. Available online. URL: www.cdc.gov/ncbddd/musculardystrophy/facts.html. Accessed June 15, 2023.

- Identify any patterns of muscle weakness and atrophy.
- Test reflex responses and coordination.
- Look for contractions.

Various laboratory tests may be used to confirm the diagnosis of MD, including the following:

- **Blood and urine tests**. These tests help detect defective genes and identify specific neuromuscular disorders.
- **Exercise tests**. These tests help detect elevated rates of certain chemicals following exercise and are used to determine the nature of the MD or other muscle disorders.
- **Genetic testing**. This testing helps look for genes known to either cause or be associated with inherited muscle disease.
- **Deoxyribonucleic acid (DNA) analysis and enzyme assays**. These can confirm the diagnosis of certain neuromuscular diseases, including MD. Genetic linkage studies can identify whether a specific genetic marker on a chromosome and a disease are inherited together. They are particularly useful in studying families with members of different generations who are affected. Advances in genetic testing include whole exome and whole genome sequencing, which will enable people to have all of their genes screened at once for disease-causing mutations, rather than have just one gene or several genes tested at a time.
- **Genetic counseling**. It can help parents who have a family history of MD determine if they are carrying one of the mutated genes that cause the disorder. Two tests can be used to help expectant parents find out if their child is affected.
- **Diagnostic imaging**. This imaging can help determine the specific nature of a disease or condition. Magnetic resonance imaging (MRI) is used to examine muscle quality, any atrophy, or abnormalities in size and fatty replacement of muscle tissue, as well as to monitor

disease progression. Other forms of diagnostic imaging for MD include the following:

- **Phosphorus magnetic resonance spectroscopy.** It measures cellular response to exercise and the amount of energy available to muscle fiber
- **Ultrasound imaging (also known as "sonography").** It uses high-frequency sound waves to obtain images inside the body.
- **Muscle biopsies.** This helps monitor the course of the disease and treatment effectiveness. Muscle biopsies can sometimes also assist in carrier testing.
- **Immunofluorescence testing.** This testing detects specific proteins such as dystrophin within muscle fibers.
- **Electron microscopy.** This helps identify changes in the subcellular components of muscle fibers. Electron microscopy can also identify changes that characterize cell death, mutations in muscle cell mitochondria, and an increase in connective tissue seen in muscle diseases such as MD.
- **Neurophysiology studies.** These studies identify physical and/or chemical changes in the nervous system.
- **Nerve conduction velocity.** This is to measure the speed and strength with which an electrical signal travels along a nerve and can help determine whether nerve damage is present.
- **Repetitive stimulation.** This is to assess the function of the neuromuscular junction by electrically stimulating a motor nerve several times in a row.
- **Electromyography (EMG).** EMG helps record muscle fiber and motor unit activity. Results may reveal electrical activity characteristic of MD or other neuromuscular disorders.

Treating Muscular Dystrophy

Available treatments are aimed at keeping people independent for as long as possible and to prevent complications that can arise from weakness, reduced mobility, and cardiac and respiratory difficulties. Treatment may involve a combination of approaches, including physical therapy, drug therapy, and surgery.

- **Assisted ventilation**. This is often needed to treat respiratory muscle weakness that accompanies many forms of MD, especially in the later stages.
  - Drug therapy may be prescribed to delay muscle degeneration.
  - The U.S. Food and Drug Administration (FDA) has approved injections of the drugs golodirsen and viltolarsen to treat individuals with DMD who have a confirmed mutation of the dystrophin gene that is amenable to exon 53 skipping. The FDA approved the injection of the drug casimersen to treat individuals who have a confirmed mutation of the DMD gene that is amenable to exon 45 skipping.
  - The FDA also approved three applications of fingolimod (Gilenya) to treat the relapsing form of MD in adults. Corticosteroids, such as prednisone, can slow the rate of muscle deterioration in DMD and help children retain strength to prolong independent walking by as much as several years. However, these medicines have side effects, such as weight gain, facial changes, loss of linear (height) growth, and bone fragility that can be especially troubling in children.
  - Immunosuppressive drugs such as cyclosporine and azathioprine can delay some damage to dying muscle cells.
  - Drugs that may provide short-term relief from myotonia (muscle spasms and weakness) include mexiletine, phenytoin, and baclofen as they are known to block signals sent from the spinal cord to contract the muscles. Dantrolene interferes with the process of muscle contraction. And quinine is another option.

- The FDA granted accelerated approval of the drug Exondys 51 to treat individuals who have a confirmed mutation of the dystrophin gene amenable to exon 15 skipping. The accelerated approval means the drug can be administered to people who meet the rare disease criteria while the company works on additional trials to learn more about the effectiveness of the drug. (Drugs for myotonia may not be effective in myotonic MD but work well for myotonia congenita, a genetic neuromuscular disorder characterized by the slow relaxation of the muscles.) Respiratory infections may be treated with antibiotics.
- **Physical therapy**. This therapy can help prevent malformation, improve movement, and keep the muscles as flexible and strong as possible.
  - Passive stretching can increase joint flexibility and prevent contractures that restrict movement and cause loss of function.
  - Regular, moderate exercise can help people with MD maintain range of motion and muscle strength, prevent muscle atrophy, and delay the development of contractures. Individuals with a weakened diaphragm can learn coughing and deep breathing exercises that are designed to keep the lungs fully expanded.
  - Postural correction is used to counter the muscle weakness, contractures, and spinal irregularities that force individuals with MD into uncomfortable positions.
  - Support aids such as wheelchairs, splints and braces, other orthopedic appliances, and overhead bed bars (trapezes) can help maintain mobility. Spinal supports can help delay scoliosis. Orthotic devices such as standing frames and swivel walkers can help people remain standing or walking.
  - Repeated low-frequency bursts of electrical stimulation to the thigh muscles may produce a slight increase in strength in some male children with DMD though this therapy has not been proven to be effective.

- **Occupational therapy**. This therapy may help some with progressive weakness and loss of mobility. Some individuals may need to learn new job skills or new ways to perform tasks, while other people may need to change careers altogether. Assistive technology (AT) may include modifications to home and workplace settings and the use of motorized wheelchairs, wheelchair accessories, and adaptive utensils.
- **Speech therapy**. This therapy may help individuals whose facial and throat muscles have weakened. They can learn to use special communication devices, such as a computer with a voice synthesizer.
- **Dietary changes**. These have not been shown to slow the progression of MD. Proper nutrition is essential, however, for overall health.
- **Feeding techniques**. These techniques may help people with MD who have a swallowing disorder.
- **Corrective surgery**. This surgery is often performed to ease complications from MD.
  - Tendon or muscle-release surgery is recommended when a contracture becomes severe enough to lock a joint or greatly impair movement.
  - Individuals with either Emery-Dreifuss or myotonic dystrophy may require a pacemaker at some point to treat cardiac problems.
  - Surgery to reduce the pain and postural imbalance caused by scoliosis may help some individuals. Scoliosis occurs when the muscles that support the spine begin to weaken and can no longer keep the spine straight.
  - People with myotonic dystrophy often develop cataracts, a clouding of the lens of the eye that blocks light, and may need cataract surgery.[6]

---

[6] "Muscular Dystrophy," National Institute of Neurological Disorders and Stroke (NINDS), January 20, 2023. Available online. URL: www.ninds.nih.gov/health-information/disorders/muscular-dystrophy#toc-how-is-muscular-dystrophy-diagnosed-and-treated. Accessed June 15, 2023.

Section 14.6 | X-Linked Agammaglobulinemia

X-linked agammaglobulinemia (XLA) is a condition that affects the immune system and occurs almost exclusively in males. It is part of a group of disorders called "primary immunodeficiencies" (or inborn errors of immunity), in which part of the immune system does not function as it should. People with XLA have very few B cells, which are specialized white blood cells (WBCs) that help protect the body against infection. B cells can mature into cells that produce special proteins called "antibodies" or "immunoglobulins." Antibodies attach to specific foreign particles and germs, marking them for destruction. Individuals with XLA are more susceptible to infections because their body makes very few antibodies.

Children with XLA are usually healthy for the first one or two months of life because they are protected by antibodies acquired before birth from their mother. After this time, the maternal antibodies are cleared from the body, and the affected child begins to develop recurrent infections. Children with XLA generally take longer to recover from infections, and infections often occur again, even in children who are taking antibiotic medications.

The most common bacterial infections that occur in people with XLA are lung infections (pneumonia and bronchitis), ear infections (otitis), pink eye (conjunctivitis), and sinus infections (sinusitis). Infections that cause chronic diarrhea are also common. Recurrent infections can lead to organ damage. Treatments that replace antibodies can help prevent infections, improving the quality of life (QOL) for people with XLA.

FREQUENCY OF X-LINKED AGAMMAGLOBULINEMIA
X-linked agammaglobulinemia occurs in approximately 1 in 200,000 newborns.

CAUSES OF X-LINKED AGAMMAGLOBULINEMIA
Variants (also called "mutations") in the *BTK* gene cause XLA. This gene provides instructions for making the BTK protein, which is important for the development of B cells and the normal

functioning of the immune system. Most variants in the *BTK* gene prevent the production of any BTK protein. The absence of functional BTK protein blocks B cell development and leads to a lack of antibodies. Without antibodies, the immune system cannot properly respond to foreign invaders and prevent infection.

INHERITANCE OF X-LINKED AGAMMAGLOBULINEMIA

This condition is inherited in an X-linked recessive pattern. The gene associated with this condition is located on the X chromosome, which is one of the two sex chromosomes. In males (who have only one X chromosome), one altered copy of the gene in each cell is sufficient to cause the condition. In females (who have two X chromosomes), a variant would have to occur in both copies of the gene to cause the disorder. Because it is unlikely that females will have two altered copies of this gene, males are affected by X-linked recessive disorders much more frequently than females.

An affected person's mother may carry one altered copy of the *BTK* gene. Individuals with only one altered copy of this gene do not have the immune system abnormalities associated with XLA, but they can pass the altered gene to their children. Fathers cannot pass X-linked traits to their sons, but they can pass them to their daughters.

About half of the affected individuals do not have a family history of XLA. In most of these cases, the affected individual has a new variant in the *BTK* gene that was not inherited from a parent.[7]

Section 14.7 | Lesch-Nyhan Syndrome

Lesch-Nyhan syndrome (LNS) is a condition that occurs almost exclusively in males. It is characterized by neurological and behavioral abnormalities and the overproduction of uric acid. Uric acid

---

[7] MedlinePlus, "X-Linked Agammaglobulinemia," National Institutes of Health (NIH), March 17, 2023. Available online. URL: https://medlineplus.gov/genetics/condition/x-linked-agammaglobulinemia/#inheritance. Accessed June 26, 2023.

is a waste product of normal chemical processes and is found in blood and urine. Excess uric acid can be released from the blood and build up under the skin and cause gouty arthritis (arthritis caused by an accumulation of uric acid in the joints). Uric acid accumulation can also cause kidney and bladder stones.

The nervous system and behavioral disturbances experienced by people with LNS include abnormal involuntary muscle movements, such as tensing of various muscles (dystonia), jerking movements (chorea), and flailing of the limbs (ballismus). People with LNS usually cannot walk, require assistance sitting, and generally use a wheelchair. Self-injury (including biting and head banging) is the most common and distinctive behavioral problem in individuals with LNS.

FREQUENCY OF LESCH-NYHAN SYNDROME

The prevalence of LNS is approximately 1 in 380,000 individuals. This condition occurs with a similar frequency in all populations.

CAUSES OF LESCH-NYHAN SYNDROME

Mutations in the *HPRT1* gene cause LNS. The *HPRT1* gene provides instructions for making an enzyme called "hypoxanthine phosphoribosyltransferase 1." This enzyme is responsible for recycling purines, a type of building block of deoxyribonucleic acid (DNA) and its chemical cousin ribonucleic acid (RNA). Recycling purines ensures that cells have a plentiful supply of building blocks for the production of DNA and RNA.

HPRT1 gene mutations that cause LNS result in a severe shortage (deficiency) or complete absence of hypoxanthine phosphoribosyltransferase 1. When this enzyme is lacking, purines are broken down but not recycled, producing abnormally high levels of uric acid. For unknown reasons, a deficiency of hypoxanthine phosphoribosyltransferase 1 is associated with low levels of a chemical messenger in the brain called "dopamine." Dopamine transmits messages that help the brain control physical movement and emotional behavior, and its shortage may play a role in the movement problems and other features of this disorder. However, it is unclear how a shortage of hypoxanthine phosphoribosyltransferase 1 causes the neurological and behavioral problems characteristic of LNS.

Some people with *HPRT1* gene mutations produce some functional enzymes. These individuals are said to have the Lesch-Nyhan variant. The signs and symptoms of the Lesch-Nyhan variant are often milder than those of LNS and do not include self-injury.

SYMPTOMS OF LESCH-NYHAN SYNDROME
The lack of HPRT causes a buildup of uric acid in all body fluids and leads to the following symptoms:
- severe gout
- poor muscle control
- moderate developmental disabilities, which appear in the first year of life

A striking feature of LNS is self-mutilating behaviors—characterized by lip and finger biting—that begin in the second year of life. Abnormally high uric acid levels can cause sodium urate crystals to form in the joints, kidneys, central nervous system, and other tissues of the body, leading to gout-like swelling in the joints and severe kidney problems. Neurological symptoms include:
- facial grimacing
- involuntary writhing
- repetitive movements of the arms and legs similar to Huntington disease (HD)

Because a lack of *HPRT* causes the body to poorly utilize vitamin B12, some males may develop a rare disorder called "megaloblastic anemia."

INHERITANCE OF LESCH-NYHAN SYNDROME
This condition is inherited in an X-linked recessive pattern. The gene associated with this condition is located on the X chromosome, which is one of the two sex chromosomes. In males (who have only one X chromosome), one altered copy of the gene in each cell is sufficient to cause the condition. Because it is unlikely

that females will have two altered copies of this gene, males are affected by X-linked recessive disorders much more frequently than females. A characteristic of X-linked inheritance is that fathers cannot pass X-linked traits to their sons.

TREATMENT FOR LESCH-NYHAN SYNDROME

Treatment for LNS is symptomatic. Gout can be treated with allopurinol to control excessive amounts of uric acid. Kidney stones may be treated with lithotripsy, a technique for breaking up kidney stones using shock waves or laser beams. There is no standard treatment for the neurological symptoms of LNS. Some may be relieved with the drugs carbidopa/levodopa, diazepam, phenobarbital, or haloperidol.[8]

[8] MedlinePlus, "Lesch-Nyhan Syndrome," National Institutes of Health (NIH), February 1, 2013. Available online. URL: https://medlineplus.gov/genetics/condition/lesch-nyhan-syndrome/#causes. Accessed June 26, 2023.

Chapter 15 | **Osteoporosis in Men**

Osteoporosis is a bone disease that develops when bone mineral density (BMD) and bone mass decrease or when the quality or structure of bone changes. This can lead to a decrease in bone strength that can increase the risk of broken bones (fractures).

Osteoporosis is a major cause of fractures in older men. These fractures can occur in any bone but are most common in bones of the hip, vertebrae in the spine, and wrist.

HOW COMMON IS OSTEOPOROSIS IN MEN?

Because osteoporosis is more common in women than in men, it is often thought of as a women's disease. But some men, especially those aged 65 and older, do develop osteoporosis. In addition, the number of fractures caused by fragile bones in men has increased in recent years.

A fracture after age 50 is an important signal that a person may have osteoporosis. Unfortunately, men are less likely than women to be evaluated for osteoporosis after a fracture. Men also are less likely to get osteoporosis treatment.

WHAT ARE THE RISK FACTORS FOR OSTEOPOROSIS IN MEN?

Men have some of the same risk factors for osteoporosis as women, including:
- chronic diseases, such as diabetes or rheumatoid arthritis (RA)

- regular use of certain medications, such as glucocorticoids
- Parkinson disease (PD) and other conditions that affect neurological function
- low levels of the sex hormones testosterone and estrogen
- unhealthy habits, such as smoking and drinking too much alcohol
- weak muscles
- being aged 70 or older

HOW DOES BONE MASS CHANGE WITH AGE?

Bone is made up of living tissue that is constantly changing, with older bone being broken down and new bone forming in its place (remodeling). Almost all bone in adults is remodeled every 10 years. Bone mass is lost when there is an imbalance between bone breakdown and bone formation—more bone is broken down than is formed. That imbalance occurs with aging and other conditions.

Bone mass is gained during growth and typically peaks in one's 20s. Peak bone mass is generally higher in men than in women. And, although both men and women lose bone mass with age, bone loss is typically slower in men than in women, in part because of the estrogen that women lose after menopause.

DO FRAGILE BONES LEAD TO FRACTURES IN MEN?

Having lower bone density and bone strength is a major risk factor for fracture in both men and women, and fractures become more common with age. But the increase in fractures that happens with aging starts later in men than in women because men have greater peak bone mass, to begin with, and bone loss is slower in men. As a result of this delay in men's as well as women's longer life spans, older men have fewer fractures due to osteoporosis. But men who have a major fracture (e.g., a hip fracture) are more likely to have complications and to die as a result than women.

HOW IS OSTEOPOROSIS DIAGNOSED?

The most common test used to measure BMD and diagnose oste-oporosis is a central dual-energy x-ray absorptiometry (DXA or DEXA). DXA uses a small amount of x-ray to measure how much calcium and other minerals are in a specific area of your bone.

The U.S. Preventive Services Task Force (USPSTF) says that not enough evidence is available to recommend routine DXA testing in men.

What Is a T-score?

If you are aged 50 or older, your BMD test result will be a T-score. A T-score is the difference between your BMD and the average BMD of a healthy young adult. A T-score less than –2.5 is usually considered to indicate osteoporosis.

Your doctor might use the fracture risk assessment tool (FRAX) along with the T-score to estimate your risk for fracture. This score uses your age, sex, medical history, country, and other factors.

What Is a Z-score?

If you are younger than 50 years of age, your BMD test result will be a Z-score. The Z-score is the difference between your BMD and the average BMD of healthy people of your age, ethnicity, and sex.

WHAT TREATMENTS ARE AVAILABLE FOR OSTEOPOROSIS?

Osteoporosis treatment strategies are the same in men and women:

- proper nutrition
- lifestyle changes
- exercise
- fall prevention to help prevent fractures
- medications

HOW CAN MEN AND WOMEN PREVENT OSTEOPOROSIS?

Weight-bearing exercise, especially if you start at a young age, is a great way to strengthen bones and help prevent osteoporosis. Exercise also helps prevent falls that lead to fractures.

Other steps that may help prevent osteoporosis and fractures are as follows:

- eating a well-balanced diet rich in calcium and vitamin D
- drinking alcohol in moderation
- quitting smoking or not starting if you do not smoke[1]

[1] "Osteoporosis in Men," National Institute of Arthritis and Musculoskeletal and Skin Diseases (NIAMS), May 2023. Available online. URL: www.niams.nih.gov/health-topics/osteoporosis-men. Accessed June 15, 2023.

Chapter 16 | **Perineal Disorders**

Chapter Contents

WHAT IS AN INGUINAL HERNIA?

An inguinal hernia is a bulging of the contents of the abdomen through a weak area in the lower abdominal wall (see Figure 16.1). Inguinal hernias can occur at either of two passages through the lower abdominal wall, one on each side of the groin. These passages are called "inguinal canals." Inguinal hernias can also occur through two deeper passages in the groin called the "femoral canals." Hernias through these passages are also known as "femoral hernias."

Inguinal hernias most often contain fat or part of the small intestine. When an inguinal hernia occurs, part of the peritoneum—the lining of the abdominal cavity—bulges through the abdominal wall and forms a sac around the hernia.

Inguinal hernias may slide in and out of the abdominal wall. A doctor can often move an inguinal hernia back inside the abdominal wall with a gentle massage.

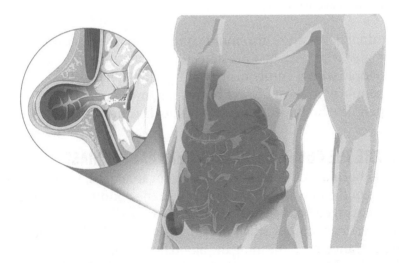

Figure 16.1. Inguinal Hernia

National Institute of Diabetes and Digestive and Kidney Diseases (NIDDK)
An inguinal hernia happens when the contents of the abdomen bulge through a weak area in the lower abdominal wall.

Inguinal hernias typically develop on one side of the groin and form on the right side more often than on the left. Some people who have an inguinal hernia on one side will have or will develop a hernia on the other side.

HOW COMMON ARE INGUINAL HERNIAS?

Inguinal hernias are relatively common. Researchers estimate that about 27 percent of men and 3 percent of women will develop an inguinal hernia at some point in their lives.

WHO IS MORE LIKELY TO HAVE AN INGUINAL HERNIA?

Inguinal hernias are more common in certain age groups.

- Among adults, the chance of having an inguinal hernia increases with age, and inguinal hernias are most common in people aged 75–80.
- Among children, inguinal hernias are most common in those between the ages of zero and five.
- Among infants, inguinal hernias are more common in premature infants.

Inguinal hernias are also more common in:
- males who have had prostatectomy
- people with a family history of inguinal hernias
- people who have a lower body mass index (BMI)
- people who have connective tissue disorders

WHAT ARE THE COMPLICATIONS OF INGUINAL HERNIAS?

Inguinal hernias may become stuck, or incarcerated, meaning the contents of the hernia that bulge through the abdominal wall cannot be massaged back inside the abdominal wall.

If a hernia becomes stuck outside the abdominal wall, it may become strangulated, meaning the blood flow to the hernia is cut off. Lack of blood flow can cause the death of tissues inside the hernia.

If a hernia that contains part of the small intestine becomes stuck and strangulated, this can lead to intestinal obstruction and death of the strangulated part of the intestine.

WHAT ARE THE SYMPTOMS OF AN INGUINAL HERNIA?

Symptoms of an inguinal hernia may include the following:
- a bulge in the groin—the area between the lower abdomen and thighs
- a bulge in the scrotum in a male
- feelings of discomfort, pain, heaviness, or burning in the groin

Your symptoms may get worse when you strain, lift, cough, or stand for a long time and may get better when you rest or lie down.

Seek Medical Help Right Away

If you have symptoms of a stuck or strangulated hernia, seek medical help right away. A strangulated hernia is a life-threatening condition.

Symptoms of stuck or strangulated hernias may include the following:
- a hernia bulge that is suddenly larger than before
- a hernia bulge that used to go back inside the abdomen but no longer does
- fever
- redness in the area of the hernia
- sudden or severe pain or tenderness in the area of the hernia
- symptoms of intestinal obstruction, such as abdominal pain, bloating, nausea, and vomiting

WHAT CAUSES INGUINAL HERNIAS?

A weak area in the muscles and connective tissue of the lower abdominal wall at the inguinal canal allows an inguinal hernia to develop. A hernia can form in different ways, causing two types of hernias.
- **Indirect inguinal hernias.** These hernias are related to a defect in the lower abdominal wall that is present at birth. In a developing fetus, the inguinal canals have openings inside the abdomen that typically close before

birth. In some cases, one or both openings remain open. Contents of the abdomen may bulge through this opening, causing a hernia. While the defect is present at birth, an indirect inguinal hernia may not occur until many years later.

- **Direct inguinal hernias.** These hernias are related to a weak area in the inguinal canal wall that develops later in life. Contents of the abdomen may bulge out through this weak area, causing a hernia. This type of hernia primarily occurs in men. Women and children rarely develop this type of hernia.

Researchers are studying other factors that might play a role in causing inguinal hernias. These factors include the following:

- connective tissue that is weaker than normal or connective tissue disorders
- genes that increase the risk of inguinal hernias
- health conditions that cause increased pressure inside the abdomen, such as chronic cough or chronic constipation
- regular or repeated activities that cause increased pressure inside the abdomen, such as heavy lifting and standing or walking for many hours each day at work

HOW DO DOCTORS DIAGNOSE INGUINAL HERNIAS?

To diagnose an inguinal hernia, your doctor will ask about your medical history and symptoms and perform a physical exam. In some cases, doctors also order imaging tests.

During a physical exam, the doctor will examine your abdomen. The doctor may ask you to stand, cough, or strain while he or she checks for a bulge caused by the hernia. The doctor may try to gently massage the contents of the hernia back into the abdomen.

What Tests Do Doctors Use to Diagnose Inguinal Hernias?

If the diagnosis is not clear after a physical exam, your doctor may order imaging tests to check for an inguinal hernia. Doctors may also use imaging tests to check for complications.

Imaging tests may include the following:
- **Ultrasound**. It uses sound waves to create an image of your organs.
- **Computed tomography (CT)**. CT uses a combination of x-rays and computer technology to create images.
- **Magnetic resonance imaging (MRI)**. MRI takes pictures of your body's internal organs and soft tissues without using x-rays.

HOW DO DOCTORS TREAT INGUINAL HERNIAS?

Most people with inguinal hernias will need surgery to repair the hernia. Several different types of open and laparoscopic hernia surgery are available. The type of surgery your doctor recommends may depend on factors such as the size of the hernia and your age, health, and medical history.

Open Hernia Surgery

In open hernia surgery, a surgeon makes a cut in your groin to view and repair the hernia. After repairing the hernia, surgeons typically use stitches and a piece of mesh to close the abdominal wall. The mesh strengthens the weak area where the hernia occurred. In some cases, surgeons may use stitches alone to close and strengthen the weak area in the abdominal wall.

Patients most often receive local anesthesia and a sedative for open hernia surgery. In some cases, doctors may give patients general anesthesia or a spinal block to make the body numb from the waist down.

Laparoscopic Hernia Surgery

In laparoscopic hernia surgery, a surgeon makes several small cuts in your lower abdomen and inserts special tools to view and repair the hernia. The surgeon uses a piece of mesh to close and strengthen the abdominal wall.

Patients most often receive general anesthesia for laparoscopic hernia surgery. Recovery time after laparoscopic surgery may be shorter than after open hernia surgery.

Watchful Waiting

Research suggests that men with inguinal hernias that cause few or no symptoms may be able to safely delay surgery, an approach called "watchful waiting." Men who delay surgery should watch for symptoms and see a doctor regularly. About 70 percent of men who delay surgery will develop new or worsening symptoms and will need surgery within five years.

HOW DO DOCTORS TREAT THE COMPLICATIONS OF INGUINAL HERNIAS?

If an inguinal hernia causes complications, such as becoming stuck or strangulated, you will need emergency surgery to repair the hernia and treat the complications.

What Could You Expect after Surgery to Treat an Inguinal Hernia?

You may have some pain or discomfort after hernia surgery. The pain is typically mild and goes away within two weeks after surgery. Your doctor will recommend medicines to relieve pain.

Talk with your doctor about when you can safely return to your usual activities after hernia surgery. Many people can go back to work and resume daily activities within three to five days after hernia surgery.

What Are the Risks of Hernia Surgery?

Surgery to repair an inguinal hernia is quite safe. However, possible complications of hernia surgery include the following:
- urinary retention
- infection
- swelling in the area you had surgery due to a buildup of blood, called a "hematoma," or a buildup of blood plasma, called a "seroma"
- chronic or severe pain
- return of the hernia, which may require another surgery

Serious complications, such as damage to blood vessels or organs, are rare.

Talk with your doctor about the risks of hernia surgery and symptoms you should watch for after surgery. For example, you should call your doctor right away if you have:

- bleeding, drainage, or redness in the area where you had surgery
- fever or chills
- nausea or vomiting
- pain or swelling in your abdomen
- pain or swelling in your groin that gets worse
- pain that is severe or does not get better when you take pain medicines
- problems breathing
- problems urinating[1]

Section 16.2 | Perineal Injury

WHAT IS THE PERINEUM, AND WHY IS IT IMPORTANT?

In males, the perineum lies just below the pelvic floor muscles, which support the bladder and bowel. The perineum protects the pelvic floor muscles and the blood vessels that supply the genitals and urinary tract. The perineum also protects the nerves used to urinate or have an erection.

WHAT IS PERINEAL INJURY?

Perineal injury is an injury to the perineum, the area of the body between the anus and the scrotum. It is a type of genital injury.

---

[1] "Inguinal Hernia," National Institute of Diabetes and Digestive and Kidney Diseases (NIDDK), September 2019. Available online. URL: www.niddk.nih.gov/health-information/digestive-diseases/inguinal-hernia. Accessed June 16, 2023.

Types of Perineal Injuries

Injuries to the perineum can happen suddenly, known as an "acute injury," or gradually, known as a "chronic injury."

Acute injuries include the following:
- straddle injuries, which can happen if you fall with your legs on each side of an object or bar and hit your perineum when you land
- impalement injuries that occur when an object punctures the perineum
- burns

Acute injuries can also happen from violent trauma, during surgery, during sexual abuse, or from some medical conditions.

Chronic injuries develop gradually from pressure on the perineum for a long time. Long-term pressure can come from certain seated activities, such as road cycling long distances.

HOW COMMON ARE PERINEAL INJURIES?

Injuries to the perineum are rare. A study found that the perineum was injured in 1 percent of motorcyclists and 3 percent of bicyclists involved in traffic accidents.

WHO IS MORE LIKELY TO HAVE A PERINEAL INJURY?

Perineal injury is more likely for men who:
- are in military combat
- have surgery in their genital region
- ride bicycles, motorcycles, or horses
- work in construction or on a farm
- engage in gymnastics
- have been sexually abused

WHAT ARE THE COMPLICATIONS OF PERINEAL INJURY?

Bladder control problems or sexual problems may develop if the blood vessels, nerves, or muscles in the perineum are damaged. Infections may develop after a burn or wound.

Bladder Control Problems

Perineal trauma can injure nerves of the pelvis, causing bladder and bowel problems. The nerves in your bladder signal when it is full, and your brain directs your bladder and pelvic floor muscles to hold or release urine. Injury to those nerves can block or interfere with the signals, causing your bladder muscles to squeeze involuntarily at the wrong time or not to squeeze at all. Damage to your pelvic floor muscles can also cause bowel control problems.

Damage to the perineum could also injure an internal part of the penis containing the urethra. The urethra may tear or become narrower, or you may experience urinary incontinence.

Sexual Problems

The perineal nerves carry signals between the genitals and the brain. Injury to those nerves can interfere with the sensations of sexual contact.

If the blood vessels in the perineum are damaged, you may develop erectile dysfunction (ED), the inability to achieve or maintain an erection firm enough for sexual intercourse. ED may also be caused by damage to the urethra.

In rare situations, a blunt injury to the perineum may burst a blood vessel inside the penis, causing a persistent partial erection that can last for days to weeks or longer. This condition is called "high-flow priapism" and, if not treated, may lead to ED.

WHAT ARE THE SIGNS AND SYMPTOMS OF PERINEAL INJURY IN MALES?

Signs of a perineal injury include the following:
- bleeding or an open wound
- object embedded in the perineum
- burned skin
- bruising
- swelling
- fresh blood in the urethral opening
- inability to urinate

Along with these signs, you may have symptoms such as pain in the genital, groin, or abdominal areas. In some cases, the pain may be severe.

Bicycle or motorcycle riders may also experience genital numbness. The level of numbness increases with longer or rougher rides.

WHAT CAUSES PERINEAL INJURY?
Acute Perineal Injuries
Causes of acute perineal injury in males include the following:

- **Perineal surgery**. A surgeon may need to cut the perineum during some types of surgery, such as:
  - surgery to remove the prostate
  - surgery to repair a stricture, or narrowing, of the portion of the urethra that runs through the perineum
  - colorectal or anal cancer surgery to remove a tumor
- **Straddle injuries**. These injuries include motorcycle- and bike-riding accidents, horseback-riding accidents, or accidental falls onto stationary objects, such as fence rails or gymnastic equipment.
- **Impalement**. These injuries may involve metal fence posts, rods, or weapons that pierce the perineum. Impalement injuries occur in combat situations or where moving equipment and pointed tools are in use, such as on farms or construction sites. Impalement can also result from a fall onto something sharp.
- **Sexual abuse**. Forceful and inappropriate sexual contact can cause perineal injury.
- **Burns**. Contact with hot objects or liquids could injure the perineum. These may occur in military combat or from contact with hot liquids or hot objects, such as personal grooming implements. Burns may also lead to infections.
- **Other conditions**. Fournier gangrene is an acute infection that occurs in the genital region and causes tissue death. It affects the perineum, scrotum, or penis in males. It is a rare disease and may be a complication from other types of urinary tract conditions, surgery, or trauma.

Chronic Perineal Injuries

Chronic perineal injuries most often result from a job- or sport-related practice—such as riding a bicycle, motorcycle, or horse.

- **Bicycle, motorcycle, and horseback riding.** Sitting on a narrow, saddle-style bike seat—which has a protruding "nose" in the front—places far more pressure on the perineum than sitting in a regular chair. In a regular chair, the flesh and bone of the buttocks partially absorb the pressure of sitting, and the pressure occurs farther toward the back than on a bike seat. The straddling position on a narrow seat pinches the perineal blood vessels and nerves, possibly causing blood vessel and nerve damage over time. Research shows wider, noseless seats reduce perineal pressure.

Cycling has many cardiovascular benefits that improve overall sexual and urinary health. There is controversy about whether long-distance cycling leads to modest, increased risk of ED. ED may be caused by repetitive pressure on blood vessels, which constricts them and results in plaque buildup in the vessels. Genital numbness has been noted in male cyclists who engage in long-distance cycling events. Cyclists should aim to ride in a way that avoids acute genital numbness. Long-distance riders should get their bike professionally fit to their body, consider using seats that minimize perineal pressure, and spend less time engaged with the saddle during long rides.

HOW DO HEALTH-CARE PROFESSIONALS DIAGNOSE PERINEAL INJURY?

Health-care professionals diagnose perineal injury based on the circumstances and severity of the injury. In general, a health-care professional will conduct a physical exam and order one or more imaging tests.

Physical Exam

During a physical exam, your health-care professional looks for wounds, swelling, or bruises and may use a digital rectal exam

(DRE) to feel for internal injuries. Your health-care professional may also conduct a neurologic exam to test skin sensation.

Imaging Tests

Your health-care professional may order one or more of the following imaging tests to check for internal injuries:

- **Computed tomography (CT) scans.** CT scans can show traumatic injury to the perineum.
- **Magnetic resonance imaging (MRI).** MRI can show damage to blood vessels and muscles.
- **Ultrasound.** This can show damage to blood vessels in the perineum.
- **X-rays.** These include the addition of a special dye that can show if your urethra is damaged.

Injury Evaluation

When health-care professionals evaluate injuries, they typically ask how the injury occurred and when was the last time you urinated. In cases of genital injuries, these questions may make you feel uncomfortable because, in addition to other causes, genital injuries can be caused by sexual abuse, and health-care professionals are required by law to report cases of sexual abuse that come to their attention.

HOW DO HEALTH-CARE PROFESSIONALS TREAT PERINEAL INJURIES IN MALES?

Treatments for perineal injury vary with the severity and type of injury. If you are bleeding, your health-care professional will take immediate steps to minimize blood loss and repair the injury. Tears or incisions may require stitches, and burns may require ointment. Traumatic or piercing injuries may require surgery to repair damaged pelvic floor muscles, blood vessels, and nerves. In case of a urethral injury, your urine may need to be collected through a tube called a "catheter." Treatment for these acute injuries may also include antibiotics to prevent infection.

After a health-care professional stabilizes an acute injury so blood loss is no longer a concern, some long-term effects of the injury, such as bladder control and sexual function problems, may persist. Injuries to the urethra could cause it to become narrower, and it may need to be treated. A health-care professional can treat high-flow priapism caused by a blunt injury to the perineum with medication or surgery.

For people with a chronic perineal injury, a health-care professional will work with you to treat the condition and any complications.

COULD YOU PREVENT A PERINEAL INJURY?

You can take steps to protect your perineum and reduce the chance of accidental injury.

- **Bicycle, motorcycle, or horseback riding**. Use seats or saddles that minimize pressure on the perineum and shift pressure to the buttocks. The National Institute for Occupational Safety and Health (NIOSH), part of the Centers for Disease Control and Prevention (CDC), recommends noseless seats for people who ride bikes as part of their job.

You can also adjust the height of the handlebars, pedals, or seat and wear padded shorts to reduce pressure and chafing of your perineum. In addition, increasing the time you stand while cycling may decrease numbness.

- **Construction, agricultural, or factory work**. Wear appropriate protective gear, such as coveralls or bodysuits if you are around moving equipment or sharp objects. Be aware of your surroundings and potential hazards.
- **Military combat and first responders**. People engaged in military combat should use pelvic personal protective equipment to limit penetration and reduce the rate of injury. Police and other first responders may want to use similar equipment as specific jobs and situations warrant.

- **Surgery.** While surgeons try to avoid procedures that can damage your blood vessels, perineal nerves, and muscles, sometimes a perineal incision may be needed to achieve the best result. Discuss the risks of any planned surgery with your health-care professional, so you can make an informed decision and understand what to expect after the operation.[2]

[2] "Perineal Injury in Males," National Institute of Diabetes and Digestive and Kidney Diseases (NIDDK), April 2020. Available online. URL: www.niddk.nih.gov/health-information/urologic-diseases/perineal-injury-males. Accessed June 16, 2023.

Chapter 17 | **Sleep Apnea**

Sleep apnea is a common condition in which your breathing stops and restarts many times while you sleep. This can prevent your body from getting enough oxygen. You may want to talk to your health-care provider about sleep apnea if someone tells you that you snore or gasp during sleep or if you experience other symptoms of poor-quality sleep, such as excessive daytime sleepiness.

The following are the two types of sleep apnea:

- **Obstructive sleep apnea (OSA).** OSA happens when your upper airway becomes blocked many times while you sleep, reducing or completely stopping airflow. This is the most common type of sleep apnea (see Figure 17.1). Anything that could narrow your airway such as obesity, large tonsils, or changes in your hormone levels can increase your risk for OSA.
- **Central sleep apnea (CSA).** CSA happens when your brain does not send the signals needed to breathe. Health conditions that affect how your brain controls your airway and chest muscles can cause CSA.

CAUSES FOR SLEEP APNEA

- Central sleep apnea is caused by problems with the way your brain controls your breathing while you sleep.
- OSA is caused by conditions that block airflow through your upper airways during sleep. For example, your tongue may fall backward and block your airway.
- Your age, family history, lifestyle habits, other medical conditions, and some features of your body can raise your risk of sleep apnea. Healthy lifestyle changes can help lower your risk.

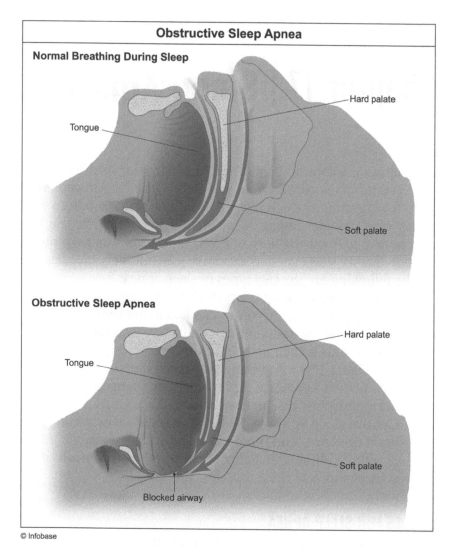

Figure 17.1. Obstructive Sleep Apnea

Infobase

WHAT RAISES THE RISK OF OBSTRUCTIVE SLEEP APNEA?

Many conditions can cause sleep apnea. Some factors such as unhealthy lifestyle habits can be changed. Other factors such as age, family history, race and ethnicity, and sex cannot be changed.

- **Age**. Sleep apnea can occur at any age, but your risk increases as you get older. As you age, fatty tissue can build up in your neck and the tongue and raise your risk of sleep apnea.
- **Endocrine disorders, or changes in your hormone levels**. Your hormone levels can affect the size and shape of your face, tongue, and airway. People who have low levels of thyroid hormones or high levels of insulin or growth hormone have a higher risk of sleep apnea.
- **Family history and genetics**. Sleep apnea can be inherited. Your genes help determine the size and shape of your skull, face, and upper airway. Also, your genes can raise your risk of other health conditions that can lead to sleep apnea, such as cleft lip, cleft palate, and Down syndrome.
- **Heart or kidney failure**. These conditions can cause fluid to build up in your neck, which can block your upper airway.
- **Large tonsils and a thick neck**. These features may cause sleep apnea because they narrow your upper airway. Also, having a large tongue and your tongue's position in your mouth can make it easier for your tongue to block your airway while you sleep.
- **Lifestyle habits**. Drinking alcohol and smoking can raise your risk of sleep apnea. Alcohol can make the muscles of your mouth and throat relax, which may close your upper airway. Smoking can cause inflammation in your upper airway, which affects breathing.
- **Obesity**. This condition is a common cause of sleep apnea. People with this condition can have increased fat deposits in their necks that can block the upper airway. Maintaining a healthy weight can help prevent or treat sleep apnea caused by obesity.
- **Sex**. Sleep apnea is more common in men than in women. Men are more likely to have serious sleep apnea and to get sleep apnea at a younger age than women.

WHAT RAISES THE RISK OF CENTRAL SLEEP APNEA?

- **Age**. As you get older, normal changes in how your brain controls breathing during sleep may raise your risk of sleep apnea.
- **Family history and genetics**. Your genes can affect how your brain controls your breathing during sleep. Genetic conditions, such as congenital central hypoventilation syndrome, can raise your risk.
- **Lifestyle habits**. Drinking alcohol and smoking can affect how your brain controls sleep or the muscles involved in breathing.
- **Opioid use**. Opioid use disorder or long-term use of prescribed opioid-based pain medicines can cause problems with how your brain controls sleep.
- **Health conditions**. Some conditions that affect how your brain controls your airway and chest muscles can raise your risk. These include heart failure, stroke, amyotrophic lateral sclerosis (ALS), and myasthenia gravis. Also, your hormone levels can affect how your brain controls your breathing.
- **Premature birth**. Babies born before 37 weeks of pregnancy have a higher risk of breathing problems during sleep. In most cases, the risk gets lower as the baby gets older.

SYMPTOMS OF SLEEP APNEA

Your partner may alert you to some of the symptoms of sleep apnea, such as:

- breathing that starts and stops during sleep
- frequent loud snoring
- gasping for air during sleep

You may also notice the following symptoms yourself:

- daytime sleepiness and tiredness, which can lead to problems learning, focusing, and reacting
- dry mouth or headaches
- sexual dysfunction or decreased libido
- waking up often during the night to urinate

Children who have sleep apnea may be overactive and may experience bedwetting, worsening asthma, and trouble paying attention in school.

Talk to your health-care provider about your symptoms.

DIAGNOSIS OF SLEEP APNEA
Your health-care provider will ask you about your symptoms, risk factors, and whether you have a family history of sleep apnea. You may need a sleep study to help diagnose sleep apnea.

Sleep Study
Your health-care provider will ask you to see a sleep specialist or go to a center for a sleep study. Sleep studies can help diagnose which type of sleep apnea you have and how serious it is.

Sleep Diary
A sleep diary can help you keep track of how long and how well you sleep and how sleepy you feel during the day. These details can help your health-care provider diagnose your condition.

Ruling Out Other Medical Conditions
Your provider may order other tests to help rule out other medical conditions that can cause sleep apnea:
- **Blood tests**. These tests check the levels of certain hormones to check for endocrine disorders that could contribute to sleep apnea.
- **Thyroid hormone tests**. These tests can rule out hypothyroidism.
- **Growth hormone tests**. These tests can rule out acromegaly.
- **Total testosterone and dehydroepiandrosterone sulfate (DHEAS) tests**. These tests can help rule out polycystic ovary syndrome (PCOS).
- **Pelvic ultrasounds**. These examine the ovaries and help detect cysts. This can rule out PCOS.

Your provider will also want to know whether you are using medicines, such as opioids, that could affect your sleep or cause breathing symptoms of sleep apnea. They may want to know whether you have traveled recently to altitudes greater than 6,000 feet because these low-oxygen environments can cause symptoms of sleep apnea for a few weeks after traveling.

TREATMENT FOR SLEEP APNEA
If a sleep study shows that you have sleep apnea, your health-care provider may talk to you about making lifelong heart-healthy lifestyle changes. You may also need breathing or oral devices or surgery to help keep your airways open while you sleep.

Healthy Lifestyle Changes
To help treat your sleep apnea, you may need to adopt lifelong healthy lifestyle changes. These include getting regular physical activity, maintaining healthy sleeping habits and a healthy weight, limiting alcohol, and quitting smoking. Your provider may also ask you to sleep on your side and not on your back. This helps keep your airway open while you sleep.

Breathing Devices
A breathing device, such as a continuous positive airway pressure (CPAP) machine, is the most common treatment for sleep apnea. A CPAP machine provides constant air pressure in your throat to keep the airway open when you breathe in.

Breathing devices work best when you also make healthy lifestyle changes. Side effects of CPAP treatment may include:
- congestion
- dry eyes
- dry mouth
- nosebleeds
- runny nose

If you experience stomach discomfort or bloating, you should stop using your CPAP machine and contact your health-care provider.

Depending on the type of sleep apnea you have, you may need another type of breathing device such as an auto-adjusting positive airway pressure (APAP) machine or a bilevel positive airway pressure (BPAP) machine.

Oral Devices

Oral devices, also called "oral appliances," are custom-fit devices that you typically wear in your mouth while you sleep. The following are the two types of oral devices that work differently to open the upper airway while you sleep. Some hybrid devices have features of both types.

- **Mandibular repositioning mouthpieces**. These devices cover the upper and lower teeth and hold the jaw in a position that prevents it from blocking the upper airway.
- **Tongue retaining devices**. These mouthpieces hold the tongue in a forward position to prevent it from blocking the upper airway.

A new type of oral device was recently approved by the U.S. Food and Drug Administration (FDA; www.fda.gov/news-events/press-announcements/fda-authorizes-marketing-novel-device-reduce-snoring-and-mild-obstructive-sleep-apnea-patients-18) for use while awake. The device delivers electrical muscle stimulation through a removable mouthpiece that sits around the tongue. You wear the mouthpiece once a day for 20 minutes at a time, for six weeks. The device stimulates the tongue muscle while awake to help prevent the tongue from collapsing backward and blocking the airway during sleep.

If you have sleep apnea, your provider may prescribe an oral device if you do not want to use CPAP or cannot tolerate CPAP. They recommend that you visit a dentist who will custom-make an appliance for you. Make sure that it is comfortable and teach you how to use it to get the best results.

Therapy for Your Mouth and Facial Muscles

Exercises for your mouth and facial muscles, also called "orofacial therapy," may help treat sleep apnea in children and adults. This therapy helps improve the position of your tongue and strengthens the muscles that control your lips, tongue, upper airway, and face.

Surgical Procedures

You may need surgery if other treatments do not work for you. Possible surgical procedures include:

- adenotonsillectomy to remove your tonsils and adenoids
- surgery to place an implant that monitors your breathing patterns and helps control certain muscles that open your airways during sleep
- surgery to remove some soft tissue from your mouth and throat, which helps make your upper airway bigger
- maxillary or jaw advancement surgery to move your upper jaw (maxilla) and lower jaw (mandible) forward, which helps make your upper airway bigger[1]

---

[1] "What Is Sleep Apnea?" National Heart, Lung, and Blood Institute (NHLBI), March 24, 2022. Available online. URL: www.nhlbi.nih.gov/health/sleep-apnea. Accessed June 15, 2023.

Chapter 18 | Cancers in Men

Chapter Contents

Section 18.1 | Cancer among Men: Some Statistics

Cancer begins in your cells, which are the building blocks of your body. Normally, your body forms new cells as you need them, replacing old cells that die. Sometimes, this process goes wrong. New cells grow even when you do not need them, and old cells do not die when they should. These extra cells can form a mass called a "tumor." Tumors can be benign or malignant. Benign tumors are not cancerous, while malignant ones are. Cells from malignant tumors can invade nearby tissues. They can also break away and spread to other parts of the body.

Cancer is not just one disease but many diseases. There are more than 100 different types of cancers. Most cancers are named for where they start. For example, lung cancer starts in the lung, and breast cancer starts in the breast. The spread of cancer from one part of the body to another is called "metastasis." Symptoms and treatment depend on the cancer type and how advanced it is. Most treatment plans may include surgery, radiation, and/or chemotherapy. Some may involve hormone therapy, immunotherapy or other types of biologic therapy, or stem cell transplantation.[1]

FAST FACTS ABOUT CANCER AND MEN

Men have higher rates of getting and dying from cancer than women. You can lower your chance of getting certain kinds of cancers.

Most cancers take years to develop. Many things can affect your chance of getting cancer. Things that raise your chance of getting cancer are called "risk factors."

You cannot control some risk factors, such as getting older. But you can control many others. In fact, there are things you can do every day to avoid getting cancer. Two of the most important things you can do are making healthy choices and getting the screening tests that are right for you.

---

[1] MedlinePlus, "Cancer," National Institutes of Health (NIH), May 18, 2017. Available online. URL: https://medlineplus.gov/cancer.html. Accessed July 6, 2023.

Healthy Choices

Quitting smoking is one of the best ways to lower your cancer risk. Smoking can cause cancer almost anywhere in the body. If you do not smoke, make sure you stay away from other people's smoke.

The link between smoking and cancer is well-known. But you may be surprised by other things that can lead to cancer.

- Ultraviolet (UV) rays from the sun or artificial sources, such as a tanning bed, booth, or sunlamp, can cause skin cancer, the most common cancer.
- Drinking alcohol raises your risk of getting five kinds of cancers, including liver cancer and colorectal cancer.
- About 40 percent of all cancers are associated with overweight and obesity.

Screening Tests

Screening means checking your body for cancer before you have symptoms. All screening tests have benefits and harms. Screening is recommended when the benefits outweigh the harms.

COLORECTAL CANCER SCREENING

If you are 45–75 years old, get screened regularly.

You should start getting screened for colorectal cancer soon after turning 45 and get screened regularly until you are 75. Several screening tests are available. Some can be done at home, and others are done in a doctor's office. Talk to your doctor about which test is right for you.

LUNG CANCER SCREENING

Screening is recommended for people who are 50–80 years old and are current or former heavy smokers.

The U.S. Preventive Services Task Force (USPSTF), a group of experts, recommends yearly lung cancer screening with low-dose computed tomography (LDCT) for people who are 50–80 years old, have a history of heavy smoking, and smoke now or quit within the past 15 years.

PROSTATE CANCER SCREENING

Middle-aged men should talk to their doctors about the possible benefits and harms of screening.

The goal of screening for prostate cancer is to find cancers that may be at high risk for spreading if not treated and to find them early before they spread. However, most prostate cancers grow slowly or not at all.

A blood test called a "prostate-specific antigen" (PSA) test is commonly used to screen for prostate cancer. If you are thinking about being screened, learn about the possible benefits and harms of screening and talk to your doctor about your personal risk factors.[2]

Section 18.2 | Breast Cancer

Breast cancer is most often found in women, but men can get breast cancer too. About 1 out of every 100 breast cancers diagnosed in the United States is found in a man.

The most common kinds of breast cancer in men are as follows:

- **Invasive ductal carcinoma**. The cancer cells begin in the ducts and then grow outside the ducts into other parts of the breast tissue. Invasive cancer cells can also spread, or metastasize, to other parts of the body.
- **Invasive lobular carcinoma**. Cancer cells begin in the lobules and then spread from the lobules to the breast tissues that are close by. These invasive cancer cells can also spread to other parts of the body.
- **Ductal carcinoma in situ (DCIS)**. It is a breast disease that may lead to invasive breast cancer. The cancer cells are only in the lining of the ducts and have not spread to other tissues in the breast.

---

[2] "Cancer and Men," Centers for Disease Control and Prevention (CDC), June 5, 2023. Available online. URL: www.cdc.gov/cancer/dcpc/resources/features/cancerandmen/index.htm. Accessed June 15, 2023.

WHAT ARE THE RISK FACTORS FOR BREAST CANCER IN MEN?

Several factors can increase a man's chance of getting breast cancer. Having risk factors does not mean you will get breast cancer.

- **Getting older.** The risk for breast cancer increases with age. Most breast cancers are found after age 50.
- **Genetic mutations.** Inherited changes (mutations) in certain genes, such as *BRCA1* and *BRCA2*, increase breast cancer risk.
- **Family history of breast cancer.** A man's risk for breast cancer is higher if a close family member has had breast cancer.
- **Radiation therapy treatment.** Men who had radiation therapy to the chest have a higher risk of getting breast cancer.
- **Hormone therapy treatment.** Drugs containing estrogen (a hormone that helps develop and maintain female sex characteristics), which were used to treat prostate cancer in the past, increase men's breast cancer risk.
- **Klinefelter syndrome (KS).** It is a rare genetic condition in which a male has an extra X chromosome. This can lead to the body making higher levels of estrogen and lower levels of androgens (hormones that help develop and maintain male sex characteristics).
- **Certain conditions that affect the testicles.** Injury to, swelling in, or surgery to remove the testicles can increase breast cancer risk.
- **Liver disease.** Cirrhosis (scarring) of the liver can lower androgen levels and raise estrogen levels in men, increasing the risk of breast cancer.
- **Overweight and obesity.** Older men who are overweight or have obesity have a higher risk of getting breast cancer than men at a normal weight.

What Can You Do to Reduce Your Risk of Breast Cancer?

If several members of your family have had breast or ovarian cancer or one of your family members has a known *BRCA1* or *BRCA2* mutation, share this information with your doctor. Your doctor may refer you for genetic counseling. In men, mutations in the *BRCA1* and *BRCA2* genes can increase the risk of breast cancer, high-grade prostate cancer, and pancreatic cancer.

If genetic testing shows that you have a *BRCA1* or *BRCA2* gene mutation, your doctor will explain what you should do to find cancer early if you get it.

All men can lower their risk by keeping a healthy weight and being physically active.

WHAT ARE THE SYMPTOMS OF BREAST CANCER IN MEN?

The most common symptoms of breast cancer in men are as follows:
- a lump or swelling in the breast
- redness or flaky skin in the breast
- irritation or dimpling of breast skin
- nipple discharge
- pulling in of the nipple or pain in the nipple area

These symptoms can happen with other conditions that are not cancer. If you have any symptoms or changes, see your doctor right away.

HOW IS BREAST CANCER TREATED?

As in women, treatment for breast cancer in men depends on how big the tumor is and how far it has spread. Treatment may include surgery, chemotherapy, radiation therapy, hormone therapy, and targeted therapy.[3]

---

[3] "Breast Cancer in Men," Centers for Disease Control and Prevention (CDC), September 26, 2022. Available online. URL: www.cdc.gov/cancer/breast/men/index.htm. Accessed June 16, 2023.

Section 18.3 | Liver Cancer

The liver is the largest organ in the human body, located on the upper right side of the body, behind the lower ribs. The liver does many jobs, including:

- storing nutrients
- removing waste products and worn-out cells from the blood
- filtering and processing chemicals in food, alcohol, and medications
- producing bile, a solution that helps digest fats and eliminates waste products

When cancer starts in the liver, it is called "liver cancer." Each year in the United States, about 25,000 men and 11,000 women get liver cancer, and about 19,000 men and 9,000 women die from the disease.

WHAT CAUSES LIVER CANCER?

Behaviors and conditions that increase the risk of getting liver cancer are as follows:

- being overweight or having obesity
- having a long-term hepatitis B virus or hepatitis C virus infection
- smoking cigarettes
- drinking alcohol
- having cirrhosis (scarring of the liver, which can also be caused by hepatitis and alcohol use)
- having nonalcoholic fatty liver disease (extra fat in the liver that is not caused by alcohol)
- having diabetes
- having hemochromatosis, a condition where the body takes up and stores more iron than it needs
- eating foods that have aflatoxin (a fungus that can grow on foods, such as grains and nuts that have not been stored properly)

WHAT ARE THE SYMPTOMS OF LIVER CANCER?

In its early stages, liver cancer may not have symptoms that can be seen or felt. However, as the cancer grows larger, people may notice one or more of the following common symptoms. It is important to remember that these symptoms could also be caused by other health conditions. If you have any of the following symptoms, talk to your doctor:

- discomfort in the upper abdomen on the right side
- a swollen abdomen
- a hard lump on the right side just below the rib cage
- pain near the right shoulder blade or in the back
- jaundice (yellowing of the skin and whites of the eyes)
- easy bruising or bleeding
- unusual tiredness
- nausea and vomiting
- loss of appetite
- weight loss for no known reason

HOW CAN YOU REDUCE YOUR RISK FOR LIVER CANCER?

You can lower your risk of getting liver cancer in the following ways:

- Keep a healthy weight.
- Get vaccinated against hepatitis B. The hepatitis B vaccine is recommended for all infants at birth and for adults who may be at increased risk.
- Get tested for hepatitis C and get medical care if you have it.
- Do not smoke or quit if you do.
- Avoid drinking too much alcohol.[4]

---

[4] "Liver Cancer," Centers for Disease Control and Prevention (CDC), November 15, 2022. Available online. URL: www.cdc.gov/cancer/liver/index.htm. Accessed July 6, 2023.

Section 18.4 | Lung Cancer

Lungs are organs in your chest that allow your body to take in oxygen from the air. They also help remove carbon dioxide (a waste gas that can be toxic) from your body.

The lungs' intake of oxygen and removal of carbon dioxide is called "gas exchange." Gas exchange is part of breathing. Breathing is a vital function of life; it helps your body work properly. Other organs and tissues also help make breathing possible.[5]

Lung cancer begins in the lungs and may spread to lymph nodes or other organs in the body, such as the brain. Cancer from other organs may also spread to the lungs. When cancer cells spread from one organ to another, they are called "metastases."

Lung cancers are usually grouped into two main types called "small cell" and "non-small cell." These types of lung cancer grow differently and are treated differently.

WHAT ARE THE RISK FACTORS FOR LUNG CANCER?

Research has found several risk factors that may increase your chances of getting lung cancer.

Smoking

Cigarette smoking is the number one risk factor for lung cancer. In the United States, cigarette smoking is linked to about 80–90 percent of lung cancer deaths. Using other tobacco products, such as cigars or pipes, also increases the risk of lung cancer. Tobacco smoke is a toxic mix of more than 7,000 chemicals. Many are poisons. At least 70 are known to cause cancer in people or animals.

People who smoke cigarettes are 15–30 times more likely to get lung cancer or die from lung cancer than people who do not smoke. Even smoking a few cigarettes a day or smoking occasionally increases the risk of lung cancer. The more years a person smokes and the more cigarette smoke each day, the higher the risk is.

---

[5] "The Lungs," National Heart, Lung, and Blood Institute (NHLBI), March 24, 2022. Available online. URL: www.nhlbi.nih.gov/health/lungs. Accessed July 18, 2023.

People who quit smoking have a lower risk of lung cancer than if they had continued to smoke, but their risk is higher than the risk for people who never smoked. Quitting smoking at any age can lower the risk of lung cancer.

Cigarette smoking can cause cancer almost anywhere in the body. Cigarette smoking causes cancer of the mouth and throat, esophagus, stomach, colon, rectum, liver, pancreas, voicebox (larynx), trachea, bronchus, kidney and renal pelvis, urinary bladder, and cervix, and it causes acute myeloid leukemia (AML).

Secondhand Smoke

Smoke from other people's cigarettes, pipes, or cigars (secondhand smoke) also causes lung cancer. When a person breathes in secondhand smoke, it is like he or she is smoking. In the United States, two out of five adults who do not smoke and half of children are exposed to secondhand smoke, and about 7,300 people who never smoked die from lung cancer due to secondhand smoke every year.

Radon

Radon is a naturally occurring gas that comes from rocks and dirt, and it can get trapped in houses and buildings. It cannot be seen, tasted, or smelled. According to the U.S. Environmental Protection Agency (EPA), radon causes about 20,000 cases of lung cancer each year, making it the second leading cause of lung cancer. Nearly 1 out of every 15 homes in the United States is thought to have high radon levels. The EPA recommends testing homes for radon and using proven ways to lower high radon levels.

Other Substances

Examples of substances found at some workplaces that increase lung cancer risk include asbestos, arsenic, diesel exhaust, and some forms of silica and chromium. For many of these substances, the risk of getting lung cancer is even higher for those who smoke.

Personal or Family History of Lung Cancer

If you are a lung cancer survivor, there is a risk that you may develop another lung cancer, especially if you smoke. Your risk of lung cancer may be higher if your parents, brothers or sisters, or children have had lung cancer. This could be true because they also smoke or they live or work in the same place where they are exposed to radon and other substances that can cause lung cancer.

Radiation Therapy to the Chest

Cancer survivors who had radiation therapy to the chest are at a higher risk of lung cancer.

Diet

Scientists are studying many different foods and dietary supplements to see whether they change the risk of getting lung cancer. There is much we still need to know. We do know that smokers who take beta-carotene supplements have an increased risk of lung cancer.

Also, arsenic in drinking water (primarily from private wells) can increase the risk of lung cancer.

WHAT ARE THE SYMPTOMS OF LUNG CANCER?

Different people have different symptoms of lung cancer. Some people have symptoms related to the lungs. Some people whose lung cancer has spread to other parts of the body (metastasized) have symptoms specific to that part of the body. Some people just have general symptoms of not feeling well. Most people with lung cancer do not have symptoms until the cancer is advanced. Lung cancer symptoms may include:

- coughing that gets worse or does not go away
- chest pain
- shortness of breath
- wheezing
- coughing up blood
- feeling very tired all the time
- weight loss with no known cause

Other changes that can sometimes occur with lung cancer may include repeated bouts of pneumonia and swollen or enlarged lymph nodes (glands) inside the chest in the area between the lungs.

These symptoms can happen with other illnesses, too. If you have some of these symptoms, talk to your doctor, who can help find the cause.

WHAT CAN YOU DO TO REDUCE YOUR RISK OF LUNG CANCER?

You can help lower your risk of lung cancer in the following ways:

- **Do not smoke.** Cigarette smoking causes about 80–90 percent of lung cancer deaths in the United States. The most important thing you can do to prevent lung cancer is to not start smoking or to quit if you smoke.
- **Avoid secondhand smoke.** Smoke from other people's cigarettes, cigars, or pipes is called "secondhand smoke." Make your home and car smoke-free.
- **Get your home tested for radon.** The EPA recommends that all homes be tested for radon.
- **Be careful at work.** Health and safety guidelines in the workplace can help workers avoid carcinogens—things that can cause cancer.

WHO SHOULD BE SCREENED FOR LUNG CANCER?

Screening means testing for a disease when there are no symptoms or history of that disease. Doctors recommend a screening test to find a disease early when treatment may work better.

The only recommended screening test for lung cancer is low-dose computed tomography (also called a "low-dose CT scan" (LDCT)). In this test, an x-ray machine scans the body and uses low doses of radiation to make detailed pictures of the lungs.

Who Should Be Screened?

The U.S. Preventive Services Task Force (USPSTF) recommends yearly lung cancer screening with LDCT for people who:

- have a history of heavy smoking
- smoke now or have quit within the past 15 years
- are between the ages of 55 and 80

Heavy smoking means a smoking history of 30 pack years or more. A pack year is smoking an average of one pack of cigarettes per day for one year. For example, a person could have a 30-pack-year history by smoking one pack a day for 30 years or two packs a day for 15 years.

Risks of Screening

Lung cancer screening has at least three risks:

- A lung cancer screening test can suggest that a person has lung cancer when no cancer is present. This is called a "false-positive result." False-positive results can lead to follow-up tests and surgeries that are not needed and may have more risks.
- A lung cancer screening test can find cases of cancer that may never have caused a problem for the patient. This is called "overdiagnosis." Overdiagnosis can lead to treatment that is not needed.
- Radiation from repeated LDCT tests can cause cancer in otherwise healthy people.

That is why lung cancer screening is recommended only for adults who have no symptoms but are at high risk for developing the disease because of their smoking history and age.

If you are thinking about getting screened, talk to your doctor. If lung cancer screening is right for you, your doctor can refer you to a high-quality screening facility.

The best way to reduce your risk of lung cancer is to not smoke and to avoid secondhand smoke. Lung cancer screening is not a substitute for quitting smoking.

When Should Screening Stop?

The USPSTF recommends that yearly lung cancer screening stop when the person being screened:

- turns 81 years of age
- has not smoked in 15 years
- develops a health problem that makes him or her unwilling or unable to have surgery if lung cancer is found

HOW IS LUNG CANCER DIAGNOSED AND TREATED?
Types of Lung Cancer
The two main types of lung cancer are small-cell lung cancer and non-small-cell lung cancer. These categories refer to what the cancer cells look like under a microscope. Non-small-cell lung cancer is more common than small-cell lung cancer.

Staging
If lung cancer is diagnosed, other tests are done to find out how far it has spread through the lungs, lymph nodes, and the rest of the body. This process is called "staging." The type and stage of lung cancer tell doctors what kind of treatment you need.

Types of Treatment
Lung cancer is treated in several ways, depending on the type of lung cancer and how far it has spread. People with non-small-cell lung cancer can be treated with surgery, chemotherapy, radiation therapy, targeted therapy, or a combination of these treatments. People with small-cell lung cancer are usually treated with radiation therapy and chemotherapy.

Complementary and Alternative Medicines
Complementary and alternative medicines are medicines and health practices that are not standard cancer treatments.
- **Complementary medicine.** This is used in addition to standard treatments. Examples include acupuncture, dietary supplements, massage therapy, hypnosis, and meditation.
- **Alternative medicine.** This is used instead of standard treatments. Examples include special diets, megadose vitamins, herbal preparations, special teas, and magnet therapy.

Many kinds of complementary and alternative medicine have not been tested scientifically and may not be safe. Talk to your doctor about the risks and benefits before you start any kind of complementary or alternative medicine.

Which Treatment Is Right for You?

Choosing the treatment that is right for you may be hard. Talk to your cancer doctor about the treatment options available for your type and stage of cancer. Your doctor can explain the risks and benefits of each treatment and their side effects. Side effects are how your body reacts to drugs or other treatments.

Sometimes, people get an opinion from more than one cancer doctor. This is called a "second opinion." Getting a second opinion may help you choose the treatment that is right for you.[6]

Section 18.5 | Kidney Cancer

Our body has two kidneys, one on each side of the body, located behind the liver and stomach. The kidneys make urine, which is how the body washes liquid waste out of the body. The kidneys also play a role in controlling blood pressure and stimulating the bone marrow to make red blood cells (RBCs).

When cancer starts in the kidney, it is called "kidney and renal pelvis cancer." It can also be called "renal cell cancer" as that is the most common type of kidney and renal pelvis cancer.

WHAT IS THE RENAL PELVIS?

The renal pelvis is in the center of the kidney and is responsible for collecting the urine and feeding it into the ureters, two tubes that connect the kidneys with the bladder. The bladder holds urine until it is peed out.

STATISTICS ON KIDNEY AND RENAL PELVIS CANCER

In 2020, the latest year for which incidence data are available, in the United States, 40,220 new cases of kidney and renal pelvis cancer

---

[6] "What Is Lung Cancer?" Centers for Disease Control and Prevention (CDC), October 25, 2022. Available online. URL: www.cdc.gov/cancer/lung/basic_info/what-is-lung-cancer.htm. Accessed July 18, 2023.

Cancers in Men

were reported among men, and 9,541 men died of this cancer. For every 100,000 men, 22 new kidney and renal pelvis cancer cases were reported, and 5 men died of this cancer. Figures 18.1 and 18.2 show the rate of prevalence of kidney and renal pelvis cancer by gender and among different races and ethnicities.

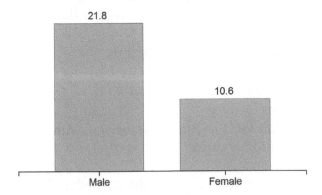

Figure 18.1. Kidney and Renal Pelvis Cancer, in Both Sexes

Centers for Disease Control and Prevention (CDC)

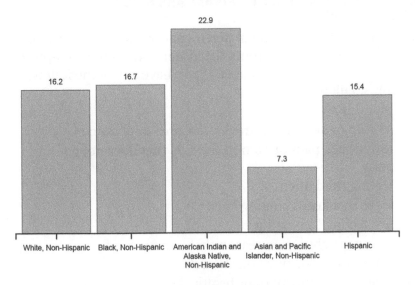

Figure 18.2. Kidney and Renal Pelvis Cancer, by Race and Ethnicity

Centers for Disease Control and Prevention (CDC)

WHAT ARE THE RISK FACTORS FOR KIDNEY AND RENAL PELVIS CANCERS?

Risk factors of kidney and renal pelvis cancers include the following:

- being overweight or having obesity
- smoking
- having high blood pressure (HBP; it is not known whether the increased risk is due to HBP itself or the medicines used to treat it)
- taking certain pain medicines for a long time
- having certain genetic conditions
- having a long-lasting infection with hepatitis C
- having kidney stones
- having sickle cell trait (SCT), which is associated with a very rare form of kidney cancer (renal medullary carcinoma)
- being exposed to a chemical called "trichloroethylene," which is used to remove grease from metal

WHAT ARE THE SYMPTOMS OF KIDNEY AND RENAL PELVIS CANCERS?

A person with kidney or renal pelvis cancer may or may not have one or more of the symptoms listed here. The same symptoms can also come from other causes. If you have any of the following symptoms, talk to your doctor.

- blood in the urine
- a lump or swelling in the kidney area or abdomen
- lower back pain or pain in the side that does not go away
- feeling tired often
- fever that keeps coming back
- not feeling like eating
- losing weight for no reason that you know of
- something blocking your bowels
- a general feeling of poor health

HOW COULD YOU REDUCE YOUR RISK FOR KIDNEY AND RENAL PELVIS CANCERS?

To lower your risk of kidney and renal pelvis cancers, do the following:

- Do not smoke or quit if you do.
- Keep a healthy weight.
- Eat a healthy diet.
- Exercise.
- Be very careful if you use certain kinds of chemicals, especially trichloroethylene. This chemical is used by workers in some jobs (e.g., those who work with metals).[7]

Section 18.6 | Bladder Cancer

The bladder (sometimes called the "urinary bladder") is a balloon-shaped organ in your lower abdomen, near the pelvis. It stores urine from the kidneys until it is passed out of the body. When cancer starts in the bladder, it is called "bladder cancer."

STATISTICS ON BLADDER CANCER

In 2020, the latest year for which incidence data are available, in the United States, 53,946 new cases of urinary bladder cancer were reported among men, and 12,064 men died of this cancer. For every 100,000 men, 30 new urinary bladder cancer cases were reported, and 7 men died of this cancer. Figures 18.3 and 18.4 show the rate of prevalence of urinary bladder cancer by gender and among different races and ethnicities.

---

[7] "Kidney Cancer," Centers for Disease Control and Prevention (CDC), July 6, 2022. Available online. URL: www.cdc.gov/cancer/kidney/index.htm. Accessed June 26, 2023.

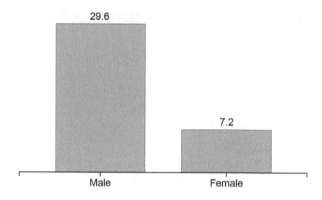

Figure 18.3. Urinary Bladder Cancer, in Both Sexes

Centers for Disease Control and Prevention (CDC)

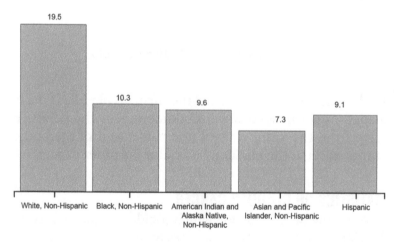

Figure 18.4. Urinary Bladder Cancer, by Race and Ethnicity

Centers for Disease Control and Prevention (CDC)

RISK FACTORS OF BLADDER CANCER

Smoking is the most important risk factor for bladder cancer. Other risk factors include the following:

- having a family history of bladder cancer
- having certain gene mutations (unusual changes made when your body's cells are dividing)

- being exposed to too much of certain workplace chemicals used in processing paint, dye, metal, and petroleum products
- taking some kinds of chemotherapy drugs
- drinking well water contaminated with arsenic
- taking the Chinese herb *Aristolochia fangchi*
- having chronic urinary tract infections (UTIs; including those caused by *Schistosoma haematobium*)

WHAT ARE THE SYMPTOMS OF BLADDER CANCER?

The most common symptom is blood in the urine. Other symptoms include:
- having to urinate often
- pain while urinating
- back pain
- pelvic pain

These symptoms can also come from other conditions. If you have any of them, talk to your doctor, which is the only way to find out what may be causing them.

HOW COULD YOU REDUCE YOUR RISK OF BLADDER CANCER?

To lower the risk of bladder cancer, do not smoke (and, if you do, quit) and be especially careful around certain kinds of chemicals.[8]

---

[8] "Bladder Cancer," Centers for Disease Control and Prevention (CDC), July 6, 2022. Available online. URL: www.cdc.gov/cancer/bladder/index.htm. Accessed June 26, 2023.

Section 18.7 | Pancreatic Cancer

Pancreatic cancer is the fourth most common cause of cancer death among men and women in the United States.[9]

The rate of new cases of pancreatic cancer was 13.3 per 100,000 men and women per year. The death rate was 11.1 per 100,000 men and women per year. These rates are age-adjusted and based on 2016–2020 cases and deaths. Approximately 1.7 percent of men and women will be diagnosed with pancreatic cancer at some point during their lifetime, based on 2017–2019 data. In 2020, there were an estimated 95,389 people living with pancreatic cancer in the United States.[10]

RISK FACTORS OF PANCREATIC CANCER

Risk factors for pancreatic cancer include tobacco use; a personal history of pancreatitis, diabetes, or obesity; and a family history of pancreatic cancer. About 10 percent of patients with pancreatic cancer have a positive family history of the disease. The differences between the populations and the burden of disease may be related to higher rates of cigarette smoking and diabetes mellitus among African-American men versus White men and higher body mass indices among African-American women versus White women.

SYMPTOMS OF PANCREATIC CANCER

Patients often remain asymptomatic or have only nonspecific symptoms such as malaise, fatigue, and loss of appetite until late in the course of the disease—often after it has spread extensively—when weight loss, jaundice, and severe abdominal pain often appear. Due to late diagnosis, approximately 80–85 percent of cases are unresectable (i.e., too advanced to permit surgical resection), and

---

[9] Effective Health Care Program, "Imaging Tests for the Diagnosis and Staging of Pancreatic Adenocarcinoma," Agency for Healthcare Research and Quality (AHRQ), January 2020. Available online. URL: https://effectivehealthcare.ahrq.gov/products/cancer-pancreas/research-protocol. Accessed July 19, 2023.

[10] Surveillance, Epidemiology, and End Results (SEER) Program, "Cancer Stat Facts: Pancreatic Cancer," National Cancer Institute (NCI), April 19, 2023. Available online. URL: https://seer.cancer.gov/statfacts/html/pancreas.html. Accessed July 19, 2023.

the median survival of patients with unresectable tumors is only 6–10 months.

Common symptoms leading to suspicion of pancreatic cancer are jaundice, epigastric pain, and weight loss. Signs and symptoms alone, however, are insufficient to diagnose pancreatic cancer.

DIAGNOSIS OF PANCREATIC CANCER

Screening for pancreatic adenocarcinoma is not recommended for the general population (e.g., the U.S. Preventive Services Task Force (USPTF) gives it a D recommendation). However, some professional organizations recommend screening those who are at high risk of developing pancreatic cancer. One report suggested that having two or more first-degree relatives with pancreatic cancer (or three or more blood relatives with pancreatic cancer, one of whom is a first-degree relative) is sufficient justification for considering a screening test. Furthermore, some genetic risk factors (e.g., Peutz-Jeghers syndrome, Lynch syndrome, and *BRCA2*, *PALB2*, and *p16* mutations) motivate testing when the patient also has had a first-degree relative with pancreatic cancer.

Imaging Tests for Diagnosing Pancreatic Cancer

Multidetector computed tomography (MDCT) scan is often the first imaging test in a patient whose symptoms suggest pancreatic adenocarcinoma. It provides three-dimensional (3D) multiplanar reconstruction images that enable the determination of tumor size, extent, and spread with a standardized pancreas protocol. The test does not always differentiate malignant from benign pancreatic lesions, and its ability to detect small tumors or small hepatic/peritoneal metastases is limited. A concern about MDCT is that the procedure exposes the patient to radiation and therefore may increase cancer risk. Also, the quality of the CT protocol, as well as the experience and expertise of the radiologist reading the CT, may influence the accuracy of MDCT for diagnosis and staging of pancreatic adenocarcinoma.

One notable type of MDCT is MDCT with angiography with or without 3D reconstruction. This technology permits more precise imaging of blood vessels than other forms of MDCT.

Other procedures and imaging tests are also used to aid the diagnosis of pancreatic adenocarcinoma, including endoscopic ultrasound-guided fine-needle aspiration (EUS-FNA), positron emission tomography-computed tomography (PET-CT), and magnetic resonance imaging (MRI).

For EUS-FNA, a specialized ultrasound probe is introduced orally and advanced via an endoscope through the upper gastrointestinal (GI) tract toward the pancreas. The probe's proximity to the pancreas allows the ultrasound to access and image the entire pancreas, the related vasculature, and associated lymph nodes. The endoscopist can take a small aspiration (FNA) of any suspicious lesions, permitting cytologic evaluation. If the biopsy is adequate, EUS-FNA can distinguish benign from malignant lesions and characterize certain types of lesions (e.g., cystic pancreatic lesions). Reported disadvantages of EUS-FNA include the procedure's invasiveness, dependence on the skill of the endoscopist, and its inability to evaluate distant metastases. The relative newness of EUS-FNA could mean a large variation in endoscopists' technical skills. Potential patient harms related to EUS-FNA include perforation and bleeding, pancreatitis, and adverse effects related to sedation.

PET is a whole-body scan whose image highlights where a radioisotope tracer concentrates and is, therefore, particularly useful for detecting distant metastases. The most commonly used radioisotope tracer is fluorodeoxyglucose 18F (FDG). FDG-PET can locate sites metabolically active, such as malignant tumors or sites with inflammation, and may help distinguish malignant tumors from benign pancreatic cysts or other masses that are not metabolically active. FDG-PET and CT can be combined to add precise anatomic localization (from CT) to functional data (from PET). The two scans are acquired concurrently, and the data from each are merged.

MRI is an alternative to MDCT as an initial imaging test for patients with a clinical suspicion of pancreatic adenocarcinoma or as a tool to evaluate the extent of the disease. During an MRI procedure, electromagnetic fields and radiofrequency radiation translate hydrogen nuclei distribution in body tissues into images of anatomic structure. Similar to MDCT, a standardized pancreas protocol is available. MRI may be helpful when characterizing small (less than 1 cm) hepatic lesions, differentiating an inflammatory pancreatic mass from pancreatic adenocarcinoma, or detecting metastases to the liver. MRI can also be used as an adjunct to CT to better detect extrahepatic disease.

STAGING OF PANCREATIC CANCER

The most commonly used system for staging pancreatic adenocarcinoma is the 2010 American Joint Committee on Cancer (AJCC) system:

- stage 0 (carcinoma in situ, with neither lymph node involvement nor metastases)
- stage IA (a less than equal to 2 cm tumor limited to the pancreas, with neither lymph node involvement nor metastases)
- stage IB (a less than 2 cm tumor limited to the pancreas, with neither lymph node involvement nor metastases)
- stage IIA (any size tumor that extends beyond the pancreas but does not involve either the celiac axis or the superior mesenteric artery (SMA) and is without lymph node involvement or metastases)
- stage IIB (the same as IIA, except the lymph nodes are involved)
- stage III (any size tumor that involves the celiac axis or SMA and lymph nodes but without metastases)
- stage IV (any size tumor, any lymph node involvement, and metastases)

An exact staging process before surgery (i.e., assigning the patient to stage I/II/III/IV) for pancreatic adenocarcinoma may not be carried out, and the patient's disease is often staged at surgery.

Resectability

Surgical resection offers the only hope of cure and is decided via multidisciplinary consultation (e.g., surgeon, gastroenterologist, radiologist, oncologist, radiation oncologist). The two key factors in assessing resectability are distant metastasis (which usually indicates unresectability) and blood vessel involvement (which sometimes indicates unresectability, depending on the degree of involvement). The major blood vessels of focus are the superior mesenteric vein (SMV), the portal vein, the celiac artery, the common hepatic artery, and the SMA. According to the guideline from the National Comprehensive Cancer Network (NCCN) on pancreatic adenocarcinoma:

- A resectable tumor shows no involvement of either the SMV or portal vein and shows "clear fat planes" around the celiac axis, hepatic artery, and SMA, and there are no distant metastases.
- An unresectable tumor has a less than 180 degree encasement of the SMA or any celiac abutment, an unreconstructible SMV/portal vein occlusion, any aortic invasion/encasement, or any distant metastases.
- A "borderline" resectable tumor fits neither of the two categories described above (e.g., some abutment of the SMV/portal vein, a less than 180-degree abutment of the SMA). For these cases, the NCCN recommends biopsy and possible neoadjuvant chemotherapy, which may shrink the tumor and permit subsequent resection.

These criteria continue to evolve, as surgical techniques advance and more tumors are deemed resectable via reconstruction of blood vessels.

Regarding the interface between stage and resectability, the AJCC and other professional organizations state that stages I and II are resectable, but stages III and IV are not. However, it is believed that minor arterial involvement (stage III) may still permit resection.

PROGNOSIS OF PANCREATIC CANCER
Pancreatic adenocarcinoma is fatal if untreated, so it is critical to choose the right imaging test and initiate therapy in a timely manner. A comparative effectiveness review (CER) on this topic can assist medical decisions in several ways.[11]

---

[11] See footnote [9].

Section 18.8 | **Penile Cancer**

Penile cancer is a disease in which malignant (cancer) cells form in the tissues of the penis.

The penis is a rod-shaped male reproductive organ that passes sperm and urine from the body. It contains the following two types of erectile tissue (spongy tissue with blood vessels that fill with blood to make an erection):

- **Corpora cavernosa**. The two columns of erectile tissue that form most of the penis.
- **Corpus spongiosum**. The single column of erectile tissue that forms a small portion of the penis. The corpus spongiosum surrounds the urethra (the tube through which urine and sperm pass from the body).

The erectile tissue is wrapped in connective tissue and covered with skin. The glans (head of the penis) is covered with loose skin called the "foreskin."

STAGES OF PENILE CANCER
Stage 0
Stage 0 is divided into stages 0is and 0a.

- **Stage 0is**. In this stage, abnormal cells are found on the surface of the skin of the penis. These abnormal cells form growths that may become cancer and spread into nearby normal tissue. Stage 0is is also called "carcinoma in situ" or "penile intraepithelial neoplasia."
- **Stage 0a**. In this stage, squamous cell cancer that does not spread is found on the surface of the skin of the penis or on the underneath surface of the foreskin of the penis. Stage 0a is also called "noninvasive localized squamous cell carcinoma."

Stage I
In stage I, cancer has formed and spread to the tissue just under the skin of the penis. Cancer has not spread to lymph vessels, blood

vessels, or nerves. The cancer cells look more like normal cells under a microscope.

Stage II

Stage II is divided into stages IIA and IIB.

In stage IIA, cancer has spread:

- to the tissue just under the skin of the penis (The cancer has spread to lymph vessels, blood vessels, and/or nerves.)
- to tissue just under the skin of the penis (Under a microscope, the cancer cells look very abnormal, or the cells are sarcomatoid.)
- into the corpus spongiosum (The spongy erectile tissue in the shaft and glans fills with blood to make an erection.)

In stage IIB, cancer has spread:

- through the layer of connective tissue that surrounds the corpus cavernosum and into the corpus cavernosum (spongy erectile tissue that runs along the shaft of the penis)

Stage III

Stage III is divided into stages IIIA and IIIB. Cancer is found in the penis.

- **Stage IIIA.** In this stage, cancer has spread to one or two lymph nodes on one side of the groin.
- **Stage IIIB.** In this stage, cancer has spread to 3 or more lymph nodes on one side of the groin or to lymph nodes on both sides of the groin.

Stage IV

In stage IV, cancer has spread:

- to tissues near the penis, such as the scrotum, prostate, or pubic bone, and may have spread to lymph nodes in the groin or pelvis

- to one or more lymph nodes in the pelvis or through the outer covering of the lymph nodes to nearby tissue
- to lymph nodes outside the pelvis or to other parts of the body, such as the lung, liver, or bone

RISK FACTORS OF PENILE CANCER

Human papillomavirus (HPV) infection may increase the risk of developing penile cancer.

Anything that increases a person's chance of getting a disease is called a "risk factor." Not every person with one or more of these risk factors will develop penile cancer, and it will develop in people who do not have any known risk factors. Talk with your doctor if you think you may be at risk.

Risk factors for penile cancer include the following:
- being uncircumcised (Circumcision may help prevent infection with the human papillomavirus (HPV). A circumcision is an operation in which the doctor removes part or all of the foreskin from the penis. Many boys are circumcised shortly after birth. Men who were not circumcised at birth may have a higher risk of developing penile cancer.)
- being age 60 or older
- having phimosis (a condition in which the foreskin of the penis cannot be pulled back over the glans)
- having poor personal hygiene
- having many sexual partners
- using tobacco products

SIGNS OF PENILE CANCER

These and other signs may be caused by penile cancer or by other conditions. Check with your doctor if you have any of the following:
- redness, irritation, or a sore on the penis
- a lump on the penis

DIAGNOSE OF PENILE CANCER

In addition to asking about your personal and family health history and doing a physical exam, your doctor may perform the following tests and procedures:

- **Physical exam of the penis**. An exam in which the doctor checks the penis for signs of disease, such as lumps or anything else that seems unusual.
- **Biopsy**. The removal of cells or tissues, so they can be viewed under a microscope by a pathologist to check for signs of cancer. The tissue sample is removed during one of the following procedures:
  - **Incisional biopsy**. The removal of part of a lump or a sample of tissue that does not look normal.
  - **Excisional biopsy**. The removal of an entire lump or area of tissue that does not look normal.

TREATMENT FOR PENILE CANCER

Different types of treatments are available for patients with penile cancer. Some treatments are standard (the currently used treatment), and some are being tested in clinical trials. A treatment clinical trial is a research study meant to help improve current treatments or obtain information on new treatments for patients with cancer. When clinical trials show that a new treatment is better than the standard treatment, the new treatment may become the standard treatment. Patients may want to think about taking part in a clinical trial. Some clinical trials are open only to patients who have not started treatment.

The following are a few types of treatments used.

Surgery

Surgery is the most common treatment for all stages of penile cancer. A doctor may remove the cancer using one of the following operations:

- **Mohs microsurgery**. A procedure in which the tumor is cut from the skin in thin layers. During the surgery, the edges of the tumor and each layer of the tumor removed are viewed through a microscope to check for cancer cells. Layers continue to be removed until no more cancer cells are seen. This type of surgery removes as little normal tissue as possible and is often used to remove cancer on the skin. It is also called "Mohs surgery."

- **Laser surgery**. A surgical procedure that uses a laser beam (a narrow beam of intense light) as a knife to make bloodless cuts in tissue or to remove a surface lesion such as a tumor.
- **Cryosurgery**. A treatment that uses an instrument to freeze and destroy abnormal tissue. This type of treatment is also called "cryotherapy."
- **Circumcision**. Surgery to remove part or all of the foreskin of the penis.
- **Wide local excision**. Surgery to remove only the cancer and some normal tissue around it.
- **Amputation of the penis**. Surgery to remove part or all of the penis. If part of the penis is removed, it is a partial penectomy. If all of the penis is removed, it is a total penectomy.

Lymph nodes in the groin may be taken out during surgery.

After the doctor removes all the cancer that can be seen at the time of the surgery, some patients may be given chemotherapy or radiation therapy after surgery to kill any cancer cells that are left. Treatment given after the surgery to lower the risk that the cancer will come back is called "adjuvant therapy."

Radiation Therapy

Radiation therapy is a cancer treatment that uses high-energy x-rays or other types of radiation to kill cancer cells or keep them from growing. The following are the two types of radiation therapy:

- **External radiation therapy**. This therapy uses a machine outside the body to send radiation toward the area of the body with cancer.

- **Internal radiation therapy.** This therapy uses a radioactive substance sealed in needles, seeds, wires, or catheters that are placed directly into or near the cancer.

The way the radiation therapy is given depends on the type and stage of the cancer being treated. External and internal radiation therapy are used to treat penile cancer.

Chemotherapy

Chemotherapy is a cancer treatment that uses drugs to stop the growth of cancer cells, either by killing the cells or by stopping them from dividing. When chemotherapy is taken by mouth or injected into a vein or muscle, the drugs enter the bloodstream and can reach cancer cells throughout the body (systemic chemotherapy). When chemotherapy is placed directly onto the skin (topical chemotherapy), the drugs mainly affect cancer cells in those areas (regional chemotherapy). The way the chemotherapy is given depends on the type and stage of the cancer being treated.

Topical chemotherapy may be used to treat stage 0 penile cancer.

Immunotherapy

Immunotherapy is a treatment that uses the patient's immune system to fight cancer. Substances made by the body or made in a laboratory are used to boost, direct, or restore the body's natural defenses against cancer. Topical immunotherapy with imiquimod may be used to treat stage 0 penile cancer.[12]

[12] "Penile Cancer Treatment (PDQ®)—Patient Version," National Cancer Institute (NCI), May 12, 2023. Available online. URL: www.cancer.gov/types/penile/patient/penile-treatment-pdq. Accessed July 18, 2023.

Section 18.9 | **Prostate Cancer**

The prostate is a part of the male reproductive system, which includes the penis, prostate, and testicles (see Figure 18.5). The prostate is located just below the bladder and in front of the rectum. It is about the size of a walnut and surrounds the urethra (the tube that empties urine from the bladder). It produces fluid that makes up a part of semen.

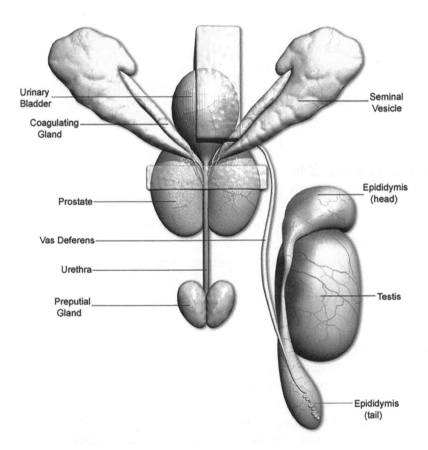

Figure 18.5. The Male Reproductive and Urinary System

National Institute of Diabetes and Digestive and Kidney Diseases (NIDDK)

As a man ages, the prostate tends to increase in size. This can cause the urethra to narrow and decrease urine flow. This is called "benign prostatic hyperplasia" (BPH), and it is not the same as prostate cancer. Men may also have other prostate changes that are not cancerous. When cancer starts in the prostate, it is called "prostate cancer." Prostate cancer is the most common cancer in American men.

WHO IS AT RISK OF PROSTATE CANCER?

All men are at risk for prostate cancer. Out of every 100 American men, about 13 will get prostate cancer during their lifetime, and about 2–3 men will die from prostate cancer.

The most common risk factor is age. The older a man is, the greater the chance of getting prostate cancer.

Some men are at increased risk for prostate cancer. You are at an increased risk of getting or dying from prostate cancer if you are African American or have a family history of prostate cancer.

African-American Men

- They are more likely to get prostate cancer than other men.
- They are more than twice as likely to die from prostate cancer than White men.
- They get prostate cancer at a younger age, tend to have more advanced disease when it is found, and tend to have a more severe type of prostate cancer than other men.

Family History

For some men, genetic factors may put them at higher risk of prostate cancer. You may have an increased risk of getting a type of prostate cancer caused by genetic changes that are inherited if:

- you have a first-degree relative (father, son, or brother) who had prostate cancer, including relatives in three generations on your mother's or father's side of the family

- you were diagnosed with prostate cancer when you were 55 years old or younger
- you were diagnosed with prostate cancer and other members of your family have been diagnosed with breast, ovarian, or pancreatic cancer

WHAT ARE THE SYMPTOMS OF PROSTATE CANCER?

Different people have different symptoms of prostate cancer. Some men do not have symptoms at all.

Some symptoms of prostate cancer are:
- difficulty starting urination
- weak or interrupted flow of urine
- frequent urination, especially at night
- difficulty emptying the bladder completely
- pain or burning during urination
- blood in the urine or semen
- pain in the back, hips, or pelvis that does not go away
- painful ejaculation

Keep in mind that these symptoms may be caused by conditions other than prostate cancer.

WHAT IS SCREENING FOR PROSTATE CANCER?

Cancer screening means looking for cancer before it causes symptoms. The goal of screening for prostate cancer is to find cancers that may be at high risk for spreading if not treated and to find them early before they spread.

If you are thinking about being screened, learn about the possible benefits and harms of screening, diagnosis, and treatment and talk to your doctor about your personal risk factors.

There is no standard test to screen for prostate cancer. The following are the two tests that are commonly used to screen for prostate cancer.

Prostate-Specific Antigen Test

A blood test called a "prostate-specific antigen" (PSA) test measures the level of PSA in the blood. PSA is a substance made by the prostate. The levels of PSA in the blood can be higher in men who have prostate cancer. The PSA level may also be elevated in other conditions that affect the prostate.

As a rule, the higher the PSA level in the blood, the more likely a prostate problem is present. But many factors, such as age and race, can affect PSA levels. Some prostate glands make more PSA than others.

Prostate-specific antigen levels can also be affected by:
- certain medical procedures
- certain medications
- an enlarged prostate
- a prostate infection

Because many factors can affect PSA levels, your doctor is the best person to interpret your PSA test results. If the PSA test is abnormal, your doctor may recommend a biopsy to find out if you have prostate cancer.

Digital Rectal Examination

Digital rectal examination (DRE) is when a health-care provider inserts a gloved, lubricated finger into a man's rectum to feel the prostate for anything abnormal such as cancer. In 2018, the U.S. Preventive Services Task Force stated that it does not recommend DRE as a screening test because of a lack of evidence on the benefits.

WHO SHOULD GET SCREENED FOR PROSTATE CANCER?

In 2018, the U.S. Preventive Services Task Force (USPSTF) made the following recommendations about prostate cancer screening:
- Men aged 55–69 should make individual decisions about being screened for prostate cancer with a PSA test.
- Before making a decision, men should talk to their doctor about the benefits and harms of screening for prostate cancer, including the benefits and harms of other tests and treatments.

- Men aged 70 and older should not be screened for prostate cancer routinely.

This recommendation applies to men who:
- are at average risk for prostate cancer
- are at increased risk for prostate cancer
- do not have symptoms of prostate cancer
- have never been diagnosed with prostate cancer

Other organizations such as the American Urological Association (AUA), the American Cancer Society (ACS), and the American College of Physicians (ACP) may have other recommendations.

Talk to Your Doctor
If you are thinking about being screened, you and your doctor should consider:
- if you have a family history of prostate cancer
- if you are African American
- if you have other medical conditions that may make it difficult for you to be treated for prostate cancer if it is found or that may make you less likely to benefit from screening
- how you value the potential benefits and harms of screening, diagnosis, and treatment

WHAT ARE THE BENEFITS AND HARMS OF PROSTATE CANCER SCREENING?
Possible Benefits of Screening
The benefits of screening for prostate cancer may include the following:
- Screening can help find prostate cancers that may be at high risk of spreading early so that they can be treated before they spread. This may lower the chance of death from prostate cancer in some men.
- Some men prefer to know if they have prostate cancer.

Possible Harms
The possible harms of screening for prostate cancer include harms from screening, diagnosis, and treatment.

POSSIBLE HARM FROM SCREENING

- **False-positive test results**. This occurs when a man has an abnormal PSA test but does not have prostate cancer. False-positive test results often lead to unnecessary tests, such as a biopsy of the prostate. They may cause men to worry about their health. Older men are more likely to have false-positive test results.

POSSIBLE HARMS FROM DIAGNOSIS

Screening finds prostate cancer in some men who would never have had symptoms from their cancer in their lifetime. Treatment of men who would not have had symptoms or died from prostate cancer can cause them to have complications from treatment, but not benefit from treatment. This is called "overdiagnosis."

Prostate cancer is diagnosed with a prostate biopsy. A biopsy is when a small piece of tissue is removed from the prostate and looked at under a microscope to see if there are cancer cells. Older men are more likely to have a complication after a prostate biopsy.

A prostate biopsy can cause:

- pain
- blood in the semen or ejaculate
- infection

POSSIBLE HARMS FROM TREATMENT

The most common treatments for prostate cancer are surgery to remove the prostate and radiation therapy.

The most common harms from prostate cancer treatment are as follows:

- **Urinary incontinence (accidental leakage of urine)**. About one out of every five men who have surgery to remove the prostate loses bladder control.
- **Erectile dysfunction (impotence)**. About two out of every three men who have surgery to remove the prostate become impotent, and about half of the men who receive radiation therapy become impotent.
- **Bowel problems**. This includes fecal incontinence (accidental leakage of bowel movements) and urgency

(sudden and uncontrollable urge to have a bowel movement). About one out of every six men who have radiation therapy has bowel problems.

HOW IS PROSTATE CANCER DIAGNOSED?

A biopsy is a procedure that can be used to diagnose prostate cancer.

A biopsy is when a small piece of tissue is removed from the prostate and looked at under a microscope to see if there are cancer cells.

A Gleason score is determined when the biopsy is looked at under the microscope. If there is cancer, the score indicates how likely it is to spread. The score ranges from 2 to 10. The lower the score, the less likely it is that cancer will spread.

A biopsy is the main tool for diagnosing prostate cancer, but a doctor can use other tools to help make sure the biopsy is made in the right place. For example, doctors may use a transrectal ultrasound when a probe the size of a finger is inserted into the rectum and high-energy sound waves (ultrasound) are bounced off the prostate to create a picture of the prostate called a "sonogram." Magnetic resonance imaging (MRI) uses magnets and radio waves to produce images on a computer. MRI does not use any radiation.

Staging

If prostate cancer is diagnosed, other tests are done to find out if cancer cells have spread within the prostate or to other parts of the body. This process is called "staging." Whether the cancer is only in the prostate or has spread outside the prostate determines your stage of prostate cancer. The stage of prostate cancer tells doctors what kind of treatment you need.

HOW IS PROSTATE CANCER TREATED?

Different types of treatment are available for prostate cancer. You and your doctor will decide which treatment is right for you. Some common treatments are as follows:

- **Expectant management**. If your doctor thinks your prostate cancer is unlikely to grow quickly, he or she may recommend that you do not treat the cancer right away. Instead, you can choose to wait and see if you get symptoms in one of two ways:

- **Active surveillance.** It involves closely monitoring prostate cancer by performing PSA and DRE tests and prostate biopsies regularly and treating cancer only if it grows or causes symptoms.
- **Watchful waiting.** No tests are done. Your doctor treats any symptoms when they develop. This is usually recommended for men who are expected to live for 10 more years or less.
- **Surgery.** A prostatectomy is an operation where doctors remove the prostate. Radical prostatectomy removes the prostate as well as the surrounding tissue.
- **Radiation therapy.** Using high-energy rays (similar to x-rays) to kill cancer. The following are the two types of radiation therapy:
  - **External radiation therapy.** A machine outside the body directs radiation at the cancer cells.
  - **Internal radiation therapy (brachytherapy).** Radioactive seeds or pellets are surgically placed into or near cancer to destroy the cancer cells.

Other therapies used in the treatment of prostate cancer that is still under investigation include the following:

- **Cryotherapy.** Placing a special probe inside or near the prostate cancer to freeze and kill the cancer cells.
- **Chemotherapy.** Using special drugs to shrink or kill cancer. The drugs can be pills you take or medicines given through your veins or, sometimes, both.
- **Biological therapy.** Working with your body's immune system to help it fight cancer or to control side effects from other cancer treatments. Side effects are how your body reacts to drugs or other treatments.
- **High-intensity focused ultrasound.** Directing high-energy sound waves (ultrasound) at cancer to kill cancer cells.

- **Hormone therapy.** Blocking cancer cells from getting the hormones they need to grow.[13]

Section 18.10 | Testicular Cancer

The testicles are two egg-shaped glands located inside the scrotum (a sac of loose skin that lies directly below the penis). The testicles are held within the scrotum by the spermatic cord, which also contains the vas deferens and vessels and nerves of the testicles.

The testicles are the male sex glands and produce testosterone and sperm. Germ cells within the testicles produce immature sperm that travel through a network of tubules (tiny tubes) and larger tubes into the epididymis (a long coiled tube next to the testicles) where the sperm mature and are stored.

WHAT IS TESTICULAR CANCER?
Almost all testicular cancers start in the germ cells. The two main types of testicular germ cell tumors are seminomas and nonseminomas. These two types grow and spread differently and are treated differently. Nonseminomas tend to grow and spread more quickly than seminomas. Seminomas are more sensitive to radiation. A testicular tumor that contains both seminoma and nonseminoma cells is treated as a nonseminoma.

Testicular cancer is the most common cancer in men aged 20–35.

RISKS OF TESTICULAR CANCER
Anything that increases a person's chance of getting a disease is called a "risk factor." Not every person with one or more of the following risk factors will develop testicular cancer, and it will

[13] "What Is Prostate Cancer?" Centers for Disease Control and Prevention (CDC), August 25, 2022. Available online. URL: www.cdc.gov/cancer/prostate/basic_info/what-is-prostate-cancer.htm. Accessed June 19, 2023.

develop in people who do not have any known risk factors. Talk with your doctor if you think you may be at risk. Risk factors for testicular cancer include:

- having had an undescended testicle
- having had abnormal development of the testicles
- having a personal history of testicular cancer
- having a family history of testicular cancer (especially in a father or brother)
- being White

SIGNS AND SYMPTOMS OF TESTICULAR CANCER

The following and other signs and symptoms may be caused by testicular cancer or by other conditions. Check with your doctor if you have any of the following:

- a painless lump or swelling in either testicle
- a change in how the testicle feels
- a dull ache in the lower abdomen or the groin
- a sudden buildup of fluid in the scrotum
- pain or discomfort in a testicle or in the scrotum

DIAGNOSIS OF TESTICULAR CANCER

The following tests and procedures may be used:

- **Physical exam and history**. An exam of the body to check general signs of health, including checking for signs of disease, such as lumps or anything else that seems unusual. The testicles will be examined to check for lumps, swelling, or pain. A history of the patient's health habits and past illnesses and treatments will also be taken.
- **Ultrasound exam of the testes**. A procedure in which high-energy sound waves (ultrasound) are bounced off internal tissues or organs and make echoes. The echoes form a picture of body tissues called a "sonogram."
- **Serum tumor marker test**. A procedure in which a sample of blood is examined to measure the amounts of certain substances released into the blood by organs,

tissues, or tumor cells in the body. Certain substances are linked to specific types of cancer when found in increased levels in the blood. These are called "tumor markers." The following tumor markers are used to detect testicular cancer:

- alpha-fetoprotein (AFP)
- beta-human chorionic gonadotropin (β-hCG)

Tumor marker levels are measured before inguinal orchiectomy and biopsy to help diagnose testicular cancer.

- **Inguinal orchiectomy**. A procedure to remove the entire testicle through an incision in the groin. A tissue sample from the testicle is then viewed under a microscope to check for cancer cells. (The surgeon does not cut through the scrotum into the testicle to remove a sample of tissue for biopsy because, if cancer is present, this procedure could cause it to spread into the scrotum and lymph nodes. It is important to choose a surgeon who has experience with this kind of surgery.) If cancer is found, the cell type (seminoma or nonseminoma) is determined in order to help plan treatment.

FACTORS AFFECTING PROGNOSIS AND TREATMENT OPTIONS

The prognosis (chance of recovery) and treatment options depend on the following:

- stage of the cancer (whether it is in or near the testicle or has spread to other places in the body and blood levels of AFP, β-hCG, and LDH)
- type of cancer
- size of the tumor
- number and size of retroperitoneal lymph nodes

Testicular cancer can usually be cured in patients who receive adjuvant chemotherapy or radiation therapy after their primary treatment.

TREATMENT FOR TESTICULAR CANCER

There are different types of treatment for patients with testicular cancer. Surgery, radiation therapy, chemotherapy, surveillance, and high-dose chemotherapy with stem cell transplant are the different types of treatments used. Treatment for testicular cancer may cause side effects, such as infertility. Follow-up tests may be needed to see how well the treatment is working.[14]

Section 18.11 | Colorectal Cancer

WHAT IS COLORECTAL CANCER?

The colon is the large intestine or large bowel. The rectum is the passageway that connects the colon to the anus. Sometimes, abnormal growths, called "polyps," form in the colon or rectum. Over time, some polyps may turn into cancer. Colorectal cancer is a disease in which cells in the colon or rectum grow out of control. Sometimes, it is called "colon cancer," for short.

Screening tests can find polyps, so they can be removed before turning into cancer. Screening also helps find colorectal cancer at an early stage when treatment works best.

WHAT ARE THE RISK FACTORS FOR COLORECTAL CANCER?

Your risk of getting colorectal cancer increases as you get older. Other risk factors include:

- inflammatory bowel disease, such as Crohn's disease or ulcerative colitis
- a personal or family history of colorectal cancer or colorectal polyps
- a genetic syndrome such as familial adenomatous polyposis (FAP) or hereditary nonpolyposis colorectal cancer (Lynch syndrome)

---

[14] "Testicular Cancer Treatment (PDQ®)—Patient Version," National Cancer Institute (NCI), May 17, 2023. Available online. URL: www.cancer.gov/types/testicular/patient/testicular-treatment-pdq#_50. Accessed June 19, 2023.

Lifestyle factors that may contribute to an increased risk of colorectal cancer include:
- lack of regular physical activity
- a diet low in fruit and vegetables
- a low-fiber and high-fat diet or a diet high in processed meats
- overweight and obesity
- alcohol consumption
- tobacco use

WHAT ARE THE SYMPTOMS OF COLORECTAL CANCER?

Colorectal polyps (abnormal growths in the colon or rectum that can turn into cancer if not removed) and colorectal cancer do not always cause symptoms, especially at first. Someone could have polyps or colorectal cancer and not know it. That is why getting screened regularly for colorectal cancer is so important.

If you have symptoms, they may include:
- a change in bowel habits
- blood in or on your stool (bowel movement)
- diarrhea, constipation, or feeling that the bowel does not empty all the way
- abdominal pain, aches, or cramps that do not go away
- weight loss and you do not know why

If you have any of these symptoms, talk to your doctor. They may be caused by something other than cancer. The only way to know what is causing them is to see your doctor.

WHAT SHOULD YOU KNOW ABOUT SCREENING?
What Is Colorectal Cancer Screening?

A screening test is used to look for a disease when a person does not have symptoms. (When a person has symptoms, diagnostic tests are used to find out the cause of the symptoms.)

Colorectal cancer almost always develops from precancerous polyps (abnormal growths) in the colon or rectum. Screening tests can find precancerous polyps so that they can be removed before they turn into cancer. Screening tests can also find colorectal cancer early when treatment works best.

Screening Recommendations

Regular screening, beginning at age 45, is the key to preventing colorectal cancer and finding it early. The U.S. Preventive Services Task Force (USPSTF) recommends that adults aged 45–75 be screened for colorectal cancer. The USPSTF recommends that adults aged 76–85 talk to their doctor about screening.

The USPSTF recommends several colorectal cancer screening strategies, including stool tests, flexible sigmoidoscopy, colonoscopy, and computed tomography (CT) colonography (virtual colonoscopy).

When Should You Begin to Get Screened?

Most people should begin screening for colorectal cancer soon after turning 45 and then continue getting screened at regular intervals. If you think you are at increased risk for colorectal cancer, speak with your doctor about:

- when to begin screening
- which test is right for you
- how often to get tested

Colorectal Cancer Screening Tests

Several screening tests can be used to find polyps or colorectal cancer. The USPSTF outlines the following colorectal cancer screening strategies. It is important to know that if your test result is positive or abnormal on some screening tests (stool tests, flexible sigmoidoscopy, and CT colonography), a colonoscopy test is needed to complete the screening process. Talk to your doctor about which test is right for you.

STOOL TESTS

- The guaiac-based fecal occult blood test (gFOBT) uses the chemical guaiac to detect blood in the stool. It is done once a year. For this test, you receive a test kit from your health-care provider. At home, you use a stick or brush to obtain a small amount of stool. You return the test kit to the doctor or a lab, where the stool samples are checked for the presence of blood.

- The fecal immunochemical test (FIT) uses antibodies to detect blood in the stool. It is also done once a year in the same way as a gFOBT.
- The FIT-DNA test (also referred to as the "stool DNA test") combines the FIT with a test that detects altered DNA in the stool. For this test, you collect an entire bowel movement and send it to a lab, where it is checked for altered DNA and for the presence of blood. It is done once every three years.

FLEXIBLE SIGMOIDOSCOPY

For this test, the doctor puts a short, thin, flexible, lighted tube into your rectum. The doctor checks for polyps or cancer inside the rectum and lower third of the colon.

This test is done every 5 years or every 10 years with an FIT every year.

COLONOSCOPY

This is similar to flexible sigmoidoscopy, except the doctor uses a longer, thin, flexible, lighted tube to check for polyps or cancer inside the rectum and the entire colon. During the test, the doctor can find and remove most polyps and some cancers. A colonoscopy is also used as a follow-up test if anything unusual is found during one of the other screening tests.

This test is done every 10 years (for people who do not have an increased risk of colorectal cancer).

COMPUTED TOMOGRAPHY COLONOGRAPHY (VIRTUAL COLONOSCOPY)

CT colonography, also called a "virtual colonoscopy," uses x-rays and computers to produce images of the entire colon, which are displayed on a computer screen for the doctor to analyze.

This test is done every five years.

Insurance and Medicare Coverage

Colorectal cancer screening tests may be covered by your health insurance policy without a deductible or co-pay. For more information about Medicare coverage, visit www.medicare.gov or call 1-800-MEDICARE (1-800-633-4227). TTY users should call 1-877-486-2048. Check your insurance plan to find out what benefits are covered for colorectal cancer screening.

WHAT CAN YOU DO TO REDUCE YOUR RISK OF COLORECTAL CANCER?

Overall, the most effective way to reduce your risk of colorectal cancer is to get screened for colorectal cancer routinely, beginning at age 45.

Almost all colorectal cancers begin as precancerous polyps (abnormal growths) in the colon or rectum. Such polyps can be present in the colon for years before invasive cancer develops. They may not cause any symptoms, especially early on.

Diet

Research is underway to find out if changes to your diet can reduce your colorectal cancer risk. Medical experts often recommend a diet low in animal fats and high in fruits, vegetables, and whole grains to reduce the risk of other chronic diseases, such as coronary artery disease (CAD) and diabetes. This diet may also reduce the risk of colorectal cancer.

Healthy Choices

Some studies suggest that people may reduce their risk of developing colorectal cancer by increasing physical activity, keeping a healthy weight, limiting alcohol consumption, and avoiding tobacco.[15]

---

[15] "What Is Colorectal Cancer?" Centers for Disease Control and Prevention (CDC), February 23, 2023. Available online. URL: www.cdc.gov/cancer/colorectal/basic_info/what-is-colorectal-cancer.htm. Accessed June 19, 2023.

Chapter 19 | Mental Health Concerns in Men

Section 19.1 | Men and Mental Health

WHY IS MEN'S MENTAL HEALTH IMPORTANT?

Mental disorders affect men and women. The prevalence of several mental disorders is lower in men than in women. However, other disorders are diagnosed at comparable rates for men and women or at higher rates for men, such as attention deficit hyperactivity disorder (ADHD). Men are also more likely to die by suicide than women, according to the Centers for Disease Control and Prevention (CDC).

Certain symptoms may also be more common in men than women, and the course of illness can be affected by a person's sex. Researchers are only now beginning to tease apart the various biological and psychosocial factors that may impact mental health.

Men are less likely to have received mental health treatment than women in the past year. Recognizing the signs that you or someone you love may have a mental disorder is the first step toward getting treatment. The earlier that treatment begins, the more effective it can be.

WHAT ARE THE SYMPTOMS OF MENTAL DISORDERS IN MEN?

Men and women can develop most of the same mental disorders and conditions, but they may experience different symptoms. Some common symptoms include the following:

- anger, irritability, or aggressiveness
- noticeable changes in mood, energy level, or appetite
- difficulty sleeping or sleeping too much
- difficulty concentrating, feeling restless, or on edge
- increased worry or feeling stressed
- misuse of alcohol, drugs, or both
- persistent sadness or feelings of hopelessness
- feeling flat or having trouble feeling positive emotions
- engaging in high-risk activities
- aches, headaches, or digestive problems without a clear cause
- obsessive thinking or compulsive behavior

- thoughts or behaviors that interfere with work, family, or social life
- unusual thinking or behaviors that concern other people
- thoughts of death or suicide or suicide attempts

Mental disorders can be treated: If you are unsure where to go for help, ask a health-care provider or visit the Help for Mental Illnesses webpage of the National Institute of Mental Health (NIMH; www.nimh.nih.gov/health/find-help). Communicating well with a health-care provider can improve your care and help you both make good choices about your health.

FEDERAL RESOURCES

- **Brother, You're on My Mind**. This National Institute on Minority Health and Health Disparities (NIMHD) initiative uses a variety of activities to raise awareness of the mental health challenges associated with depression and stress that affect African-American men and their families.
- **Men's Health**. MedlinePlus of the National Library of Medicine (NLM) offers resources on the unique health issues men experience.
- **Preventing Suicide Among Men in the Middle Years**. Recommendations for Suicide Prevention Programs: The Suicide Prevention Resource Center created this resource to help state and community suicide prevention programs design and implement projects to prevent suicide among men in the middle years (ages 35–64).
- **Substance Abuse and Mental Health Services Administration (SAMHSA)**. SAMHSA offers publications addressing the specific needs of men.
- **Why We Need to Talk About Men's Mental Health**. This resource from the Office on Women's Health (OWH) of the U.S. Department of Health and Human Services (HHS) discusses the importance of supporting men's mental health.

HEALTH HOTLINES

- **988 Suicide & Crisis Lifeline.** The lifeline provides free and confidential emotional support to people in suicidal crisis or emotional distress 24 hours a day, 7 days a week, across the United States. Call or text 988 to connect with a trained crisis counselor. Support is also available via live chat.
- **Disaster Distress Hotline.** This helpline from the SAMHSA provides immediate crisis counseling for people experiencing emotional distress related to any natural or human-caused disaster. The helpline is free, multilingual, confidential, and available 24 hours a day, 7 days a week. Call or text 800-985-5990.
- **Veterans Crisis Line.** This helpline is a free, confidential resource for veterans of all ages and circumstances. Call 800-273-8255, press 1; text 838255; or chat online to connect with 24/7 support.
- **NIH Health Info Lines.** This helpline provides information on various types of mental disorders and chronic illnesses. [1]

Section 19.2 | Depression

Depression (also known as "major depression," "major depressive disorder," or "clinical depression") is a common but serious mood disorder. It causes severe symptoms that affect how a person feels, thinks, and handles daily activities, such as sleeping, eating, or working.

To be diagnosed with depression, the symptoms must be present for at least two weeks.

There are different types of depression, some of which develop due to specific circumstances.

---

[1] "Men and Mental Health," National Institute of Mental Health (NIMH), May 2023. Available online. URL: www. nimh.nih.gov/health/topics/men-and-mental-health. Accessed June 15, 2023.

- **Major depression.** It includes symptoms of depressed mood or loss of interest, most of the time for at least two weeks, that interfere with daily activities.
- **Persistent depressive disorder (also called "dysthymia" or "dysthymic disorder").** This type of disorder consists of less severe symptoms of depression that last much longer, usually for at least two years.
- **Seasonal affective disorder (SAD).** SAD is a kind of depression that comes and goes with the seasons, with symptoms typically starting in the late fall and early winter and going away during the spring and summer.
- **Depression with symptoms of psychosis.** This is a severe form of depression in which a person experiences psychosis symptoms, such as delusions (disturbing, false fixed beliefs) or hallucinations (hearing or seeing things others do not hear or see).

People with bipolar disorder (formerly called "manic depression" or "manic-depressive illness") also experience depressive episodes, during which they feel sad, indifferent, or hopeless, combined with a very low activity level. But a person with bipolar disorder also experiences manic (or less severe hypomanic) episodes, or unusually elevated moods, in which they might feel very happy, irritable, or "up," with a marked increase in activity level.

Other types of depressive disorders found in the *Diagnostic and Statistical Manual of Mental Disorders, Fifth Edition* (DSM-5) include disruptive mood dysregulation disorder (diagnosed in children and adolescents) and premenstrual dysphoric disorder (that affects women around the time of their period).

WHO GETS DEPRESSION?
Depression can affect people of all ages, races, ethnicities, and genders.

Women are diagnosed with depression more often than men, but men can also be depressed. Because men may be less likely to recognize, talk about, and seek help for their feelings or emotional problems, they are at greater risk of depression symptoms being undiagnosed or undertreated.

Studies also show higher rates of depression and an increased risk for the disorder among members of the lesbian, gay, bisexual, transgender, queer or questioning, intersex, asexual, and more (LGBTQIA+) community.

WHAT ARE THE RISK FACTORS FOR DEPRESSION?

Research suggests that genetic, biological, environmental, and psychological factors play a role in depression.

Depression can happen at any age, but it often begins in adulthood. Depression is now recognized as occurring in children and adolescents although children may express more irritability than sadness. Many chronic mood and anxiety disorders in adults begin as high levels of anxiety in childhood.

Depression, especially in midlife or older age, can co-occur with other serious medical illnesses, such as diabetes, cancer, heart disease, and Parkinson disease (PD). These conditions are often worse when depression is present, and research suggests that people with depression and other medical illnesses tend to have more severe symptoms of both illnesses.

The Centers for Disease Control and Prevention (CDC) has also recognized that having certain mental disorders, including depression and schizophrenia, can make people more likely to get severely ill from COVID-19.

Sometimes, a physical health problem, such as thyroid disease, or medications taken for a physical illness cause side effects that contribute to depression. A health-care provider experienced in treating these complicated illnesses can help work out the best treatment strategy.

Other risk factors for depression include the following:
- personal or family history of depression
- major negative life changes, trauma, or stress

WHAT ARE THE SIGNS AND SYMPTOMS OF DEPRESSION?

If you have been experiencing some of the following signs and symptoms, most of the day, nearly every day, for at least two weeks, you may be suffering from depression:

- persistent sad, anxious, or "empty" mood
- feelings of hopelessness or pessimism
- feelings of irritability, frustration, or restlessness
- feelings of guilt, worthlessness, or helplessness
- loss of interest or pleasure in hobbies and activities
- decreased energy, fatigue, or feeling slowed down
- difficulty concentrating, remembering, or making decisions
- difficulty sleeping, waking early in the morning, or oversleeping
- changes in appetite or unplanned weight changes
- physical aches or pains, headaches, cramps, or digestive problems that do not have a clear physical cause and do not go away with treatment
- thoughts of death or suicide or suicide attempts

Not everyone who is depressed experiences all these symptoms. Some people experience only a few symptoms, while others experience many symptoms. Symptoms associated with depression interfere with day-to-day functioning and cause significant distress for the person experiencing them.

Depression can also involve other changes in mood or behavior that include the following:

- increased anger or irritability
- feeling restless or on edge
- becoming withdrawn, negative, or detached
- increased engagement in high-risk activities
- greater impulsivity
- increased use of alcohol or drugs
- isolating from family and friends
- inability to meet the responsibilities of work and family or ignoring other important roles
- problems with sexual desire and performance

Depression can look different in men and women. Although men, women, and people of all genders can feel depressed, how they express those symptoms and the behaviors they use to cope with them may differ. For example, some men (as well as women) may show symptoms other than sadness, instead seeming angry or irritable. And, although increased use of alcohol or drugs can be a coping strategy for any person with depression, men may be more likely to use alcohol or drugs to help them cope.

In some cases, mental health symptoms appear as physical problems, for example, a racing heart, a tightened chest, ongoing headaches, or digestive issues. Men are often more likely to see a health-care provider about these physical symptoms than their emotional ones.

Because depression tends to make people think more negatively about themselves and the world, some people may also have thoughts of suicide or self-harm.

Several persistent symptoms, in addition to low mood, are required for a diagnosis of depression, but people with only a few symptoms may also benefit from treatment. The severity and frequency of symptoms and how long they last will vary depending on the person, the illness, and the stage of the illness.

If you experience signs or symptoms of depression and they persist or do not go away, talk to a health-care provider. If you see signs or symptoms of depression in someone you know, encourage them to seek help from a mental health professional.

HOW IS DEPRESSION TREATED?

Depression, even the most severe cases, can be treated. The earlier treatment begins, the more effective it is. Depression is usually treated with medication, psychotherapy, or a combination of the two.

Some people may experience treatment-resistant depression (TRD), which occurs when a person does not get better after trying at least two antidepressant medications. If treatments, such as medication and psychotherapy, do not reduce depressive symptoms or the need for rapid relief from symptoms is urgent, brain stimulation therapy may be an option to explore.

No two people are affected the same way by depression, and there is no "one-size-fits-all" treatment. Finding the treatment that works best for you may take trial and error.

Medications

Antidepressants are medications commonly used to treat depression. They work by changing how the brain produces or uses certain chemicals involved in mood or stress. You may need to try several different antidepressants before finding the one that improves your symptoms and has manageable side effects. A medication that has helped you or a close family member in the past will often be considered first.

Antidepressants take time—usually four to eight weeks—to work, and problems with sleep, appetite, and concentration often improve before mood lifts. It is important to give a medication a chance to work before deciding whether it is the right one for you.

New medications, such as intranasal esketamine, can have rapidly acting antidepressant effects, especially for people with TRD. Esketamine is a medication approved by the U.S. Food and Drug Administration (FDA) for TRD. Delivered as a nasal spray in a doctor's office, clinic, or hospital, it acts rapidly, typically within a couple of hours, to relieve depression symptoms. People who use esketamine will usually continue taking an oral antidepressant to maintain the improvement in their symptoms.

Another option for TRD is to take an antidepressant alongside a different type of medication that may make the antidepressant more effective, such as an antipsychotic or anticonvulsant medication. Further research is needed to identify the best role of these newer medications in routine practice.

If you begin taking an antidepressant, do not stop taking it without talking to a health-care provider. Sometimes, people taking antidepressants feel better and stop taking the medications on their own, and their depression symptoms return. When you and your health-care provider have decided it is time to stop a medication, usually after a course of 9–12 months, the provider will help you slowly and safely decrease your dose. Abruptly stopping a medication can cause withdrawal symptoms.

Note: In some cases, children, teenagers, and young adults under 25 years may experience an increase in suicidal thoughts or behavior when taking antidepressants, especially in the first few weeks after starting or when the dose is changed. The FDA advises that patients of all ages taking antidepressants be watched closely, especially during the first few weeks of treatment.

Psychotherapies

Several types of psychotherapy (also called "talk therapy" or "counseling") can help people with depression by teaching them new ways of thinking and behaving and how to change habits that contribute to depression. Evidence-based approaches to treating depression include cognitive-behavioral therapy (CBT) and interpersonal therapy (IPT).

The growth of telehealth for mental health services, which offers an alternative to in-person therapy, has made it easier and more convenient for people to access care in some cases. For people who may have been hesitant to look for mental health care in the past, telemental health services might be an easier first step than traditional mental health services.

Brain Stimulation Therapies

If medication or psychotherapy does not reduce symptoms of depression, brain stimulation therapy may be an option to explore. There are now several types of brain stimulation therapy, some of which have been authorized by the FDA to treat depression. Other brain stimulation therapies are experimental and still being investigated for treating mental disorders like depression.

Although brain stimulation therapies are less frequently used than medication and psychotherapy, they can play an important role in treating mental disorders in people who do not respond to other treatments. These therapies are used for most mental disorders only after medication and psychotherapy have been tried and usually continue to be used alongside these treatments.

Brain stimulation therapies act by activating or inhibiting the brain with electricity. The electricity is given directly through electrodes implanted in the brain or indirectly through electrodes placed on the scalp. The electricity can also be induced by applying magnetic fields to the head.

The brain stimulation therapies with the largest bodies of evidence include the following:

- electroconvulsive therapy (ECT)
- repetitive transcranial magnetic stimulation (rTMS)
- vagus nerve stimulation (VNS)
- magnetic seizure therapy (MST)
- deep brain stimulation (DBS)

ECT and rTMS are the most widely used brain stimulation therapies, with ECT having the longest history of use. The other therapies are newer and, in some cases, still considered experimental. Other brain stimulation therapies may also hold promise for treating specific mental disorders.

ECT, rTMS, and VNS have authorization from the FDA to treat severe TRD. They can be effective for people who have not been able to feel better with other treatments or for whom medications cannot be used safely and in severe cases where a rapid response is needed, such as when a person is catatonic, suicidal, or malnourished.

Whereas ECT involves using electricity to induce seizures, in rTMS, a magnet is used to activate the brain. Unlike ECT, in which stimulation is more generalized, in rTMS, the stimulation is targeted to a specific brain site. Both procedures are noninvasive and do not require surgery to perform. In contrast, VNS is usually a surgical procedure that involves implanting a device under the skin to activate the vagus nerve.

Additional types of brain stimulation therapy are being investigated for treating depression and other mental disorders.

Alternative Treatments

The FDA has not approved any natural products for depression. Although research is ongoing, some people use natural products, including vitamin D and the herbal dietary supplement St. John's wort, for depression. However, these products can come with risks. For instance, dietary supplements and natural products can limit the effectiveness of some medications or interact in dangerous or even life-threatening ways with them.

Do not use vitamin D, St. John's wort, or other dietary supplements or natural products without talking to a health-care provider. Rigorous studies must be conducted to test whether these and other natural products are safe and effective.

Daily morning light therapy is a common treatment choice for people with SAD. Light therapy devices are much brighter than ordinary indoor lighting and considered safe, except for people with certain eye diseases or taking medications that increase sensitivity to sunlight. As with all interventions for depression, evaluation, treatment, and follow-up by a health-care provider are strongly recommended. Research into the potential role of light therapy in treating nonseasonal depression is ongoing.[2]

Section 19.3 | Anxiety

Anxiety is a normal part of life. Many people worry about things such as health, money, or family problems. But anxiety disorders involve more than temporary worry or fear. For people with an anxiety disorder, the anxiety does not go away and can get worse over time. The symptoms can interfere with daily activities, such as job performance, schoolwork, and relationships.

There are several types of anxiety disorders, including generalized anxiety disorder (GAD), panic disorder, social anxiety disorder (SAD), and various phobia-related disorders.[3]

---

[2] "Depression," National Institute of Mental Health (NIMH), April 2023. Available online. URL: www.nimh.nih.gov/health/topics/depression. Accessed June 26, 2023.
[3] "Anxiety Disorders," National Institute of Mental Health (NIMH), April 2023. Available online. URL: www.nimh.nih.gov/health/topics/anxiety-disorders. Accessed June 26, 2023.

WHO IS AT RISK FOR ANXIETY DISORDERS?

The risk factors for the different types of anxiety disorders can vary. For example, GAD and phobias are more common in women, but social anxiety affects men and women equally. The following are some general risk factors for all types of anxiety disorders:

- certain personality traits, such as being shy or withdrawn when you are in new situations or meeting new people
- traumatic events in early childhood or adulthood
- family history of anxiety or other mental disorders
- some physical health conditions, such as thyroid problems or arrhythmia[4]

WHAT ARE THE SIGNS AND SYMPTOMS OF ANXIETY?
Generalized Anxiety Disorder

GAD usually involves a persistent feeling of anxiety or dread, which can interfere with daily life. It is not the same as occasionally worrying about things or experiencing anxiety due to stressful life events. People living with GAD experience frequent anxiety for months, if not years.

Symptoms of GAD include the following:

- feeling restless, wound up, or on edge
- being easily fatigued
- having difficulty concentrating
- being irritable
- having headaches, muscle aches, stomachaches, or unexplained pains
- difficulty controlling feelings of worry
- having sleep problems, such as difficulty falling or staying asleep

Panic Disorder

People with panic disorder have frequent and unexpected panic attacks. Panic attacks are sudden periods of intense fear, discomfort,

[4] MedlinePlus, "Anxiety," National Institutes of Health (NIH), May 22, 2020. Available online. URL: https://medlineplus.gov/anxiety.html. Accessed June 26, 2023.

or sense of losing control even when there is no clear danger or trigger. Not everyone who experiences a panic attack will develop panic disorder.

During a panic attack, a person may experience:
- pounding or racing heart
- sweating
- trembling or tingling
- chest pain
- feelings of impending doom
- feelings of being out of control

People with panic disorder often worry about when the next attack will happen and actively try to prevent future attacks by avoiding places, situations, or behaviors they associate with panic attacks. Panic attacks can occur as frequently as several times a day or as rarely as a few times a year.

Social Anxiety Disorder

SAD is an intense, persistent fear of being watched and judged by others. For people with SAD, the fear of social situations may feel so intense that it seems beyond their control. For some people, this fear may get in the way of going to work, attending school, or doing everyday things.

People with social anxiety disorder may experience:
- blushing, sweating, or trembling
- pounding or racing heart
- stomachaches
- rigid body posture or speaking with an overly soft voice
- difficulty making eye contact or being around people they do not know
- feelings of self-consciousness or fear that people will judge them negatively

Phobia-Related Disorders

A phobia is an intense fear of—or aversion to—specific objects or situations. Although it can be realistic to be anxious in some circumstances, the fear people with phobias feel is out of proportion to the actual danger caused by the situation or object.

People with a phobia:
- may have an irrational or excessive worry about encountering the feared object or situation
- take active steps to avoid the feared object or situation
- experience immediate intense anxiety upon encountering the feared object or situation
- endure unavoidable objects and situations with intense anxiety

The following are a few types of phobias and phobia-related disorders:
- **Specific phobias (sometimes called "simple phobias").** As the name suggests, people who have a specific phobia have an intense fear of, or feel intense anxiety about, specific types of objects or situations. Some examples of specific phobias include the fear of:
  - flying
  - heights
  - specific animals, such as spiders, dogs, or snakes
  - receiving injections
  - blood
- **Social anxiety disorder (previously called "social phobia").** People with SAD have a general intense fear of, or anxiety toward, social or performance situations. They worry that actions or behaviors associated with their anxiety will be negatively evaluated by others, leading them to feel embarrassed. This worry often causes people with social anxiety to avoid social situations. Social anxiety disorder can manifest in a range of situations, such as within the workplace or the school environment.
- **Agoraphobia.** People with agoraphobia have an intense fear of two or more of the following situations:
  - using public transportation
  - being in open spaces
  - being in enclosed spaces

- standing in line or being in a crowd
- being outside of the home alone

People with agoraphobia often avoid these situations, in part, because they think being able to leave might be difficult or impossible in the event they have panic-like reactions or other embarrassing symptoms. In the most severe form of agoraphobia, an individual can become housebound.

- **Separation anxiety disorder**. Separation anxiety is often thought of as something that only children deal with. However, adults can also be diagnosed with separation anxiety disorder. People with separation anxiety disorder fear being away from the people they are close to. They often worry that something bad might happen to their loved ones while they are not together. This fear makes them avoid being alone or away from their loved ones. They may have bad dreams about being separated or feel unwell when separation is about to happen.[5]

HOW ARE ANXIETY DISORDERS DIAGNOSED?

To diagnose anxiety disorders, your health-care provider will ask about your symptoms and medical history. You may also have a physical exam and lab tests to make sure that a different health problem is not the cause of your symptoms.

If you do not have another health problem, you will get a psychological evaluation. Your provider may do it, or you may be referred to a mental health professional to get one.

WHAT ARE THE TREATMENTS FOR ANXIETY DISORDERS?

The main treatments for anxiety disorders are psychotherapy (talk therapy), medicines, or both:

- **Cognitive-behavioral therapy (CBT)**. It is a type of psychotherapy that is often used to treat anxiety disorders. CBT teaches you different ways of thinking

---

[5] See footnote [3].

and behaving. It can help you change how you react to the things that cause you to feel fear and anxiety. It may include exposure therapy. This focuses on having you confront your fears so that you will be able to do the things that you had been avoiding.

- **Medicines.** Antianxiety medicines and certain antidepressants are used to treat anxiety disorders. Some types of medicines may work better for specific types of anxiety disorders. You should work closely with your health-care provider to identify which medicine is best for you. You may need to try more than one medicine before you can find the right one.[6]

Section 19.4 | Posttraumatic Stress Disorder

Posttraumatic stress disorder (PTSD) is a mental health problem. PTSD can only develop after you go through or see a life-threatening event. It is normal to have stress reactions to these types of events, and most people start to feel better after a few weeks or months.

It is normal to have upsetting memories, feel on edge, or have trouble sleeping after a traumatic event (also called "trauma"). At first, it may be hard to do the daily activities you are used to doing, such as going to work, going to school, or spending time with people you care about. But most people start to feel better after a few weeks or months. For some people, PTSD symptoms may start later, or they may come and go over time.

If it has been longer than a few months and thoughts and feelings from the trauma are upsetting you or causing problems in your life, you may have PTSD.

---

[6] See footnote [4].

WHO DEVELOPS POSTTRAUMATIC STRESS DISORDER?

Anyone can develop PTSD at any age. Some factors can increase the chance that someone will have PTSD, many of which are not under that person's control. For example, having a very intense or long-lasting traumatic event or getting injured during the event can make it more likely that a person will develop PTSD. PTSD is also more common after certain types of trauma, such as combat and sexual assault.

Personal factors—such as previous traumatic exposure, age, and gender—can affect whether or not a person will develop PTSD. What happens after a traumatic event is also important. Stress can make PTSD more likely, while social support can make it less likely.

WHAT ARE THE SYMPTOMS OF POSTTRAUMATIC STRESS DISORDER?

Posttraumatic stress disorder symptoms usually start soon after the traumatic event, but they may not appear until months or years later. They may also come and go over many years. If the symptoms last longer than four weeks, cause you great distress, or interfere with your work or home life, you might have PTSD.

The following are the four types of PTSD symptoms, but they may not be exactly the same for everyone. Each person experiences symptoms in their own way.

- **Reliving the event (also called "reexperiencing symptoms").** Memories of the traumatic event can come back at any time. They can feel very real and scary. The following are a few examples:
  - You may have nightmares.
  - You may feel like you are going through the event again. This is called a "flashback."
  - You may see, hear, or smell something that causes you to relive the event. This is called a "trigger." News reports, seeing an accident, or hearing fireworks are examples of triggers.
- **Avoiding things that remind you of the event.** You may try to avoid situations or people who remind

335

you of the trauma event. You may even avoid talking or thinking about the event. The following are a few examples:

- You may avoid crowds because they feel dangerous.
- You may avoid driving if you were in a car accident or if your military convoy was bombed.
- If you were in an earthquake, you may avoid watching movies about earthquakes.
- You may keep very busy or avoid getting help, so you do not have to think or talk about the event.

- **Having more negative thoughts and feelings than before the event**. The way you think about yourself and others may become more negative because of the trauma. The following are a few examples:
  - You may feel numb—unable to have positive or loving feelings toward other people—and lose interest in things you used to enjoy.
  - You may forget about parts of the traumatic event or not be able to talk about them.
  - You may think the world is completely dangerous, and no one can be trusted.
  - You may feel guilt or shame about the event, wishing you had done more to keep it from happening.

- **Feeling on edge or keyed up (also called "hyperarousal")**. You may be jittery or always alert and on the lookout for danger. You might suddenly become angry or irritable. The following are a few examples:
  - You may have a hard time sleeping.
  - You may find it hard to concentrate.
  - You may be startled by a loud noise or surprise.
  - You might act in unhealthy ways, such as smoking, abusing drugs or alcohol, or driving aggressively.

DO PEOPLE WITH POSTTRAUMATIC STRESS DISORDER GET BETTER?

After a traumatic event, it is normal to think, act, and feel differently than usual—but most people start to feel better after a few weeks or months. Talk to a doctor or mental health-care provider (such as a psychiatrist, psychologist, or social worker) if your symptoms:

- last longer than a few months
- are very upsetting
- disrupt your daily life

"Getting better" means different things to different people. There are many different treatment options for PTSD. For many people, these treatments can get rid of symptoms altogether. Others find they have fewer symptoms or feel that their symptoms are less intense. Your symptoms do not have to interfere with your everyday activities, work, and relationships.

WHAT TREATMENTS ARE AVAILABLE?

Both trauma-focused psychotherapy (sometimes called "counseling" or "talk therapy") and medication are proven to treat PTSD. Sometimes, people combine psychotherapy and medication.

Trauma-Focused Psychotherapy

Trauma-focused psychotherapy is the most highly recommended treatment for PTSD. "Trauma-focused" means that the treatment focuses on the memory of the traumatic event or its meaning. The three most effective types of trauma-focused psychotherapy are as follows:

- **Cognitive processing therapy (CPT).** During this therapy, you learn skills to understand how trauma changed your thoughts and feelings. Changing how you think about the trauma can change how you feel.
- **Prolonged exposure (PE).** During this therapy, you talk about your trauma repeatedly until memories are no longer upsetting. This will help you get more control over your thoughts and feelings about the trauma. You also go to places or do things that are safe but that you have been staying away from because they remind you of the trauma.
- **Eye movement desensitization and reprocessing (EMDR).** EMDR involves focusing on sounds or hand

movements while you talk about the trauma. This helps your brain work through the traumatic memories.

Medications for Posttraumatic Stress Disorder

Certain medications can be effective for treating PTSD symptoms. Some specific selective serotonin reuptake inhibitors (SSRIs) and serotonin-norepinephrine reuptake inhibitors (SNRIs), which are used for depression, also work for PTSD. These include sertraline, paroxetine, fluoxetine, and venlafaxine.[7]

Section 19.5 | Schizophrenia

Schizophrenia is a serious mental illness that affects how a person thinks, feels, and behaves. People with schizophrenia may seem like they have lost touch with reality, which can be distressing for them and for their family and friends. The symptoms of schizophrenia can make it difficult to participate in usual, everyday activities, but effective treatments are available. Many people who receive treatment can engage in school or work, achieve independence, and enjoy personal relationships.

WHAT ARE THE RISK FACTORS FOR SCHIZOPHRENIA?

Several factors may contribute to a person's risk of developing schizophrenia.

- **Genetics.** Schizophrenia sometimes runs in families. However, just because one family member has schizophrenia, it does not mean that other members of the family will also have it. Studies suggest that many different genes may increase a person's chances

---

[7] National Center for Posttraumatic Stress Disorder (NCPTSD), "PTSD Basics," U.S. Department of Veterans Affairs (VA), November 9, 2022. Available online. URL: www.ptsd.va.gov/understand/what/ptsd_basics.asp. Accessed June 15, 2023.

of developing schizophrenia but that no single gene causes the disorder by itself.

- **Environment**. Research suggests that a combination of genetic factors and aspects of a person's environment and life experiences may play a role in the development of schizophrenia. These environmental factors may include living in poverty, stressful or dangerous surroundings, and exposure to viruses or nutritional problems before birth.
- **Brain structure and function**. Research shows that people with schizophrenia may be more likely to have differences in the size of certain brain areas and in connections between brain areas. Some of these brain differences may develop before birth. Researchers are working to better understand how brain structure and function may relate to schizophrenia.

WHAT ARE THE SIGNS AND SYMPTOMS OF SCHIZOPHRENIA?

It is important to recognize the symptoms of schizophrenia and seek help as early as possible. People with schizophrenia are usually diagnosed between the ages of 16 and 30 after the first episode of psychosis. Starting treatment as soon as possible following the first episode of psychosis is an important step toward recovery. However, research shows that gradual changes in thinking, mood, and social functioning often appear before the first episode of psychosis. Schizophrenia is rare in younger children.

Schizophrenia symptoms can differ from person to person, but they generally fall into three main categories: psychotic, negative, and cognitive.

Psychotic symptoms include changes in the way a person thinks, acts, and experiences the world. People with psychotic symptoms may lose a shared sense of reality with others and experience the world in a distorted way. For some people, these symptoms come and go. For others, the symptoms become stable over time. Psychotic symptoms include the following:

- **Hallucinations**. When a person sees, hears, smells, tastes, or feels things that are not actually there. Hearing voices is common for people with schizophrenia. People who hear voices may hear them for a long time before family or friends notice a problem.

- **Delusions.** When a person has strong beliefs that are not true and may seem irrational to others. For example, individuals experiencing delusions may believe that people on the radio and television are sending special messages that require a certain response, or they may believe that they are in danger or that others are trying to hurt them.
- **Thought disorder.** When a person has ways of thinking that are unusual or illogical. People with thought disorder may have trouble organizing their thoughts and speech. Sometimes, a person will stop talking in the middle of a thought, jump from topic to topic, or make up words that have no meaning.
- **Movement disorder.** When a person exhibits abnormal body movements. People with movement disorder may repeat certain motions over and over.

Negative symptoms include loss of motivation, loss of interest or enjoyment in daily activities, withdrawal from social life, difficulty showing emotions, and difficulty functioning normally.

Negative symptoms include the following:
- having trouble planning and sticking with activities, such as grocery shopping
- having trouble anticipating and feeling pleasure in everyday life
- talking in a dull voice and showing limited facial expression
- avoiding social interaction or interacting in socially awkward ways
- having very low energy and spending a lot of time in passive activities (In extreme cases, a person might stop moving or talking for a while, which is a rare condition called "catatonia.")

These symptoms are sometimes mistaken for symptoms of depression or other mental illnesses.

Cognitive symptoms include problems in attention, concentration, and memory. These symptoms can make it hard to follow a conversation, learn new things, or remember appointments. A person's level of cognitive functioning is one of the best predictors of their day-to-day functioning. Health-care providers evaluate cognitive functioning using specific tests.

Cognitive symptoms include the following:
- having trouble processing information to make decisions
- having trouble using information immediately after learning it
- having trouble focusing or paying attention

The Centers for Disease Control and Prevention (CDC) has recognized that having certain mental disorders, including depression and schizophrenia, can make people more likely to get severely ill from COVID-19.

HOW IS SCHIZOPHRENIA TREATED?

Current treatments for schizophrenia focus on helping people manage their symptoms, improve day-to-day functioning, and achieve personal life goals, such as completing education, pursuing a career, and having fulfilling relationships.

Antipsychotic Medications

Antipsychotic medications can help make psychotic symptoms less intense and less frequent. These medications are usually taken every day in pill or liquid forms. Some antipsychotic medications are given as injections once or twice a month.

If a person's symptoms do not improve with usual antipsychotic medications, they may be prescribed clozapine. People who take clozapine must have regular blood tests to check for a potentially dangerous side effect that occurs in 1–2 percent of patients.

People respond to antipsychotic medications in different ways. It is important to report any side effects to a health-care provider.

Many people taking antipsychotic medications experience side effects, such as weight gain, dry mouth, restlessness, and drowsiness when they start taking these medications. Some of these side effects may go away over time, while others may last.

Shared decision-making between health-care providers and patients is the recommended strategy for determining the best type of medication or medication combination and the right dose. To find the latest information about antipsychotic medications, talk to a health-care provider and visit the U.S. Food and Drug Administration (FDA) website (www.fda.gov).

Psychosocial Treatments

Psychosocial treatments help people find solutions to everyday challenges and manage symptoms while attending school, working, and forming relationships. These treatments are often used together with antipsychotic medication. People who participate in regular psychosocial treatment are less likely to have symptoms reoccur or to be hospitalized.

Examples of this kind of treatment include types of psychotherapy, such as cognitive-behavioral therapy (CBT), behavioral skills training, supported employment, and cognitive remediation interventions.

Education and Support

Educational programs can help family and friends learn about symptoms of schizophrenia, treatment options, and strategies for helping loved ones with the illness. These programs can help friends and family manage their distress, boost their own coping skills, and strengthen their ability to provide support.

Coordinated Specialty Care

Coordinated specialty care (CSC) programs are recovery-focused programs for people with first-episode psychosis, an early stage of schizophrenia. Health-care providers and specialists work together as a team to provide CSC, which includes psychotherapy, medication, case management, employment and education support, and family education and support. The treatment team works collaboratively with the individual to make treatment decisions, involving family members as much as possible.

Compared with typical care, CSC is more effective at reducing symptoms, improving quality of life (QOL), and increasing involvement in work or school.

Assertive Community Treatment

Assertive community treatment (ACT) is designed especially for people with schizophrenia who are likely to experience multiple hospitalizations or homelessness. ACT is usually delivered by a team of health-care providers who work together to provide care to patients in the community.

Treatment for Drug and Alcohol Misuse

It is common for people with schizophrenia to have problems with drugs and alcohol. A treatment program that includes treatment for both schizophrenia and substance use is important for recovery because substance use can interfere with treatment for schizophrenia.[8]

[8] "Schizophrenia," National Institute of Mental Health (NIMH), May 2023. Available online. URL: www.nimh.nih.gov/health/topics/schizophrenia. Accessed June 15, 2023.

Chapter 20 | Male-Pattern Baldness

Androgenetic alopecia is a common form of hair loss in both men and women. In men, this condition is also known as "male-pattern baldness." Hair is lost in a well-defined pattern, beginning above both temples. Over time, the hairline recedes to form a characteristic "M" shape. Hair also thins at the crown (near the top of the head), often progressing to partial or complete baldness.

Androgenetic alopecia in men has been associated with several other medical conditions, including coronary heart disease (CHD) and enlargement of the prostate. Additionally, prostate cancer, disorders of insulin resistance (such as diabetes and obesity), and high blood pressure (HBP; hypertension) have been related to androgenetic alopecia.

FREQUENCY OF MALE-PATTERN BALDNESS

Androgenetic alopecia is a frequent cause of hair loss in both men and women. This form of hair loss affects an estimated 50 million men and 30 million women in the United States. Androgenetic alopecia can start as early as a person's teens and risk increases with age; more than 50 percent of men over age 50 have some degree of hair loss.

CAUSES OF MALE-PATTERN BALDNESS

A variety of genetic and environmental factors likely play a role in causing androgenetic alopecia. Although researchers are studying risk factors that may contribute to this condition, most of these factors remain unknown. Researchers have determined that this form of hair loss is related to hormones called "androgens," particularly an androgen called "dihydrotestosterone." Androgens are important for normal male sexual development before birth and during puberty. Androgens also have other important functions in both males and females, such as regulating hair growth and sex drive.

Hair growth begins under the skin in structures called "follicles." Each strand of hair normally grows for two to six years, goes into a resting phase for several months, and then falls out. The cycle starts over when the follicle begins growing a new hair. Increased levels of androgens in hair follicles can lead to a shorter cycle of hair growth and the growth of shorter and thinner strands of hair. Additionally, there is a delay in the growth of new hair to replace strands that are shed.

Although researchers suspect that several genes play a role in androgenetic alopecia, variations in only one gene, *AR*, have been confirmed in scientific studies. The *AR* gene provides instructions for making a protein called an "androgen receptor." Androgen receptors allow the body to respond appropriately to dihydrotestosterone and other androgens. Studies suggest that variations in the *AR* gene lead to increased activity of androgen receptors in hair follicles. It remains unclear, however, how these genetic changes increase the risk of hair loss in men.

Researchers continue to investigate the connection between androgenetic alopecia and other medical conditions, such as coronary heart disease (CHD) and prostate cancer in men. They believe that some of these disorders may be associated with elevated androgen levels, which may help explain why they tend to occur with androgen-related hair loss. Other hormonal, environmental, and genetic factors that have not been identified may also be involved.

INHERITANCE PATTERN OF MALE-PATTERN BALDNESS

The inheritance pattern of androgenetic alopecia is unclear because many genetic and environmental factors are likely to be involved.

Male-Pattern Baldness

This condition tends to cluster in families, however, and having a close relative with patterned hair loss appears to be a risk factor for developing the condition.[1]

[1] MedlinePlus, "Androgenetic Alopecia," National Institutes of Health (NIH), August 1, 2015. Available online. URL: https://medlineplus.gov/genetics/condition/androgenetic-alopecia/#inheritance. AccessedJuly 17, 2023.

Part 3 | **Sexual and Reproductive Health**

Chapter 21 | Men's Sexual Health: Key Considerations

Chapter Contents

Section 21.1 | Erections, Ejaculation, and More

Erections, ejaculation, and wet dreams are part of a person's life, and teens may experience any or all these biological events during puberty. Since there are a lot of misconceptions about masturbation, ejaculation, and wet dreams floating around, everyone must know about the body's basic functioning.

WHAT IS AN ERECTION?

An erection is a natural enlargement of the penis that occurs when blood flows into the sponge-like tissue inside the penis, causing it to stand away from the body. Erections are typical in a man's body and occur throughout their life span, particularly during puberty. They naturally subside on their own or after ejaculation—a process of releasing semen.

Causes of an Erection

Though erections can occur randomly for no reason, they typically happen when a boy is sexually excited due to:
- watching pornographic materials
- sexual fantasies
- hormone fluctuations

Controlling an Erection

Erections are usually not controllable, and unfortunately, there is not much teens can do about it. Some teens masturbate when they have an erection, while it subsides over time for others. The frequency of erections decreases once teens have advanced through puberty.

Frequency of Erections

As every guy is different, there is no "normal" number of erections. Factors such as hormones, sexual maturity, and the amount of sleep a teen gets determine the number of erections he has per day. Hence, some teens may experience more erections every day than others of his age.

If there is no discomfort or pain during an erection, teens need not worry about the frequency of erections in a day.

WHAT IS EJACULATION?

Ejaculation is the process that involves the discharge of semen from the penis. It happens during orgasm, the final stage of male sexual stimulation.

There is no fixed number of times one needs to ejaculate each day, week, or month. Instead, teens can listen to their bodies.

There is a claim that ejaculation reduces the risk of prostate cancer. There is no unambiguous evidence about it based on several studies. Before we conclude, more research is needed on this concept.

WHAT IS MASTURBATION?

Masturbation is the process of stimulating one's genitals for sexual pleasures among both sexes, with ejaculation being the result of masturbation. Most teens feel embarrassed talking about masturbation, and some think that masturbation is nasty or dirty. This guilt or shame about masturbation can make teens think badly about themselves, affecting their mental health. They should understand that masturbation is a normal part of human sexuality.

Myths and Facts about Masturbation

- **Myth**: Masturbation will make you go blind.
  Fact: Masturbation will not make you go blind as there is no medical evidence to prove the same.
- **Myth**: Masturbation will make you mentally ill.
  Fact: Masturbation has many mental health benefits, such as reducing stress and improving mood.
- **Myth**: Masturbation reduces the sperm count and makes it hard to have children.
  Fact: There is no proper medical evidence to support this myth.

- **Myth**: You will get sexually transmitted disease (STD) from masturbation.
  Fact: No, you will not get any STD from masturbation. Masturbation is the safest sexual activity.

WHAT ARE WET DREAMS?

Wet dreams, also known as "nocturnal emission," are involuntary ejaculations that happen at sleep, primarily due to erotic dreams. Sometimes, teens wake up from a wet dream, but they sleep through it most times. Though wet dreams are typically associated with boys, they are common for both sexes in the puberty phase.

Facts of Wet Dreams

- Wet dreams do not reduce sperm count.
- Having wet dreams does not reduce immunity.
- Wet dreams are more common in puberty, but they also occur during adulthood.
- Wet dreams do not reduce the size of the penis.
- It is also common in some people to never have wet dreams.
- Wet dreams can be more frequent when a person sleeps on their stomach.

Preventing Wet Dreams

There are no scientific ways to prevent wet dreams; however, adopting a few techniques may help reduce the frequency of wet dreams by:

- doing meditation, yoga, or a few relaxation techniques before bed
- consulting with a psychologist or counselor about dreams

References

Barrell, Amanda. "What Is Female Ejaculation?" Medical News Today, January 20, 2020. Available online. URL: www.medicalnewstoday.com/articles/323953. Accessed August 7, 2023.

Fletcher, Jenna. "Everything You Need to Know about Wet Dreams," Medical News Today, January 16, 2020.

Available online. URL: www.medicalnewstoday.com/
articles/321351#facts-and-myths. Accessed August 7, 2023.

Watson, Stephanie. "Masturbation FAQ," *WebMD*, October 31,
2021. Available online. URL: https://teens.webmd.com/boys/
masturbation-faq. Accessed August 7, 2023.

"What Is the Deal with Erections, Ejaculation, and Wet
Dreams?" Planned Parenthood Federation of America Inc.,
n.d. Available online. URL: www.plannedparenthood.org/
learn/teens/puberty/whats-deal-erections-ejaculation-and-
wet-dreams. Accessed August 7, 2023.

Section 21.2 | Reproductive Health: An Overview

Reproductive health is an important component of men's overall
health and well-being. Too often, males have been overlooked in
discussions of reproductive health, especially when reproductive
issues, such as contraception and infertility, have been perceived
as female-related. Every day, men, their partners, and health-care
providers can protect their reproductive health by ensuring effective contraception, avoiding sexually transmitted diseases (STDs),
and preserving fertility.

Common issues in male reproductive health include the
following:

- contraception
- avoiding STDs
- infertility/fertility

AN OVERVIEW ON MEN'S REPRODUCTIVE HEALTH
How Can Men Protect Their Reproductive Health and the Health of Their Partners?

It is important for men to protect their reproductive health and
that of their partners by:

- using contraception carefully, consistently, and
correctly

- minimizing the risk of STDs
- addressing factors that may reduce fertility and seeking treatment when required

Men should consult with their health-care provider to discuss which contraceptive method is best for the couple, based on overall health, age, frequency of sexual activity, number of partners, desire to have children in the future, and family history of certain diseases. Contraceptive methods work best when they are used correctly and consistently. Using contraception incorrectly or inconsistently increases the risk of pregnancy and, in some cases, also increases the risk of STDs.

It is important to discuss the risk factors for STDs with a health-care provider and ask about getting tested. It is possible to have an STD and not know it because many STDs do not cause symptoms. Men with STDs need to ask a health-care provider about treatment to address symptoms, reduce the progression of the STDs, and decrease or eliminate the risk of transmitting an STD to your partner.

If you and your partner are interested in having children but have difficulty conceiving, it is important for both the male and the female partner to consult with a health-care provider to assess fertility. Over one-third of infertility cases are caused by male reproductive issues, alone or in combination with female reproductive issues. However, treatments are available to address many of the causes of male infertility.

How Effective Is Male Contraception?

Not all contraceptive methods are appropriate for all situations, and individuals should consult their health-care providers to determine which method of birth control is best for them. For men, methods of contraception include male condoms and sterilization (vasectomy).

- **Male condom**. It is a thin sheath that covers the penis to collect sperm and prevent it from entering the woman's body. Male condoms are generally made of latex or polyurethane, but a natural alternative is lambskin (made from the intestinal membrane of lambs). Latex or polyurethane condoms reduce the risk of spreading STDs. Lambskin condoms do not prevent STDs. Male condoms are disposable after a single use.

- **Vasectomy**. It is a surgical procedure that cuts, closes, or blocks the vas deferens. This procedure blocks the path between the testes and the urethra. The sperm cannot leave the testes and cannot reach the egg. It can take as long as three months for the procedure to be fully effective. A backup method of contraception is used until tests confirm that there is no sperm in the semen. Although vasectomy can sometimes be reversed, it is not always possible. Vasectomy, like other sterilization procedures, is considered a permanent form of birth control.

Different methods of contraception have different rates of effectiveness in preventing pregnancy.

Contraception is most effective when used correctly and consistently. The failure rate increases if a method of contraception is used incorrectly.

According to the U.S. Department of Health and Human Services (HHS), male condoms have a failure rate of 11–16 percent (i.e., 11–16 women would be expected to get pregnant within one year if 100 women and their partners relied solely on male condoms for birth control). Male sterilization procedures have a failure rate of less than 1 percent if a backup method is used for the first several months after the procedure.

How Can Men Reduce the Risk of Getting a Sexually Transmitted Disease?

Men can take the following measures to avoid STDs:

- Know your partner's STD and health history.
- Talk to your health-care provider about your risk and get tested for STDs.
- Practice safe sex (such as using latex condoms correctly and consistently).

- Get vaccinated against hepatitis A virus, hepatitis B virus, and human papillomavirus (HPV).

According to the HHS, the male latex condom is the best method for protecting against STDs, including human immunodeficiency virus (HIV)/acquired immunodeficiency syndrome (AIDS). Polyurethane condoms are an effective alternative if either partner has a latex allergy. Natural/lambskin condoms do not prevent the spread of STDs because of the presence of tiny pores (holes) that may allow viruses, such as HIV, hepatitis B, and herpes to spread.

It is important to know that male condoms cannot completely protect you and your partner from contracting an STD. For example, the most common STD is the HPV. No method of contraception can fully prevent the transmission of HPV because it can infect areas not covered by a condom. However, using a condom with every sex act can lower the risk of transmission.

See your health-care provider for treatment as soon as possible after receiving a diagnosis of an STD. Notify all recent sex partners and advise them to see their health-care providers and be treated. All sexual partners should be treated at the same time to prevent reinfection. All partners should avoid sex until treatment is complete and your health-care provider advises that it is safe to resume.

Many STDs have significant health consequences. Infections from STDs can cause infertility in both men and women. Some STDs can increase the risk of some forms of cancer. A person with an STD other than HIV is two to five times more likely to contract HIV than a person without an STD. If a person is already HIV-positive, having another STD increases the chances that they will pass HIV on to their sexual partner.

How Common Is Male Infertility, and What Are Its Causes?

Infertility is defined clinically in women and men who cannot achieve pregnancy after one year of having intercourse without using birth control and in women who have two or more failed pregnancies. Studies suggest that after one year of having unprotected sex, 15 percent of couples are unable to conceive, and after two years, 10 percent of couples still have not had a successful pregnancy. In couples younger than the age of 30 who are generally healthy, 20–37 percent are able to conceive in the first three months.

Many different medical conditions and other factors can contribute to fertility problems, and an individual case may have a single cause, several causes, or—in some cases—no identifiable cause. Overall, one-third of infertility cases are caused by male reproductive issues, one-third by female reproductive issues, and one-third by both male and female reproductive issues or by unknown factors.

To conceive a child, a man's sperm must combine with a woman's egg. The testicles make and store sperm, which are ejaculated by the penis to deliver sperm to the female reproductive tract during sexual intercourse. The most common issues that lead to infertility in men are problems that affect how the testicles work. Other problems are hormone imbalances or blockages in the male reproductive organs. In about 50 percent of cases, the cause of male infertility cannot be determined.

A complete lack of sperm occurs in about 10–15 percent of men who are infertile. A hormone imbalance or blockage of sperm movement can cause a lack of sperm. In some cases of infertility, a man produces less sperm than normal. The most common cause of this condition is varicocele, an enlarged vein in the testicle. Varicocele is present in about 40 percent of men with infertility problems.

What Treatment Options Are Available for Male Infertility?

Other than the inability to conceive within a stated period of time or the inability to deliver a live-born infant, in most cases, infertility has no other outward symptoms.

The evaluation of a man's fertility includes looking for signs of hormone deficiency, such as increased body fat, decreased muscle mass, and decreased facial and body hair. The evaluation also includes questions about the man's health history, including past injury to the testicles or penis, recent high fevers, and childhood diseases such as mumps. A physical examination allows for the identification of problems, such as infection, hernia, or varicocele. A health-care provider may also ask a man to provide a semen sample to assess the health and quality of his sperm. Other tests may include measurement of hormones in the blood, a biopsy of the testicle, or genetic screening.

Treatments for male infertility may be based on the underlying cause of the problem, or in the case of no identified problem, evidence-based treatments that improve fertility may be recommended. Treatments include surgery to correct or repair anatomic abnormalities or damage to reproductive organs, use of medical procedures to deliver sperm to the woman, fertilization of the egg in a laboratory, and using a third party for donating sperm or eggs and/or carrying a pregnancy. Medication can treat some issues that affect male fertility, including hormone imbalances and erectile dysfunction (ED). Surgery can be effective for repairing blockages in the tubes that transport sperm. Surgery can also be used for repair of varicocele. Assistive reproductive technologies (ARTs), such as in vitro fertilization (IVF), can be effective if other treatments do not restore fertility (www.nichd.nih.gov/health/topics/infertility).[1]

[1] "Men's Reproductive Health," *Eunice Kennedy Shriver* National Institute of Child Health and Human Development (NICHD), July 3, 2020. Available online. URL: www.nichd.nih.gov/health/topics/factsheets/menshealth. Accessed June 16, 2023.

Chapter 22 | **Penile Health and Concerns**

Chapter Contents

Section 22.1 | Circumcision

Circumcision is the surgical procedure to remove the foreskin, the tissue that covers the tip of the penis. This procedure can be done at any age, but it is commonly done in infants, shortly after birth. Circumcision has both medical pros and cons, according to the American Academy of Pediatrics (AAP).

HOW IS CIRCUMCISION DONE?

If circumcision is required for medical reasons, a physician may refer them to a specialist who may be a general or pediatric surgeon. There are three ways in which the procedure can be done: the Gomco clamp, the Plastibell device, and the Mogen clamp.

First, blood circulation to the foreskin is cut off to reduce bleeding before the doctor cuts the foreskin.

- **Gomco clamp.** In this method, the baby's foreskin is stretched over a metal device with a bell-shaped end, and the clamp is tightened over his foreskin.
- **Plastibell.** A cut in the foreskin is done before placing the plastic device between the penis and the foreskin. A sterile string is tied over the foreskin and around the machine to cut blood flow before circumcision.
- **Mogen clamp.** A hinge-shaped metal device where the baby's foreskin is pulled forward through the hinge of the clamp is used. The clamp is locked for about 90 seconds to decrease bleeding in the foreskin.

After the operation, the wound is treated with petroleum jelly before covering it with gauze.

COMPLICATIONS OF CIRCUMCISION IN TEENS

Complications from circumcision are rare, and a few of them are listed as follows:

- bleeding
- infection

- insufficient foreskin removed
- excessive foreskin removed
- adhesions/skin bridges
- inclusion cysts
- abnormal healing
- urinary retention
- mastitis (inflammation and redness at the tip of the penis)
- meatal stenosis (a condition where the opening at the penis tip becomes narrower)
- phimosis (a situation where the foreskin cannot retract over the head of the penis)
- necrosis of the penis (a rare complication after circumcision due to collateral blood circulation)
- amputation of the glans

BENEFITS OF CIRCUMCISION
Some of the medical benefits of circumcision include:
- decreased risk of urinary tract infections (UTIs)
- easier hygiene
- lower risk of sexually transmitted diseases (STDs) and penile cancer

References
"CDC Provides Information to Male Patients and Parents," Centers for Disease Control and Prevention (CDC), September 1, 2018. Available online. URL: www.cdc.gov/nchhstp/newsroom/docs/factsheets/MC-for-HIV-Prevention-Fact-Sheet_508.pdf. Accessed August 7, 2023.

"Circumcision," Mayo Foundation for Medical Education and Research (MFMER), September 21, 2021. Available online. URL: www.mayoclinic.org/tests-procedures/circumcision/about/pac-20393550. Accessed August 7, 2023.

Krans, Brian. "Circumcision," Healthline, September 17, 2018. Available online. URL: www.healthline.com/health/circumcision. Accessed August 7, 2023.

Section 22.2 | **Balanitis**

Balanitis is an inflammation of the foreskin on head of the penis (glans) that causes the skin to become reddish and itchy. Although it rarely occurs among circumcised adult males, it affects approximately 3.3 percent of uncircumcised males at some point in their lives, as well as 4 percent of all boys under the age of four. A related condition, posthitis, involves inflammation of the foreskin that covers the head of the penis in uncircumcised males. When both the glans and foreskin are affected, the condition is known as "balanoposthitis."

CAUSES AND RISK FACTORS OF BALANITIS

Balanitis has many possible causes, ranging from skin conditions and allergic reactions that affect the penis to sexually transmitted infections (STIs) and poor hygiene. Men with phimosis—a condition in which the foreskin is tight and difficult to retract—are particularly susceptible to balanitis. Diabetes also increases the risk of developing balanitis because glucose in the urine can remain on the penis, creating a favorable environment for bacteria to grow. Some of the main causes of balanitis include the following:

- skin conditions such as eczema, psoriasis, or lichen planus
- dermatitis (inflammation of the skin) due to contact with an irritant or allergen, such as latex condoms, lubricants, spermicides, medicated ointments, detergents, fabric softeners, or perfumed bath products
- irritation or minor trauma to the skin of the penis from friction, sexual intercourse, excessive washing with harsh soap, or vigorous drying with an abrasive towel
- candida (also known as "yeast infection" or "thrush")
- STIs, such as genital herpes, chlamydia, or syphilis
- bacterial infection from poor hygiene practices, such as infrequent washing of the glans or failure to dry the tissue beneath the foreskin after washing

SYMPTOMS OF BALANITIS

The primary symptoms of balanitis include:
- swelling, redness, and tenderness of the glans
- skin irritation or rash on the end of the penis
- itching and discomfort
- thick, lumpy discharge under the foreskin
- unpleasant smell
- painful urination
- difficulty retracting the foreskin (phimosis)

DIAGNOSIS AND TREATMENT FOR BALANITIS

To make a diagnosis of balanitis, a doctor merely needs to observe inflammation of the glans. In order to treat the condition effectively, however, the doctor must also determine the underlying cause. This process may involve examining the skin for evidence of eczema, psoriasis, or other skin conditions that may affect the penis. The doctor may also advise the patient to avoid potential skin irritants or allergens, such as lubricants or perfumed bath products, to see whether the balanitis resolves itself. Finally, the doctor may order diagnostic tests—such as blood tests, urine tests, or a swab of the glans—to see whether the patient has diabetes, a yeast infection, or an STI.

If the balanitis appears to be related to a skin condition, the patient will likely be referred to a dermatologist for treatment. For balanitis caused by an allergic reaction, the patient may be prescribed a mild topical steroid cream, such as 1 percent hydrocortisone, to help relieve the swelling and other symptoms. If the cause is candida, the recommended treatment will include an antifungal cream—such as clotrimazole or miconazole—for both the patient and his sex partner. For balanitis caused by a bacterial infection, the patient will likely be prescribed an oral antibiotic, such as penicillin or erythromycin. If no infection or irritant can be identified, treatment may include astringent compresses with diluted vinegar or potassium permanganate. In rare cases, if the patient has phimosis and the balanitis recurs frequently, the doctor may recommend circumcision (surgery to remove the foreskin).

PREVENTION OF BALANITIS

Left untreated, chronic balanitis can lead to health complications, including:

- phimosis (the condition where the foreskin cannot be retracted over the inflamed glans, which may require surgery to correct)
- balanitis xerotica obliterans (chronic dermatitis affecting the glans and foreskin)
- scarring and narrowing of the opening of the penis
- reduction in blood supply to the tip of the penis
- increased risk of penile cancer

Good hygiene is key to preventing the occurrence or recurrence of balanitis. Doctors recommend washing the penis daily with warm water, making sure to pull back the foreskin to expose the glans. Although regular soap may cause irritation, aqueous cream or other nonsoap cleansers may be used as long as it is completely rinsed off. It is important to dry the head of the penis thoroughly before replacing the foreskin because moisture promotes the growth of bacteria. Men who tend to develop balanitis following sexual intercourse should wash the penis after sex. Finally, men who are prone to balanitis should avoid contact with potential irritants such as lubricants, detergents, or other chemicals.

References

Nordqvist, Christian. "Balanitis: Causes, Symptoms, and Treatments," Medical News Today, September 28, 2015. Available online. URL: www.medicalnewstoday.com/ articles/184715.php. Accessed August 7, 2023.

Ngan, Vanessa. "Balanitis," DermNet™, 2016. Available online. URL: https://dermnetnz.org/topics/balanitis. Accessed August 7, 2023.

Sobol, Jennifer. "Balanitis," MedlinePlus, August 31, 2015. Available online. URL: https://medlineplus.gov/ency/ article/000862.htm. Accessed August 7, 2023.

Section 22.3 | Penile Intraepithelial Neoplasia

Penile intraepithelial neoplasia (PEIN) is precancerous condition in which abnormal cell growth occurs in the outer layer of skin on the penis. Intraepithelial refers to the layer of cells that forms the surface or lining of an organ, while neoplasia refers to cystic lesions or tumors. PEIN is also called "erythroplasia of Queyrat," "Bowen disease of the penis," "squamous intraepithelial lesion," or "squamous cell carcinoma in situ of the penis." If left untreated, PEIN can lead to the development of penile cancer.

RISK FACTORS OF PENILE INTRAEPITHELIAL NEOPLASIA

Penile cancer is rare in the United States, with only about 2,000 new cases diagnosed each year. Some studies suggest that human papillomavirus (HPV) infection in the genital area, which also causes genital warts, is a significant risk factor in the development of penile intraepithelial cancer. As a result, many developed nations have instituted immunization programs aimed at vaccinating both boys and girls against HPV.

Other risk factors include having a weak immune system, maintaining a poor genital hygiene, smoking, inability to retract the foreskin of the glans penis, and exposure to harmful chemicals and ultraviolet (UV) rays.

Some studies suggest that being circumcised reduced the chances of developing penile cancer.

SYMPTOMS AND DIAGNOSIS OF PENILE INTRAEPITHELIAL NEOPLASIA

The main symptom of PEIN is the presence of one or more lesions, growths, or tumors on the glans or foreskin of the penis. The surface of these lesions may appear smooth, velvety, crusty, scaly, or bumpy. Men with PEIN may also experience inflammation, redness, itching, or pain in the area. In advanced stages, PEIN may cause bleeding, discharge, difficulty retracting the foreskin, or difficulty with urination.

Some of the symptoms of PEIN may resemble other conditions, such as balanitis or dermatitis, so a skin biopsy should be performed to confirm the diagnosis and rule out invasive squamous cell carcinoma.

TREATMENT FOR PENILE INTRAEPITHELIAL NEOPLASIA

Penile intraepithelial neoplasia can be treated with medications, surgery, or both. In addition to practicing good genital hygiene, men with PEIN may benefit from the use of topical medications such as 5-fluorouracil cream, which destroys abnormal skin cells, or imiquimod cream, which stimulates the immune system's response to abnormal cells. The lesions may also be removed using a variety of techniques, such as cryotherapy, curettage and cautery, excision, laser vaporization, Mohs micrographic surgery, photodynamic therapy, and radiotherapy. Since up to 10 percent of patients may experience a recurrence of PEIN following successful treatment, it is important to maintain a regular schedule of follow-up examinations.

Patients diagnosed with PEIN should undergo treatment promptly to prevent the precancerous lesions from becoming cancerous. Although penile cancer is highly curable in its early stages, the prognosis declines sharply for more advanced stages. Finally, sexual partners of patients with PEIN should be screened for related conditions—such as cervical, vulvar, and anal cancer—which can also be caused by the HPV.

References

Ngan, Vanessa. "Penile Intraepithelial Neoplasia," DermNet™, April 25, 2016. Available online. URL: www.dermnetnz.org/site-age-specific/penile-intraepithelial-neoplasia.html. Accessed August 7, 2023.

"Penile Cancer Treatment," National Cancer Institute (NCI), February 18, 2016. Available online. URL: www.cancer.gov/types/penile/hp/penile-treatment-pdq#section/_1. Accessed August 7, 2023.

Section 22.4 | **Penile Trauma**

Penile trauma can describe any sort of injury or wound that affects the penis. Trauma to the penis usually occurs when the penis is in its erect state or from penile injuries that may occur during sexual intercourse. Although most types of penile trauma will heal with appropriate treatment, many men resist seeking medical attention for penis injuries. Left untreated, however, penile trauma may result in pain, swelling, infection, sexual dysfunction, or permanent curvature of the penis (Peyronie disease).

CAUSES OF PENILE TRAUMA

Although most cases of penile trauma are related to sexual intercourse, injuries to the penis may result from a variety of other causes. The following are some of the most common types of injuries and associated causes:

- **Blunt force trauma.** Sports-related injuries—such as being hit in the groin by a ball, stick, foot, or knee—are a leading cause of blunt force trauma to the penis, which can result in pain, swelling, and bruising. Other common sources of blunt force trauma to the penis include automobile accidents and industrial accidents.
- **Cuts, abrasions, and burns.** Penis abrasion can result from vigorous, repetitive exercise, chafing from coarse fabrics, or rug burns. Minor cuts and bruises to the penis may occur from being caught in a zipper or from using a penile pump or other stretching device in an effort to enlarge the penis. Burns to the penis can result from hot liquids being spilled or clothing catching on fire.
- **Punctures.** Inserting objects into the tip of the penis can damage the urethra (the tube that carries urine and semen out of the penis). Bleeding from the penis or blood in the urine are indications of a serious injury to the urethra.
- **Severe trauma or amputation.** Part or all of the penis may be damaged or severed as a result of gunshot wounds, automobile accidents, or industrial accidents. In addition,

placing a rubber tube, metal ring, or other constricting device around the base of the penis can block blood flow and cause lasting damage to the organ.

- **Penis "fracture."** The most common form of penile trauma occurs when an erect penis is bent sharply, resulting in a tear or rupture in the tube-like structures (tunica albuginea) that carry blood to the penis. It usually occurs during sexual intercourse as a result of vigorous thrusting. Men who experience this type of injury typically feel a sharp pain and hear a popping or cracking sound. Discoloration and swelling usually occur as blood collects under the skin of the penis. Although urologists often refer to this particular injury as a penile fracture, the term is somewhat misleading since there is no bone in the penis.

DIAGNOSIS AND TREATMENT FOR PENILE TRAUMA

To diagnose an injury to the penis, a urologist will discuss the patient's medical history and conduct a physical examination, checking the organ carefully for bruises, cuts, abrasions, dents, sensitive areas, or bleeding. The urologist may also order blood and urine tests as well as diagnostic tests, such as an ultrasound or magnetic resonance imaging (MRI) exam, to determine the extent of damage to the penis. Another diagnostic tool involves inserting a tiny fiber optic camera into the urethra. Finally, the urologist may perform a retrograde urethrogram—an x-ray study that is performed by injecting a special dye into the urethra and checking to see whether it leaks out.

Treatment of penile trauma varies depending on the type and extent of injury. Many minor injuries can be treated with rest and anti-inflammatory medications. The usual treatment for penile fracture is surgery to repair tears or ruptures in the tunica albuginea and remove any blood clots. Studies have shown that surgery offers the lowest rates of penile scarring, curvature, and sexual dysfunction. The typical procedure is performed under general anesthesia. It involves making an incision around the shaft near the head of the penis and retracting the skin to locate and repair tissue damage. Afterward, the area is bandaged, and a catheter is placed in the urethra to drain urine from the bladder and allow the penis to heal. Most patients remain in the hospital under observation for one to two days and take antibiotics and pain relievers for one to two weeks after returning home.

Surgery is also the preferred option for patients with severe penile trauma or amputation. In cases where part or all of the penis has been severed, surgical reattachment may be possible for up to 16 hours if the organ is wrapped in gauze, placed in a plastic bag containing a sterile salt solution, and stored in a cooler of ice-cold water. Surgical reconstruction of the penis may also be possible following massive injuries although the extent of the damage will determine how much function the organ retains afterward.

References

"What Is Penile Trauma?" Urology Care Foundation, 2016. Available online. URL: www.urologyhealth.org/urologic-conditions/penile-trauma. Accessed August 7, 2023.

"Your Guide to Penis Pain and Injury," Herbal Love, 2016. Available online. URL: www.herballove.com/guide/your-guide-penis-pain-injury. Accessed August 7, 2023.

Section 22.5 | Priapism

Priapism is a rare but serious medical condition in which an erection lasts more than four hours. This persistent erection is not caused by sexual stimulation, and it does not dissipate after ejaculation. Instead, it occurs when blood becomes trapped in the penis due to problems with nerves or blood vessels. Left untreated, priapism can cause permanent damage to the penis and result in sexual dysfunction. There are three main types of priapism:

- **Low blood flow or ischemic priapism.** This is the most common form of priapism that occurs due to blockage of a blood vessel that prevents blood from flowing normally through the penis. The blockage prevents oxygen- and nutrient-rich blood from reaching the penile tissue, which can cause permanent damage if not treated promptly.

- **High blood flow priapism.** This rare condition occurs when a blood vessel ruptures, causing excessive blood to flow into the penile tissue. It usually results from an injury to the genital area.
- **Stuttering or episodic priapism.** This condition involves recurring, painful erections that last between two and three hours. They may occur during sleep or before or after sexual stimulation, and their frequency may increase over time. The causes and risk factors are usually similar to low blood flow priapism.

CAUSES OF PRIAPISM

Priapism can have a number of underlying causes, including the following:

- prescription medications that are commonly used to treat high blood pressure, attention deficit hyperactivity disorder (ADHD), depression, schizophrenia, and hormone imbalances
- injectable medications that are used to treat erectile dysfunction (ED)
- illegal drugs such as marijuana, ecstasy, cocaine, or methamphetamine (crystal meth)
- sickle cell disease (an inherited condition in which the body produces abnormally shaped red blood cells that can interfere with the function of blood vessels)
- blood cancers, such as leukemia and multiple myeloma
- injuries or medical conditions that affect the nervous system, brain, or spinal cord
- tumors of the prostate, bladder, or kidney
- infections in the genital area

DIAGNOSIS AND TREATMENT OF PRIAPISM

In addition to taking a medical history and performing a physical examination, a urologist or other practitioner will likely order blood tests and diagnostic tests to determine the type of priapism. These tests may include blood gas analysis of blood taken from the penile tissue, color duplex ultrasound to measure blood flow in the penis, or magnetic resonance imaging (MRI) to detect possible tumors or blood clots.

To relieve the immediate symptoms of priapism and restore normal blood flow, applying ice packs to the penis and perineum or exercising vigorously may be helpful. In other cases, a doctor may need to drain the trapped blood manually by inserting a needle into the penis. A vasoconstrictor medication may also be injected to help reduce the size of blood vessels and improve blood flow.

The recommended treatment for priapism depends on the underlying cause. If priapism occurs as a side effect of medication, the doctor may recommend stopping the medication and trying an alternative prescription. For stuttering priapism, a medication called "phenylephrine" may be prescribed to help control blood flow to the penis and prevent further episodes. For priapism resulting from a blood clot, surgery may be needed to remove the clot. High blood flow priapism resolves itself without treatment in about two-thirds of men, while the remaining cases require surgery to repair the ruptured blood vessels. If priapism causes tissue damage, resulting in sexual dysfunction, the patient may require surgery to implant a penile prosthesis.

References

"Priapism," myDr, June 25, 2016. Available online. URL: www.mydr.com.au/sexual-health/priapism. Accessed August 7, 2023.

"What to Know about Priapism," Medical News Today, August 1, 2017. Available online. URL: www.medicalnewstoday.com/articles/318737#outlook. Accessed August 7, 2023.

Section 22.6 | **Peyronie Disease**

WHAT IS PEYRONIE DISEASE?

Peyronie disease is a disorder in which scar tissue, called "plaque," forms under the skin of the penis—the male organ used for urination and sex.

The plaque builds up inside the penis, in the thick elastic membrane called the "tunica albuginea." The tunica albuginea helps keep the penis stiff during an erection. The plaque can develop anywhere along the penis.

As it develops, the plaque pulls on the surrounding tissues and causes the penis to curve or bend, usually during an erection. Curves in the penis can make erections painful and may make sexual intercourse painful, difficult, or impossible.

The plaque that develops in Peyronie disease is:

- caused by injury to your penis or by an autoimmune disease
- not the same plaque that can develop in a person's arteries
- benign—not cancerous and not a tumor

Peyronie disease occurs in two phases.

Acute Phase

During the acute phase, the plaque forms, and this phase can last up to 18 months. During this phase, the following changes occur:

- Inflammation may occur, and plaque forms on your penis.
- Your penis starts to curve.
- Your penis may hurt without an erection.
- Erections may become painful when scars develop.

Chronic Phase

The chronic phase occurs after the plaque has formed. Usually, the chronic phase begins 12–18 months after your symptoms first appear. During this phase, the following changes occur:

- Plaque and penile curvature may stabilize and not get worse.

- The pain in your penis may lessen.
- Erectile dysfunction (ED) may develop or become worse.

HOW COMMON IS PEYRONIE DISEASE?

Approximately 1 in 100 men in the United States over the age of 18 has been diagnosed with Peyronie disease. However, based on studies of men who reported having symptoms of Peyronie disease, researchers estimate that the actual number of men who have Peyronie disease is more than 1 in 10.

The chance of developing Peyronie disease increases with age. It is less common for men in their 20s and 30s to have Peyronie disease.

WHO IS MORE LIKELY TO HAVE PEYRONIE DISEASE?

You may be at higher risk of developing Peyronie disease if you:
- engage in vigorous sexual or nonsexual activities that cause micro-injuries to the penis
- have certain connective tissue and autoimmune disorders
- have a family history of Peyronie disease
- are older
- have diabetes and ED
- have a history of prostate cancer treatment with surgery

Vigorous Sexual and Nonsexual Activities

Men whose sexual or nonsexual activities (such as sports) cause micro-injuries to the penis are more likely to develop Peyronie disease.

Connective Tissue and Autoimmune Disorders

If you have certain connective tissue or autoimmune disorders, you may have a higher chance of developing Peyronie disease.

Connective tissue is a specialized tissue that supports, joins, or separates different types of tissues and organs in your body.

Connective tissue disorders may affect your joints, muscles, and skin. Some disorders associated with Peyronie disease include the following:

- **Dupuytren disease**. It is also known as "Dupuytren contracture." In this condition, the connective tissue in the palms of the hands shortens and thickens. This results in the permanent bending of the outer fingers. It is not clear why men with Peyronie disease are more likely to develop Dupuytren disease.
- **Plantar fasciitis**. It is the inflammation of the thick tissue on the bottom of the foot that creates the arch of the foot.
- **Scleroderma**. It is the abnormal growth of thick, hard patches of connective tissue. Scleroderma can also cause swelling or pain in muscles and joints.

In autoimmune disorders, the body's immune system attacks the body's own cells and organs. Autoimmune disorders associated with Peyronie disease include the following:

- **Systemic lupus erythematosus (SLE)**. SLE causes inflammation and damage to various body tissues including the joints, skin, kidneys, heart, lungs, blood vessels, and brain.
- **Sjögren syndrome**. This syndrome causes inflammation and damage to the glands that make tears and saliva.
- **Behçet disease**. This disease causes inflammation of the blood vessels.

Family History of Peyronie Disease
Medical experts believe that Peyronie disease may run in some families. For example, if your father or brother has Peyronie disease, you may have an increased chance of getting the disease too.

Aging
Your chance of getting Peyronie disease increases with age. Age-related changes in the tissues of the penis may cause it to be more easily injured and less likely to heal well.

Diabetes with Erectile Dysfunction

Men with diabetes-associated ED have a four to five times higher chance of developing Peyronie disease than the general population.

Prostate Cancer Treatment with Surgery

Your chance of getting Peyronie disease increases after surgery for prostate cancer. Medical experts believe this is related to ED developed after surgery for prostate cancer.

WHAT ARE THE COMPLICATIONS OF PEYRONIE DISEASE?

Complications of Peyronie disease may include the following:
- the inability to have sexual intercourse due to penile curvature
- ED
- emotional distress, depression, or anxiety about sexual abilities or the appearance of the penis
- stress in a relationship with a sexual partner
- problems fathering a child because intercourse is difficult

WHAT ARE THE SIGNS AND SYMPTOMS OF PEYRONIE DISEASE?

The signs and symptoms of Peyronie disease may include the following:
- hard lumps on one or more sides of the penis
- pain during sexual intercourse or during an erection
- a curve in the penis with or without an erection
- changes in the shape of the penis, such as narrowing or shortening
- ED

These may develop slowly or appear quickly and can be mild to severe. In many cases, the pain decreases over time although the curve in the penis may remain. Problems with intercourse or ED can occur during either phase.

WHAT CAUSES PEYRONIE DISEASE?

Medical experts do not know the exact cause of Peyronie disease but believe that it may be the result of:

- acute or chronic injury to the penis
- autoimmune disease

Peyronie disease is not contagious or caused by any known transmittable disease.

Injury to the Penis

Medical experts believe that hitting or bending the penis may injure the tissues inside. These injuries can happen during sex, athletic activity, or an accident. It can happen once, an acute injury, or repeatedly over time, a chronic injury.

The injury may cause bleeding and swelling inside the elastic membrane in the penis, or the tunica albuginea. When the injury heals, scar tissue may form, and a plaque can develop. The hard plaque pulls at the surrounding tissues and causes the penis to curve.

You may not be aware of micro-injuries to your penis when they occur. Researchers have found that many patients are unable to recall a specific incident just before symptoms started.

Autoimmune Disease

Men who have an autoimmune disease may develop Peyronie disease if the immune system attacks cells in the penis. This can lead to inflammation in the penis. Scar tissue may form and develop into plaque.

HOW DO HEALTH-CARE PROFESSIONALS DIAGNOSE PEYRONIE DISEASE?

Men with Peyronie disease are usually referred to a urologist—a doctor who specializes in sexual and urinary problems.

A urologist diagnoses Peyronie disease based on your medical and family history and a physical exam.

Imaging tests are usually not necessary to diagnose Peyronie disease but may be used to gather additional information about the plaque.

HOW DO HEALTH-CARE PROFESSIONALS TREAT PEYRONIE DISEASE?

The goal of treatment is to reduce pain, attain a straight or close-to-straight penis, and restore and maintain the ability to have intercourse.

Not all men with Peyronie disease need treatment. In a very few cases, Peyronie disease goes away without treatment.

Also, you may not need treatment if you have:
- small plaques
- little or no curve to your penis
- no pain
- no problems with sexual intercourse
- no urinary problems

If you need treatment, your urologist may recommend nonsurgical treatments or surgery depending on the severity of your symptoms, how much your penis curves, and whether your Peyronie disease is in the acute or chronic phase.

Your urologist will discuss your treatment options with you and review possible side effects and outcomes.

Besides treatment, your urologist may recommend lifestyle changes to reduce the risk of ED associated with Peyronie disease.

Nonsurgical Treatments

Nonsurgical treatments include injections, oral medicines, and medical therapies. They may be used when Peyronie disease is in the acute phase.
- **Injections**. Injecting a medicine directly into plaques, called "intralesional injections," can be done in the acute phase. The injection site is often numbed before the shot. These treatments can be done in the doctor's office.
  - **Collagenase**. Intralesional collagenase injections (Xiaflex) are currently the only treatment approved

by the U.S. Food and Drug Administration (FDA) for Peyronie disease. Collagenase is an enzyme that helps break down the substances that make up plaques. Breaking down the plaques reduces penile curving and improves erectile function. This treatment is approved for men with penises curving more than 30 degrees.

- **Verapamil**. It is used to treat high blood pressure (HBP) and may reduce penis pain and curving when injected into the plaque.
- **Interferon alpha-2b**. Interferon is a protein made by white blood cells (WBCs). Studies show that it reduces pain, penile curving, and plaque size.
- **Oral medicines**. There are no oral medicines that effectively treat penile curvature at this time. However, potassium para-aminobenzoate is used to treat Dupuytren contracture and may reduce plaque size. It has no effect on penile curving.

If you feel pain, your urologist may suggest you take nonsteroidal anti-inflammatory drugs (NSAIDs).

- **Nondrug medical therapies**. Other medical therapies to treat Peyronie disease are still being studied to see if they work. These therapies include the following:
  - **Mechanical traction and vacuum devices.** These are aimed at stretching or bending the penis to reduce curving.
  - **Shock wave therapy.** Focused, low-intensity electroshock waves directed at the plaque may be used to reduce pain.

Surgery

A urologist may recommend surgery to remove plaque or help straighten the penis during an erection. Surgery may be recommended for men who have Peyronie disease when:

- symptoms have not improved
- erections or intercourse, or both, is painful
- the curve in the penis prevents sexual intercourse

Medical experts recommend you do not have surgery until your plaque and penis curving stabilize.

Several types of surgeries treat Peyronie disease. Your urologist will examine the plaque on your penis and consider the best type of surgery for you. An ultrasound will show the exact location and size of the plaque.

Some men may develop complications after surgery, and sometimes, surgery does not correct some effects of Peyronie disease such as the shortening of the penis.

- **Grafting**. In this surgery, your urologist will remove the plaque and replace it with a patch of tissue that was taken from another part of your body, such as skin or a vein from your leg; grown in a laboratory; or taken from organ donors.
  This procedure may straighten the penis and restore some length that was lost due to Peyronie disease.
  Some men may experience numbness of the penis and ED after the procedure.
- **Plication**. In plication surgery, your urologist will remove or pinch a piece of the tunica albuginea from the side of the penis opposite the plaque to help straighten the penis.
  This procedure is less likely to cause numbness or ED.
  Plication cannot restore the length or girth of the penis, and the penis may become shorter.
- **Device implantation**. Penile implants may be considered if a man has both Peyronie disease and ED.
  A urologist implants a device into the penis that can cause an erection. The device may help straighten the penis during an erection.
  In some cases, the implant alone will straighten the penis adequately. If the implant alone does not straighten the penis, a urologist may combine implantation with one of the other two surgeries.

HOW COULD YOU PREVENT PEYRONIE DISEASE?

Researchers do not know how to prevent Peyronie disease. At this time, diet and nutrition have not been found to play a role in preventing Peyronie disease.[1]

Section 22.7 | Phimosis and Paraphimosis

Phimosis and paraphimosis are two distinct conditions related to the retraction of the foreskin of the penis. Phimosis primarily occurs in boys, whereas paraphimosis occurs in uncircumcised men.

WHAT IS PHIMOSIS?

The foreskin typically starts to loosen between the age of five and ten, allowing it to naturally retract the glans (the head of the penis). When this fails to occur, it is referred to as "phimosis." Phimosis is categorized into two types: physiologic and pathologic phimosis. Physiologic phimosis occurs in boys and usually resolves on its own, and pathologic phimosis, on the other hand, is a chronic inflammatory condition of the foreskin known as "balanitis xerotica obliterans" (BXO) or "lichen sclerosus," which leads to the formation of white, inflammatory, hypopigmented lesions on the foreskin.

CAUSES OF PHIMOSIS

Phimosis can result from various factors, including the following:
- **Forceful retraction.** The foreskin might cause slight damage and scarring, keeping the skin attached tightly to the glans.

---

[1] "Penile Curvature (Peyronie's Disease)," National Institute of Diabetes and Digestive and Kidney Diseases (NIDDK), August 2019. Available online. URL: www.niddk.nih.gov/health-information/urologic-diseases/penile-curvature-peyronies-disease. Accessed June 16, 2023.

- **Poor hygiene.** Poor genital hygiene may lead to smegma, a white, cheesy substance formed on the glans. This accumulation may result in infection and subsequent phimosis.
- **Balanitis.** Inflammation of the foreskin causes balanitis that tightens the skin and leads to phimosis.
- **Skin conditions.** Diseases affecting the glans, such as psoriasis, eczema, lichen sclerosus, and lichen planus, can cause scarring leading to phimosis.

SYMPTOMS OF PHIMOSIS
The symptoms of phimosis include the following:
- inability to retract the foreskin
- burning sensation or bleeding during urination
- discomfort and straining during urination
- urge to urinate even when the bladder is empty
- bulging of the foreskin during urination
- lower abdominal pain
- pus formation or pain in the foreskin
- pain during erection
- presence of white ring in the foreskin resembling scar tissue

DIAGNOSIS OF PHIMOSIS
Phimosis is diagnosed through a physical examination, often accompanied by a urine test to detect urinary tract infections. Swab tests may also be done to check for related infections.

TREATMENT OF PHIMOSIS
Phimosis is managed using the following methods:
- Topical steroid cream or gel is given to loosen the foreskin, which helps separate the foreskin from the glans.
- For cases when ointments do not work or if the condition is recurrent, circumcision is done.

WHAT IS PARAPHIMOSIS?

Paraphimosis occurs when the foreskin is retracted and becomes trapped behind the glans, preventing it from returning to its original position. This can lead to a constricting band that restricts blood flow to the glans, causing pain and discomfort.

CAUSES OF PARAPHIMOSIS

Paraphimosis is caused under the following circumstances:
- **Injury or infection**. As a result of surgery, piercings, scarring from infections, injury, or insect bites, the foreskin may not return to the original position causing paraphimosis.
- **Mishandling**. Paraphimosis is caused in cases where the foreskin is not pulled back after cleaning, catheterization, sex, or medical examination.
- **Partial circumcision**. Paraphimosis occurs in those who have had partial or no circumcision at all.
- **Diabetes**. Those with diabetes are more likely to get affected by chronic inflammation of the penis.

SYMPTOMS OF PARAPHIMOSIS

The symptoms of paraphimosis include the following:
- inability of the foreskin to return to the normal position
- swelling of the glans and foreskin
- pain and discomfort in the penis
- dark red, blue, or purple coloration of the glans
- tenderness of the penis

DIAGNOSIS OF PARAPHIMOSIS

Paraphimosis is diagnosed by physical examination. Visualization can identify the condition where a band-like structure, discoloration, or swelling is visible. Based on the other symptoms experienced, the diagnosis is made without any tests.

TREATMENT OF PARAPHIMOSIS

The following methods are used to treat paraphimosis:

- Topical gels or solutions are applied to reduce the inflammation of the foreskin.
- Needles are used to remove the blood and pus from the foreskin.
- Antibiotics are prescribed in case of infections.
- Circumcision is done if the condition is recurrent.
- When circumcision is not required, an incision or a dorsal slit is made on the foreskin to remove tightness or tension in the foreskin.
- An enzyme injection treatment or a bandage wrap on the penis is done to help ease swelling of the foreskin.

RISKS OF PHIMOSIS AND PARAPHIMOSIS

Phimosis can lead to severe conditions such as gangrene or penile cancer. If paraphimosis is not treated, it can result in permanent damage to the penile tissue.

References

Ellis, Mary Ellen. "Paraphimosis," Healthline, January 11, 2016. Available online. URL: www.healthline.com/health/paraphimosis. Accessed July 21, 2023.

"Paraphimosis," Cleveland Clinic, November 22, 2021. Available online. URL: https://my.clevelandclinic.org/health/diseases/22244-paraphimosis. Accessed July 21, 2023.

Roland, James. "Everything You Should Know about Phimosis," Healthline, September 29, 2018. Available online. URL: www.healthline.com/health/mens-health/phimosis. Accessed July 21, 2023.

"Tight Foreskin (Phimosis)," National Health Service (NHS), April 11, 2022. Available online. URL: www.nhs.uk/conditions/phimosis. Accessed July 21, 2023.

Section 22.8 | **Testicular Torsion**

WHAT IS TESTICULAR TORSION?

The spermatic cord consists of various blood vessels, ducts, and nerves that descend from the abdomen to the testicles. It supplies blood to the testicles and keeps them suspended within the scrotum. When the spermatic cords rotate and twist, failing to return to their normal position, blood flow is compromised, leading to testicular torsion. This condition is prevalent among males aged 12 and 18 and typically affects a single testicle. Only 2 percent of cases involve both testicles, often in those who have inherited the condition.

CAUSES OF TESTICULAR TORSION

Testicular torsion can occur due to an injury in the scrotum, vigorous exercise, or rapid growth of testicles during puberty. The condition may even happen during sleep. Those with a bell clapper deformity are particularly susceptible to testicular torsion. The bell clapper condition is when the testicles sway freely in the scrotum, allowing the cords to rotate and get twisted, resulting in testicular torsion.

SYMPTOMS OF TESTICULAR TORSION

Those affected with testicular torsion may experience sudden and intense pain, swelling, or a lump in the affected testicle. The intense pain may also radiate to the stomach, making walking uncomfortable. Noticeable asymmetry of the testicles is another symptom. Additional signs include red, purple, brown, or black discoloration, tenderness of the scrotum, frequent urination, and blood in the semen. Additionally, those with this condition may experience nausea, dizziness, fever, and vomiting.

DIAGNOSIS OF TESTICULAR TORSION

A doctor initially does a physical examination for swelling and discoloration and asks the patient about the other symptoms experienced. They may also perform a cremasteric reflex test by stroking the inner side of the thigh downward; a lack of testicular shrinkage or reflex response suggests torsion.

To confirm the diagnosis, an ultrasound is done to assess the flow of blood; reduced blood flow indicates torsion. A urine test is also done to check for infections. Prompt treatment is recommended to avoid reduced fertility or testicle loss due to inadequate blood flow.

TREATMENT OF TESTICULAR TORSION

It is crucial to inform the health-care provider immediately after symptoms occur, as torsion may eventually entirely cut off the blood flow to the testicles. Therefore, if the condition is not treated within four to six hours, it may result in the removal of the affected testicle.

In most cases, surgery is the primary treatment. The procedure requires a cut in the scrotum to untwist the cord, followed by attaching the testicle to the scrotum to prevent recurrence. This procedure is called "orchiopexy."

In rare cases, the doctor may attempt to untwist the spermatic cord by pushing the scrotum through manual detorsion. However, even if successful, a minor surgery is usually done to attach the cord within the scrotum to prevent future torsion.

In severe cases where the testicle is damaged, an orchiectomy is performed, which involves the removal of the affected testicle. This procedure is performed only when no other option is left.

It is essential to take care of oneself after surgery. The initial days after surgery might be painful, so it is important to refrain from carrying heavyweights and avoid vigorous exercise or activities for at least one month. Any postoperative swelling, bleeding, pain, or fever should prompt a follow-up appointment with a health-care provider.

References
Newman, Tim. "What Is Testicular Torsion?" Medical News Today, January 26, 2022. Available online. URL: www.

medicalnewstoday.com/articles/190514. Accessed
August 2, 2023.

"Testicular Torsion," Cleveland Clinic, February 27, 2023.
Available online. URL: https://my.clevelandclinic.org/
health/diseases/15382-testicular-torsion. Accessed
August 2, 2023.

"Testicular Torsion," Healthline, March 26, 2018. Available
online. URL: www.healthline.com/health/testicular-
torsion#treatment. Accessed August 2, 2023.

"Testicular Torsion," Urology Care Foundation, May 15,
2015. Available online. URL: www.urologyhealth.org/
urologic-conditions/testicular-torsion. Accessed August 2,
2023.

Section 22.9 | Erectile Dysfunction

Erectile dysfunction (ED) is a condition in which you are unable
to get or keep an erection firm enough for satisfactory sexual intercourse. ED can be a short- or long-term problem.

Health-care professionals, such as primary care providers and
urologists, can often treat ED. Although ED is very common, it is
not a normal part of aging. Talk with a health-care professional if
you have any ED symptoms. ED could be a sign of a more serious
health problem.

You may find it embarrassing and difficult to talk with a health-
care professional about ED. However, remember that a healthy
sex life can improve your quality of life (QOL) and is part of a
healthy life overall. Health-care professionals, especially urologists, are trained to speak to people about many kinds of sexual
problems.

DOES ERECTILE DYSFUNCTION HAVE ANOTHER NAME?

Erectile dysfunction is sometimes called "impotence," but health-
care professionals use this term less often.

HOW COMMON IS ERECTILE DYSFUNCTION?
Erectile dysfunction is very common. It affects about 30 million men in the United States.

WHO IS MORE LIKELY TO DEVELOP ERECTILE DYSFUNCTION?
You are more likely to develop ED if you:
- are older
- have certain diseases or conditions
- take certain medicines
- have certain psychological or emotional issues
- have certain health-related factors or behaviors, such as being overweight or smoking

CAUSES OF ERECTILE DYSFUNCTION
Many different factors affecting your vascular system, nervous system, and endocrine system can cause or contribute to ED.

Although you are more likely to develop ED as you age, aging does not cause ED. ED can be treated at any age.

Certain Diseases and Conditions
The following diseases and conditions can lead to ED:
- type 2 diabetes
- heart and blood vessel disease
- atherosclerosis
- high blood pressure (HBP)
- chronic kidney disease (CKD)
- multiple sclerosis (MS)
- Peyronie disease
- injury from treatments for prostate cancer, including radiation therapy and prostate surgery
- injury to the penis, spinal cord, prostate, bladder, or pelvis
- surgery for bladder cancer

Men who have diabetes are two to three times more likely to develop ED than men who do not have diabetes.

Taking Certain Medicines

ED can be a side effect of many common medicines, such as:
- blood pressure medicines
- antiandrogens—medicines used for prostate cancer therapy
- antidepressants
- tranquilizers, or prescription sedatives—medicines that make you calmer or sleepy
- appetite suppressants, or medicines that make you less hungry
- ulcer medicines

Certain Psychological or Emotional Issues

Psychological or emotional factors may make ED worse. You may develop ED if you have one or more of the following:
- fear of sexual failure
- anxiety
- depression
- guilt about sexual performance or certain sexual activities
- low self-esteem
- stress—about sexual performance, or stress in your life in general

Certain Health-Related Factors and Behaviors

The following health-related factors and behaviors may contribute to ED:
- smoking
- drinking too much alcohol
- using illegal drugs
- being overweight
- not being physically active

SYMPTOMS OF ERECTILE DYSFUNCTION

Symptoms of ED include the following:
- being able to get an erection sometimes, but not every time you want to have sex

- being able to get an erection, but not having it last long enough for sex
- being unable to get an erection at any time

ED is often a symptom of another health problem or health-related factor.

WHAT ARE THE COMPLICATIONS OF ERECTILE DYSFUNCTION?
Complications of ED may include the following:
- an unfulfilled sex life
- a loss of intimacy between you and a partner, resulting in a strained relationship
- depression, anxiety, and low self-esteem
- being unable to get a partner pregnant

DIAGNOSIS OF ERECTILE DYSFUNCTION
A doctor, such as a urologist, diagnoses ED with a medical and sexual history and a mental health and physical exam. You may find it difficult to talk with a health-care professional about ED. However, remember that a healthy sex life is part of a healthy life. The more your doctor knows about you, the more likely he or she can help treat your condition.

Medical and Sexual History
Taking a medical and sexual history is one of the first things a doctor will do to help diagnose ED. He or she will ask you to provide information, such as:
- how you would rate your confidence that you can get and keep an erection
- how often your penis is firm enough for intercourse when you have erections from sexual stimulation
- how often you are able to maintain an erection during sexual intercourse
- how often you find sexual intercourse satisfying
- if you have an erection when you wake up in the morning
- how you would rate your level of sexual desire

- how often you are able to climax, or orgasm, and ejaculate
- any surgeries or treatments that may have damaged your nerves or blood vessels near the penis
- any prescription or over-the-counter (OTC) medicines you take
- if you use illegal drugs, drink alcohol, or smoke

This information will help your doctor understand your ED problem. The medical history can reveal diseases and treatments that lead to ED. Reviewing your sexual activity can help your doctor diagnose problems with sexual desire, erection, climax, or ejaculation.

Mental Health and Physical Exam
A health-care professional may ask you some personal questions and use a questionnaire to help diagnose any psychological or emotional issues that may be leading to ED. The health-care professional may also ask your sexual partner questions about your relationship and how it may affect your ED.

He or she will also perform a physical exam to help diagnose the causes of ED. During the physical exam, a health-care professional most often checks your:
- penis to find out if it is sensitive to touch (If the penis lacks sensitivity, a problem in the nervous system may be the cause.)
- penis's appearance for the source of the problem (e.g., Peyronie disease causes the penis to bend or curve when erect.)
- body for extra hair or breast enlargement (which can point to hormonal problems)
- blood pressure
- pulse in your wrist and ankles (to see if you have a problem with circulation)

Lab Tests
Blood tests can uncover possible causes of ED, such as diabetes, atherosclerosis, CKD, and hormonal problems.

Imaging Tests

A technician most often performs a Doppler ultrasound in a doctor's office or an outpatient center. The ultrasound can detect poor blood flow through your penis. The technician passes a handheld device lightly over your penis to measure blood flow. Color images on a computer screen show the speed and direction blood is flowing through a blood vessel. A radiologist or urologist interprets the images. During this exam, a health-care professional may inject medicine into your penis to create an erection.

Other Tests

- **Nocturnal erection test.** During a nocturnal, or nighttime, erection test, you wear a plastic, ring-like device around your penis to test whether you have erections during the night while you sleep. This test usually takes place at home or in a special sleep lab. A more involved version of this test uses an electronic monitoring device that will record how firm the erections are, the number of erections, and how long they last. Each night during deep sleep, a man normally has three to five erections. If you have erections during either type of test, it shows that you are physically able to have an erection and that the cause of your ED is more likely a psychological or emotional issue. If you do not have an erection during either test, your ED is more likely due to a physical cause.
- **Injection test.** During an injection test, also called "intracavernosal injection," a health-care professional will inject a medicine into your penis to cause an erection. In some cases, a health-care professional may insert the medicine into your urethra instead. The health-care professional will evaluate how full your penis becomes and how long your erection lasts. Either test helps the health-care professional find the cause for your ED. The tests most often take place in a health-care professional's office.

TREATMENT FOR ERECTILE DYSFUNCTION

You can work with a health-care professional to treat an underlying cause of your ED. Choosing an ED treatment is a personal decision. However, you may also benefit from talking with your partner about which treatment is best for you as a couple.

Lifestyle Changes

Your health-care professional may suggest that you make lifestyle changes to help reduce or improve ED. You can do the following:

- Quit smoking.
- Limit or stop drinking alcohol.
- Increase physical activity and maintain a healthy body weight.
- Stop illegal drug use.

You can seek help from a health professional if you have trouble making these changes on your own.

Counseling

Talk with your doctor about going to a counselor if psychological or emotional issues are affecting your ED. A counselor can teach you how to lower your anxiety or stress related to sex. Your counselor may suggest that you bring your partner to counseling sessions to learn how to support you. As you work on relieving your anxiety or stress, a doctor can focus on treating the physical causes of ED.

HOW DO DOCTORS TREAT ERECTILE DYSFUNCTION?
Change Your Medicines

If a medicine you need for another health condition is causing ED, your doctor may suggest a different dose or different medicine. Never stop taking a medicine without speaking with your doctor first.

Prescribe Medicines You Take by Mouth

A health-care professional may prescribe you an oral medicine, or medicine you take by mouth, such as one of the following, to help you get and maintain an erection:

- sildenafil (Viagra)
- vardenafil (Levitra and Staxyn)
- tadalafil (Cialis)
- avanafil (Stendra)

All of these medicines work by relaxing smooth muscles and increasing blood flow in the penis during sexual stimulation. You should not take any of these medicines to treat ED if you are taking nitrates to treat a heart condition. Nitrates widen and relax your blood vessels. The combination can lead to a sudden drop in blood pressure, which may cause you to become faint or dizzy, or fall, leading to possible injuries.

Also, talk to your health-care professional if you are taking alpha-blockers to treat prostate enlargement. The combination of alpha-blockers and ED medicines could also cause a sudden drop in blood pressure.

A health-care professional may prescribe testosterone if you have low levels of this hormone in your blood. Although taking testosterone may help your ED, it is often unhelpful if your ED is caused by circulatory or nerve problems. Taking testosterone may also lead to side effects, including a high red blood cell (RBC) count and problems urinating.

Testosterone treatment also has not been proven to help ED associated with age-related or late-onset hypogonadism. Do not take testosterone therapy that has not been prescribed by your doctor. Testosterone therapy can affect how your other medicines work and can cause serious side effects.

Prescribe Injectable Medicines and Suppositories

Many men get stronger erections by injecting a medicine called "alprostadil" into the penis, causing it to become filled with blood. Oral medicines can improve your response to sexual stimulation, but they do not trigger an automatic erection like injectable medicines do.

Instead of injecting a medicine, some men insert a suppository of alprostadil into the urethra. A suppository is a solid piece of medicine that you insert into your body where it dissolves. A health-care professional will prescribe a prefilled applicator for you to insert the pellet about an inch into your urethra. An erection will begin within 8–10 minutes and may last 30–60 minutes.

Discuss Alternative Medicines

Some men say certain alternative medicines taken by mouth can help them get and maintain an erection. However, not all "natural" medicines or supplements are safe. Combinations of certain prescribed and alternative medicines could cause major health problems. To help ensure coordinated and safe care, discuss your use of alternative medicines, including use of vitamin and mineral supplements, with a health-care professional. Also, never order a medicine online without talking with your doctor.

HOW WILL SIDE EFFECTS OF ERECTILE DYSFUNCTION MEDICINES AFFECT YOU?

Erectile dysfunction medicines that you take by mouth, through an injection, or as a pellet in the urethra can have side effects, including a lasting erection known as "priapism." Call a health-care professional right away if an erection lasts four hours or longer.

A small number of men have vision or hearing loss after taking oral ED medicines. Call your health-care professional right away if you develop these problems.

PREVENTION OF ERECTILE DYSFUNCTION

You can help prevent many of the causes of ED by following these steps:

- **Quit smoking**. If you smoke, get help quitting. Smoking is linked to heart and blood vessel disease, which can lead to ED. Even when heart and blood vessel disease and other possible causes of ED are taken into account, smoking still increases the chances that you will have ED.

- **Follow a healthy eating plan**. To help maintain erectile function, choose whole-grain foods, low-fat dairy foods, fruits and vegetables, and lean meats. Avoid foods high in fat, especially saturated fat, and sodium. Follow a healthy eating plan to help aim for a healthy weight and control your blood pressure and diabetes. Controlling your blood pressure and diabetes may help prevent ED. Also, avoid drinking too much alcohol. If you are having trouble cutting out alcohol, see a counselor who has expert knowledge in treating people who drink too much.

- **Maintain a healthy weight to prevent diabetes and high blood pressure**. Maintaining a healthy weight can also help delay the start of diabetes and keep your blood pressure down. Talk with your doctor about how to prevent diabetes—or manage the disease if you already have it. Get regular checkups to measure your blood pressure. If you need to lose weight, talk with your health-care provider about how to lose weight safely. Ask for a referral to a dietitian who can help you plan healthy meals to lose weight. Losing weight may help reduce inflammation, increase testosterone levels, and increase self-esteem, all of which may help prevent ED. If you are at a healthy weight for your height, maintain that weight through healthy eating and physical activity.

- **Be physically active**. Physical activity increases blood flow through your body, including the penis. Talk with a health-care professional before starting new activities. Beginners should start slow, with easier activities such as walking at a normal pace or gardening. You can gradually work up to harder activities, such as walking briskly or swimming. Aim for at least 30 minutes of activity most days of the week.

- **Avoid using illegal drugs**. Using illegal drugs may prevent you from getting or keeping an erection. For instance, some illegal drugs may prevent you from becoming aroused or feeling other sensations. Using illegal drugs may mask other psychological, emotional, or physical factors that may be causing your ED. Talk with your health-care provider if you think you need help with drug abuse.[2]

[2] "Erectile Dysfunction (ED)," National Institute of Diabetes and Digestive and Kidney Diseases (NIDDK), January 11, 2017. Available online. URL: www.niddk.nih.gov/health-information/urologic-diseases/erectile-dysfunction. Accessed July 4, 2023.

Chapter 23 | Disorders of the Scrotum and Testicles

Chapter Contents

Section 23.1 | Epididymitis

WHAT IS EPIDIDYMITIS?

Acute epididymitis is a clinical syndrome causing pain, swelling, and inflammation of the epididymis and lasting less than six weeks. Sometimes, a testicle is also involved, a condition referred to as "epididymo-orchitis." A high index of suspicion for spermatic cord (testicular) torsion should be maintained among men who have a sudden onset of symptoms associated with epididymitis because this condition is a surgical emergency.

Acute epididymitis can be caused by sexually transmitted infections (STIs; e.g., *Chlamydia trachomatis*, *Neisseria gonorrhoeae*, or *Mycoplasma genitalium*) or enteric organisms (i.e., *Escherichia coli*). Acute epididymitis caused by an STI is usually accompanied by urethritis, which is frequently asymptomatic. Acute epididymitis caused by sexually transmitted enteric organisms might also occur among men who are the insertive partner during anal sex.

Nonsexually transmitted acute epididymitis caused by genitourinary pathogens typically occurs with bacteriuria secondary to bladder outlet obstruction (e.g., benign prostatic hyperplasia (BPH)). Among older men, nonsexually transmitted acute epididymitis is also associated with prostate biopsy, urinary tract instrumentation or surgery, systemic disease, or immunosuppression. Uncommon infectious causes of nonsexually transmitted acute epididymitis (e.g., Fournier gangrene) should be managed in consultation with a urologist.

Chronic epididymitis is characterized by a history of six or more weeks of symptoms of discomfort or pain in the scrotum, testicle, or epididymis. Chronic infectious epididymitis is most frequently observed with conditions associated with a granulomatous reaction.

Mycobacterium tuberculosis (TB) is the most common granulomatous disease affecting the epididymis and should be suspected, especially among men with a known history of or recent exposure to TB. The differential diagnosis of chronic noninfectious epididymitis, sometimes termed "orchialgia" or "epididymalgia," is broad (e.g., trauma, cancer, autoimmune conditions, or idiopathic

405

conditions). Men with this diagnosis should be referred to a urologist for clinical management.

DIAGNOSTIC CONSIDERATIONS

Men who have acute epididymitis typically have unilateral testicular pain and tenderness, hydrocele, and palpable swelling of the epididymis. Although inflammation and swelling usually begin in the tail of the epididymis, it can spread to the rest of the epididymis and testicle. The spermatic cord is usually tender and swollen. Spermatic cord (testicular) torsion, a surgical emergency, should be considered in all cases; however, it occurs more frequently among adolescents and men without evidence of inflammation or infection. For men with severe unilateral pain with sudden onset, for those whose test results do not support a diagnosis of urethritis or urinary tract infection (UTI), or for whom diagnosis of acute epididymitis is questionable, immediate referral to a urologist for evaluation for testicular torsion is vital because testicular viability might be compromised.

Bilateral symptoms should increase suspicion of other causes of testicular pain. Radionuclide scanning of the scrotum is the most accurate method for diagnosing epididymitis, but it is not routinely available. Ultrasound should be used primarily for ruling out torsion of the spermatic cord in cases of acute, unilateral, painful scrotal swelling. However, because partial spermatic cord torsion can mimic epididymitis on scrotal ultrasound, differentiation between spermatic cord torsion and epididymitis when torsion is not ruled out by ultrasound should be made on the basis of clinical evaluation. Although ultrasound can demonstrate epididymal hyperemia and swelling associated with epididymitis, it provides minimal diagnostic usefulness for men with a clinical presentation consistent with epididymitis. A negative ultrasound does not rule out epididymitis and, thus, does not alter clinical management. Ultrasound should be reserved for men if torsion of the spermatic cord is suspected or for those with scrotal pain who cannot receive an accurate diagnosis by history, physical examination, and objective laboratory findings.

All suspected cases of acute epididymitis should be evaluated for objective evidence of inflammation by one of the following point of care (POC) tests:

- Gram, methylene blue (MB), or gentian violet (GV) stain of urethral secretions demonstrating two or more white blood cells (WBCs) per oil immersion field (These stains are preferred POC diagnostic tests for evaluating urethritis because they are highly sensitive and specific for documenting both urethral inflammation and the presence or absence of gonococcal infection. Gonococcal infection is established by documenting the presence of WBC-containing intracellular gram-negative or purple diplococci on urethral Gram, MB, or GV stain.)
- positive leukocyte esterase test on first-void urine
- microscopic examination of sediment from a spun first-void urine demonstrating 10 or more WBCs/highest possible frequency (HPF)

All suspected cases of acute epididymitis should be tested for *C. trachomatis* and *N. gonorrhoeae* by nucleic acid amplification test (NAAT). Urine is the preferred specimen for NAAT for men. Urine cultures for chlamydial and gonococcal epididymitis are insensitive and are not recommended. Urine bacterial cultures should also be performed for all men to evaluate for the presence of genitourinary organisms and to determine antibiotic susceptibility.

TREATMENT

To prevent complications and transmission of STIs, presumptive therapy for all sexually active men is indicated at the time of the visit before all laboratory test results are available. Selection of presumptive therapy is based on risk for chlamydial and gonococcal infections or enteric organisms. Treatment goals for acute epididymitis are microbiologic infection cure, improvement of signs and symptoms, prevention of transmission of chlamydia and gonorrhea to others, and decreased potential for chlamydial or gonococcal epididymitis complications (e.g., infertility or chronic pain). Although the majority of men with acute epididymitis can be treated on an outpatient basis, referral to a specialist and hospitalization should be considered when severe pain or fever indicates other diagnoses (e.g., torsion, testicular infarction, abscess, or necrotizing fasciitis) or when men are unable to comply with an antimicrobial regimen. Age, history of diabetes, fever, and elevated C-reactive protein can indicate more severe disease requiring hospitalization.

Recommended Regimens for Epididymitis

- for acute epididymitis most likely caused by chlamydia or gonorrhea: ceftriaxone 500 mg* IM in a single dose and doxycycline 100 mg orally two times/day for 10 days
- for acute epididymitis most likely caused by chlamydia, gonorrhea, or enteric organisms (men who practice insertive anal sex): ceftriaxone 500 mg* IM in a single dose and levofloxacin 500 mg orally once daily for 10 days
- for acute epididymitis most likely caused by enteric organisms only: levofloxacin 500 mg orally once daily for 10 days

For persons weighing 150 kg and more, 1 g of ceftriaxone should be administered.

Levofloxacin monotherapy should be considered if the infection is most likely caused by enteric organisms only and gonorrhea has been ruled out by Gram, MB, or GV stain. This includes men who have undergone prostate biopsy, vasectomy, and other urinary tract instrumentation procedures. Treatment should be guided by bacterial cultures and antimicrobial susceptibilities. As an adjunct to therapy, bed rest, scrotal elevation, and nonsteroidal anti-inflammatory drugs are recommended until fever and local inflammation have subsided. Complete resolution of discomfort might not occur for a few weeks after completion of the antibiotic regimen.

OTHER MANAGEMENT CONSIDERATIONS

Men who have acute epididymitis confirmed or suspected to be caused by *N. gonorrhoeae* or *C. trachomatis* should be advised to abstain from sexual intercourse until they and their partners have been treated and symptoms have resolved. All men with acute epididymitis should be tested for human immunodeficiency virus (HIV) and syphilis.

FOLLOW-UP
Men should be instructed to return to their health-care providers if their symptoms do not improve within 72 hours after treatment. Signs and symptoms of epididymitis that do not subside in less than three days require reevaluation of the diagnosis and therapy. Men who experience swelling and tenderness that persist after completion of antimicrobial therapy should be evaluated for alternative diagnoses, including tumor, abscess, infarction, testicular cancer, TB, and fungal epididymitis.

MANAGEMENT OF SEX PARTNERS
Men who have acute sexually transmitted epididymitis confirmed or suspected to be caused by *N. gonorrhoeae* or *C. trachomatis* should be instructed to refer all sex partners during the previous 60 days before symptom onset for evaluation, testing, and presumptive treatment. If the last sexual intercourse was more than 60 days before the onset of symptoms or diagnosis, the most recent sex partner should be evaluated and treated. Arrangements should be made to link sex partners to care. Expedited partner therapy (EPT) is an effective strategy for treating sex partners of men who have or are suspected of having chlamydia or gonorrhea for whom linkage to care is anticipated to be delayed. Partners should be instructed to abstain from sexual intercourse until they and their sex partners are treated and symptoms have resolved.

SPECIAL CONSIDERATIONS
Drug Allergy, Intolerance, and Adverse Reactions
The risk for penicillin cross-reactivity is negligible between all third-generation cephalosporins (e.g., ceftriaxone).

Alternative regimens have not been studied; therefore, clinicians should consult an infectious disease specialist if such regimens are required.

Human Immunodeficiency Virus Infection

Men with HIV infection who have uncomplicated acute epididymitis should receive the same treatment regimen as those who do not have HIV. Other etiologic agents have been implicated in acute epididymitis among men with HIV, including cytomegalovirus (CMV), salmonella, toxoplasmosis, *Ureaplasma urealyticum*, *Corynebacterium* species, *Mycoplasma* species, and *Mima polymorpha*.[1]

Section 23.2 | Orchitis

WHAT IS ORCHITIS?

Orchitis refers to the painful swelling of one or both testicles caused by bacterial or viral infections. Although it can occur at any age, it most commonly affects boys after puberty.

CAUSES OF ORCHITIS

Several factors can cause orchitis:

- **Bacterial infections**. Bacteria such as *Escherichia coli*, *Streptococcus* species, and *Staphylococcus* species contribute to orchitis. They can spread from other parts of the body such as the urinary tract or epididymis.
- **Viral infections**. The most common viral infection that leads to orchitis is mumps, which affects males shortly after puberty. Those not vaccinated against mumps are more vulnerable. Other viral infections that lead to orchitis include rubella, chicken pox, cytomegalovirus, and hand, foot, and mouth disease.
- **Sexually transmitted infections (STIs)**. Certain STIs, such as syphilis, chlamydia, and gonorrhea, cause orchitis by spreading from the urethra to the testicles.

---

[1] "Epididymitis—STI Treatment Guidelines," Centers for Disease Control and Prevention (CDC), July 22, 2021. Available online. URL: www.cdc.gov/std/treatment-guidelines/epididymitis.htm. Accessed June 16, 2023.

They primarily affect men between the ages of 19 and 35.

- **Urinary tract infections (UTIs)**. Men with congenital or recurring UTIs are at a higher risk of getting orchitis.
- **Bladder outlet obstruction**. Conditions such as urethral stricture and benign prostatic hyperplasia (BPH) contribute to orchitis. While urethral stricture is the condition of scarring in the urethra that reduces the flow of urine, leading to inflammation, BPH is the condition of an enlarged prostate gland that causes a block in the flow of urine, resulting in orchitis.
- **Surgeries**. Men who have undergone urinary tract surgery and those who use Foley catheter long term may have greater risk of testicle inflammation and orchitis.

SYMPTOMS OF ORCHITIS
Orchitis is characterized by several symptoms, including:
- fever and chills
- nausea and vomiting
- fatigue and muscle pain
- swelling and tenderness in the affected testicle
- pain during urination and ejaculation
- blood in semen and unusual urine discharge
- pain in the groin

DIAGNOSIS OF ORCHITIS
A physical examination is done to check for tenderness, redness, or swelling of the testicles. Complete blood count, urine test, urine culture, urethral smear, and swab tests are done to screen for STIs. Finally, a testicular ultrasound is performed to rule out testicular torsion and confirm the presence of orchitis.

TREATMENT OF ORCHITIS
Treatment for orchitis is based on the underlying cause, as there is no specific method. Only the symptoms can be managed until

the condition subsides. Applying ice on the affected area or taking anti-inflammatory medicines and pain relievers helps reduce swelling and pain.

Antibiotics are prescribed for orchitis caused by bacteria and STIs. The patient's partner should also receive treatment for the STI if this is the cause.

Bed rest is recommended with the scrotum in an elevated position to provide relief. It is also recommended to avoid heavy lifting.

It is essential to complete the entire course of antibiotics, even if the symptoms improve, to prevent recurrence or complications.

PREVENTION OF ORCHITIS

Getting vaccinated against mumps is important to prevent the development of orchitis. Maintaining genital hygiene and practicing safe sex can also help prevent the condition. However, congenital urinary tract issues may not be preventable.

COMPLICATIONS OF ORCHITIS

While most men recover from orchitis without major complications, rare cases might lead to the following:

- **Testicular atrophy**. Orchitis caused by mumps may lead to the shrinking of the testicles.
- **Scrotal abscess**. Orchitis may lead to the formation of a painful blister in the scrotum.
- **Testicular infarction**. Orchitis could lead to the death of the testicular tissue.
- **Infertility**. When both testicles are affected, men may have a decreased sperm count leading to infertility, though this is rare.

References

"Orchitis," Cleveland Clinic, July 8, 2021. Available online. URL: https://my.clevelandclinic.org/health/diseases/21658-orchitis. Accessed August 3, 2023.

"Orchitis (Inflammation of the Testicle)," WebMD. September 18, 2022. Available online. URL: www.webmd.

com/men/inflammation-testicle-orchitis. Accessed August 3, 2023.

"Orchitis," Mayo Clinic, December 1, 2022. Available online. URL: www.mayoclinic.org/diseases-conditions/orchitis/symptoms-causes/syc-20375860. Accessed August 3, 2023.

"Orchitis," MedlinePlus, January 1, 2023. Available online. URL: https://medlineplus.gov/ency/article/001280.htm. Accessed August 3, 2023.

Roth, Erica. "Orchitis," Healthline, December 7, 2018. Available online. URL: www.healthline.com/health/orchitis. Accessed August 3, 2023.

Section 23.3 | Varicocele

WHAT IS VARICOCELE?

Swelling or enlargement of pampiniform plexus caused by the pooling of blood is known as "varicocele." Pampiniform plexus is the network of veins in the scrotum or scrotal sacs, which regulate the blood flow and temperature of the testicles. Varicocele mainly affects the left scrotal sac and is rare in both sacs. It affects 10–15 percent of men and occurs in 40 percent of infertile men. Varicocele typically begins during puberty and is often painless.

CLASSIFICATION OF VARICOCELE

Varicoceles are classified based on size and palpability into three grades:

- **Grade 0 (subclinical).** These varicoceles cannot be felt by touch but are visible on ultrasound. Treatment might not be necessary unless fertility issues or discomfort arise.
- **Grade I.** They can only be felt while performing the Valsalva maneuver technique. Treatment might not be required, but over-the-counter (OTC) medicines can alleviate swelling or itching.

- **Grade II.** The veins can be felt but not seen. If it is accompanied by pain, OTC medicines or nonsurgical treatment are options.
- **Grade III.** The veins are prominently visible. Based on the severity of the condition, surgery is considered.

SYMPTOMS OF VARICOCELE

Mild varicoceles might not show any symptoms and could be too small to feel, but large varicoceles may be accompanied by any of the following symptoms:

- different-sized testicles (shrunk or swollen)
- a lump in the scrotum
- dull, recurring pain
- visible twisted veins in the scrotum
- infertility

DIAGNOSIS OF VARICOCELE

To diagnose varicocele, a physical examination is done after reviewing the medical history of the patient. Following this, a Valsalva maneuver is performed. It is the process in which the patient holds his breath, closes his mouth, and forcefully blows air out so that the scrotal sac gets tightened, which makes it easier to feel the veins.

Further tests are done to confirm the diagnosis. A pelvic ultrasound is performed to visualize the veins in the testicles. The ultrasound results are positive if the flow of blood is in the wrong direction and the veins are above 3 mm.

Semen analysis is done to check the health of the sperm since varicocele decreases motility and sperm count. Finally, a blood test is done to check the hormone levels such as testosterone and follicle-stimulating hormone (FSH). Low testosterone levels and high FSH levels confirm the diagnosis.

TREATMENT OPTIONS FOR VARICOCELE

Appropriate treatment is given based on the grade in which varicocele is categorized after the diagnosis.

Treatment may not be required when the condition is mild and no discomfort is experienced. In other cases, pain or itching can be relieved using OTC medicines and by applying ice on the area where it is swollen.

When surgery is unnecessary, a nonsurgical treatment known as "embolization" is done. It is the process in which the blood flow is diverted away from the affected vein.

When surgery is the only option left, it is done through microscopic varicocelectomy and laparoscopic varicocelectomy, where the affected vein is blocked to prevent the flow of blood. Recovery takes almost six weeks.

References
Herndon, Jaime. "Varicocele," Healthline, January 31, 2022. Available online. URL: www.healthline.com/health/varicocele. Accessed July 26, 2023.

Leslie, Stephen W.; Hussain, Sajjad; and Siref, Larry E. "Varicocele," National Library of Medicine (NLM), May 30, 2023. Available online. URL: www.ncbi.nlm.nih.gov/books/NBK448113. Accessed July 25, 2023.

"Varicocele," Cleveland Clinic, March 30, 2023. Available online. URL: https://my.clevelandclinic.org/health/diseases/15239-varicocele. Accessed July 25, 2023.

"Varicocele," Mayo Clinic, March 3, 2022. Available online. URL: www.mayoclinic.org/diseases-conditions/varicocele/symptoms-causes/syc-20378771. Accessed July 26, 2023.

"What Are Varicoceles?" Urology Care Foundation, July 16, 2019. Available online. URL: www.urologyhealth.org/urology-a-z/v/varicoceles. Accessed July 26, 2023.

Section 23.4 | Hydrocele

A hydrocele is a generally harmless, painless buildup of fluid around one or both testicles that causes swelling in the scrotum. Hydroceles can be described as primary or secondary. Primary hydroceles occur from an imbalance in the absorption and secretion of fluids in the testis membranes. The accumulation of fluid leads to hydrocele formation. Secondary hydroceles occur due to an underlying medical condition that affects the male reproductive organs, injury to the genital area, or cancer.

Congenital hydroceles may form in newborns when the abdominal fluid drains into the scrotum, thus causing swelling. In the majority of the cases, the passage from the abdomen to the scrotum closes on its own. In some newborns, however, the sac fails to close, which causes a route to the abdominal cavity to remain open. This is called a "communicating hydrocele" since it allows the passage of fluid between the abdomen and scrotum. A noncommunicating hydrocele, on the other hand, develops when the sac closes but traps some fluid in the scrotum. Congenital hydroceles are found in about 10 percent of newborns and may regress spontaneously within the first two years of life.

Hydroceles may also affect adolescents and adults, most often men over 40. In these cases, the hydrocele may be caused by a condition in which the passage from the abdomen to the scrotum either has not closed all the way or has reopened. Other causes of hydroceles in adults include injury to the scrotum or inflammation resulting from an infection.

SYMPTOMS OF HYDROCELE

A hydrocele commonly presents as an enlargement of the scrotum, just below the testes, and is usually painless unless there is infection or some other underlying cause of discomfort. In the case of communicating hydroceles, the size of the swelling may vacillate during the day, typically growing larger with coughing, straining, crying, or any activity that raises intra-abdominal pressure.

DIAGNOSIS OF HYDROCELE

A simple physical examination involving palpation (feeling with the hand) is the first step in diagnosing a hydrocele. The doctor may also use a technique called transillumination, in which a bright light is focused on the scrotum. The presence of clear fluid allows transmission of light, and the scrotum "lights up," revealing the presence of a hydrocele or other testicular abnormalities. The doctor may also recommend blood and urine tests or a scrotal ultrasound to confirm the initial diagnosis.

TREATMENT FOR HYDROCELE

Hydroceles generally do not require treatment unless they attain a critical size and the patient experiences discomfort or difficulty moving. However, it is prudent to check with your health-care provider to rule out other complications, such as infection, testicular tumor, or inguinal hernia. An inguinal hernia, one of the most common risks associated with hydrocele, develops when a loop of the intestine protrudes into the scrotum and may require surgical intervention.

When medical intervention is required, the following are some possible treatments for hydrocele:

- **Needle aspiration**. The safest, cheapest, and most noninvasive treatment option involves drainage of fluid from the hydrocele using a syringe. While this procedure is often successful in providing symptomatic relief in large hydroceles, it carries a high likelihood of recurrence and is most often recommended when surgery is not an option.
- **Sclerotherapy**. This form of treatment is often used in conjunction with aspiration to prevent or delay the recurrence of a hydrocele. Sclerotherapy involves the injection of medication after the fluid has been drained.
- **Hydrocelectomy**. It is a surgical repair that is used to correct large, painful, recurring hydroceles. If the hydrocele is uncomplicated, the surgery generally takes less than an hour and is typically performed on an outpatient basis under either general or local

anesthesia. An incision is made in the scrotum or lower abdomen. The hydrocele sac is drained of its fluid and is partially or totally removed. Related conditions, such as inguinal hernia, may also be corrected during hydrocelectomy. Some surgeons use laparoscopy—a minimally invasive procedure using a camera-tipped instrument called a laparoscope—to repair hydroceles. Hydrocelectomy is generally considered safe, and most patients experience minimal complications and have a successful long-term outcome.

References

"Hydrocele," Mayo Clinic, October 9, 2014. Available online. URL: www.mayoclinic.org/diseases-conditions/hydrocele/basics/definition/con-20024139. Accessed August 7, 2023.

"Hydrocele—Topic Overview," *WebMD*, November 14, 2014. Available online. URL: www.webmd.com/parenting/baby/tc/hydrocele-topic-overview. Accessed August 7, 2023.

Parks, Kelly and Leung, Lawrence. "Recurrent Hydrocoele," National Center for Biotechnology Information (NCBI), 2013. Available online. URL: www.ncbi.nlm.nih.gov/pmc/articles/PMC3894005. Accessed August 7, 2023.

Section 23.5 | Spermatocele

WHAT IS A SPERMATOCELE?

A spermatocele—often called a "spermatic cyst"—is a benign fluid-filled mass within the scrotum. The cyst is an accumulation of fluid and sperm cells that typically arises from the caput (head) of the epididymis, a tightly coiled tube located above each testicle that collects and transports sperm. Spermatoceles are common and generally do not require treatment. However, discomfort, pain, or a bothersome enlargement may require surgical intervention.

Spermatoceles are found in an estimated 30 percent of adult men. They are usually asymptomatic, do not affect fertility, and are most often discovered during self-examination or in an imaging test carried out for other conditions.

CAUSES OF SPERMATOCELE

The exact cause of spermatoceles is unknown although a number of possible etiologies have been proposed:
- They could be caused by an obstruction in the epididymal ducts.
- Sperm may accumulate in the head of the epididymis and lead to the formation of a cyst.
- Although they usually form spontaneously without any preceding injury, infection, or inflammation, they could result from a previous medical condition.

SYMPTOMS OF SPERMATOCELE

Symptoms of spermatoceles include the following:
- a lump or mass in the scrotum
- enlarged scrotum
- pain, swelling, or redness of the scrotum
- pressure felt at the base of the penis

DIAGNOSIS OF SPERMATOCELE

A spermatocele can be felt as a firm, smooth lump by palpating (feeling) the scrotum during a medical examination or self-exam.

Diagnosis can be confirmed by a transillumination exam, in which a doctor shines a light behind each testicle. An ultrasound may be used for further confirmation, and a sonogram can help determine if the lump is a spermatocele or a benign or cancerous tumor. If the lump is painful, a blood count and urinalysis may be required to detect infection or inflammation.

TREATMENT FOR SPERMATOCELE

Spermatoceles are not dangerous, and if the cyst is small and does not change in size, treatment may not be needed. However, treatment might be required for pain alleviation or, in rare cases, if there is decreased blood supply to the penis.

Oral analgesics are often prescribed for symptomatic pain relief. If the pain and discomfort are caused by underlying epididymitis— inflammation of the epididymis—antibiotics may be prescribed.

If the spermatocele becomes larger and causes considerable discomfort, a procedure to remove it surgically, known as a spermatocelectomy, may be carried out. Needle aspiration, often used to treat other types of cysts, is contraindicated in spermatoceles because it could result in infection due to spillage of sperm within the scrotum.

Spermatocelectomy is generally an outpatient surgical procedure, performed under anesthesia. A postoperative evaluation is done after two to six weeks to ensure that the incision is healing properly and that there are no complications. Spermatocelectomy has an excellent outcome and prognosis, with a 94 percent recovery rate.

References

Mayo Clinic Staff, "Diseases and Conditions: Spermatocele," Mayo Clinic, December 16, 2014. Available online. URL: www.mayoclinic.org/diseases-conditions/spermatocele/basics/definition/con-20024190. Accessed August 7, 2023.

Paris, Vernon M. "Spermatocele Treatment & Management," Medscape, October 15, 2015. Available online. URL: http://emedicine.medscape.com/article/443432-treatment#d9. Accessed August 7, 2023.

"Spermatoceles," Urology Care Foundation, n.d. Available online. URL: www.urologyhealth.org/urologic-conditions/spermatoceles. Accessed August 7, 2023.

Thomson, Gregory E. and Wood, Christopher G. "Spermatocele (Epididymal Cyst)," *Web*MD, November 14, 2014. Available online. URL: www.webmd.com/men/tc/spermatocele-epididymal-cyst-topic-overview. Accessed August 7, 2023.

Chapter 24 | Sexually Transmitted Diseases

Chapter Contents

Section 24.1 | What Are Sexually Transmitted Diseases?

Sexually transmitted diseases (STDs)/sexually transmitted infections (STIs) are a group of illnesses that are passed from person to person during sexual intercourse, oral sex, or certain types of sex play. These diseases can be caused by bacteria, viruses, or parasites and are spread through intimate sexual contact involving the penis, mouth, or anus or contact with any of the membranes that line the urinary and/or genital tracts. STDs/STIs are also called "venereal diseases."

Health-care providers often use the term "infection" rather than "disease" because it is possible for a person to have no symptoms but still have the infection and require treatment. Scientists have identified more than 20 different STIs.

WHAT ARE SOME TYPES OF SEXUALLY TRANSMITTED DISEASES OR SEXUALLY TRANSMITTED INFECTIONS?

Approximately 20 different infections are known to be transmitted through sexual contact. Some common STIs are:

- chlamydia
- gonorrhea
- genital herpes
- human immunodeficiency virus (HIV)/acquired immunodeficiency syndrome (AIDS)
- human papillomavirus (HPV)
- syphilis
- bacterial vaginosis
- trichomoniasis
- viral hepatitis
- Zika

WHAT CAUSES SEXUALLY TRANSMITTED DISEASES OR SEXUALLY TRANSMITTED INFECTIONS?

The following are the three major causes of STDs/STIs:

- bacteria, including chlamydia, gonorrhea, and syphilis
- viruses, including HIV/AIDS, herpes simplex virus (HSV), HPV, hepatitis B virus, cytomegalovirus (CMV), and Zika

- parasites, such as trichomonas vaginalis, or insects, such as crab lice or scabies mites

Any STI can be spread through sexual activity, including sexual intercourse, and some STIs are also spread through oral sex and other sexual activity. Ejaculation does not have to occur for an STI to pass from person to person.

In addition, sharing contaminated needles, such as those used to inject drugs, or using contaminated body piercing or tattooing equipment can also transmit some infections, such as HIV, hepatitis B, and hepatitis C. A few infections can be sexually transmitted but are also spread through nonsexual, close contact. Some of these infections, such as CMV, are not considered STIs even though they can be transmitted through sexual contact.

Regardless of how a person is exposed, once a person is infected by an STI, he or she can spread the infection to other people through oral, vaginal, or anal sex, even if he or she has no symptoms.

WHAT ARE THE SYMPTOMS OF SEXUALLY TRANSMITTED DISEASES OR SEXUALLY TRANSMITTED INFECTIONS?

People with STDs/STIs may feel ill and notice some of the following signs and symptoms:

- unusual discharge from the penis or vagina
- sores or warts on the genital area
- painful or frequent urination
- itching and redness in the genital area
- blisters or sores in or around the mouth
- abnormal vaginal odor
- anal itching, soreness, or bleeding
- abdominal pain
- fever

In some cases, people with STIs have no symptoms. Over time, any symptoms that are present may improve on their own. It is also possible for a person to have an STI with no symptoms and then pass it on to others without knowing it.

If you are concerned that you or your sexual partner may have an STI, talk to your health-care provider. Even if you do not have symptoms, it is possible you may have an STI that needs treatment to ensure your and your partners' sexual health.

HOW DO HEALTH-CARE PROVIDERS DIAGNOSE A SEXUALLY TRANSMITTED DISEASE OR SEXUALLY TRANSMITTED INFECTION?

Any person who is sexually active should discuss his or her risk factors for STDs/STIs with a health-care provider and ask about getting tested. If you are sexually active, it is important to remember that you may have an STD/STI and not know it because many STDs/STIs do not cause symptoms. You should get tested and have regular checkups with a health-care provider who can help assess and manage your risk, answer your questions, and diagnose and treat an STD/STI if needed.

Some STDs/STIs may be diagnosed during a physical exam or through microscopic examination of a sore or fluid swabbed from the penis or anus. This fluid can also be cultured over a few days to see whether infectious bacteria or yeast can be detected. Blood tests are used to detect infections, such as hepatitis A, B, and C, or HIV/AIDS.

Because STDs are passed from person to person and can have serious health consequences, the health department notifies people if they have been exposed to certain STDs/STIs. Not all STDs/STIs are reported, though. If you receive a notice, it is important to see a health-care provider, be tested, and start treatment right away.

WHAT ARE THE TREATMENTS FOR SEXUALLY TRANSMITTED DISEASES AND SEXUALLY TRANSMITTED INFECTIONS?

Sexually transmitted diseases and STIs caused by bacteria or parasites can be treated with antibiotics. These antibiotics are most often given by mouth (orally). However, sometimes, they are injected or applied directly to the affected area.

The treatments, complications, and outcomes for viral STIs depend on the particular virus (HIV, genital herpes, HPV, hepatitis, or CMV). Treatments can reduce the symptoms and the progression of most of these infections. For example, medications are available to limit the frequency and severity of genital herpes outbreaks while reducing the risk that the virus will be passed on to other people.

Individuals with HIV need to take special antiretroviral drugs that control the amount of virus they carry. These drugs, called "highly active antiretroviral therapy" (HAART), can help people live longer, healthier lives and can prevent onward transmission of HIV to others.

Whatever the infection and regardless of how quickly the symptoms resolve after beginning treatment, the infected person and their partner(s) must take all of the medicines prescribed by the health-care provider to ensure that the STI is completely treated. Likewise, they should follow health-care provider recommendations about how long to abstain from sex after the treatment is completed to avoid passing the infection back and forth.

IS THERE A CURE FOR SEXUALLY TRANSMITTED DISEASES AND SEXUALLY TRANSMITTED INFECTIONS?

Viruses such as HIV, genital herpes, HPV, hepatitis, and CMV cause STDs/STIs that cannot be cured. People with an STI caused by a virus will be infected for life and will always be at risk of infecting their sexual partners. However, treatments for these viruses can significantly reduce the risk of passing on the infection and can reduce or eliminate symptoms. STIs caused by bacteria, yeast, or parasites can be cured using appropriate medication.[1]

[1] "Sexually Transmitted Diseases (STDs)," *Eunice Kennedy Shriver* National Institute of Child Health and Human Development (NICHD), January 31, 2017. Available online. URL: www.nichd.nih.gov/health/topics/stds. Accessed June 20, 2023.

Section 24.2 | Chlamydia

WHAT IS CHLAMYDIA?
Chlamydia is a common sexually transmitted disease (STD). It is caused by bacteria called "*Chlamydia trachomatis*." Anyone can get chlamydia. It often does not cause symptoms, so people may not know that they have it. Antibiotics can cure it. But, if it is not treated, chlamydia can cause serious health problems.

HOW DOES CHLAMYDIA SPREAD?
You can get chlamydia during oral, vaginal, or anal sex with someone who has chlamydia.

If you have had chlamydia and were treated in the past, you can get reinfected if you have unprotected sex with someone who has it.

WHO IS MORE LIKELY TO GET CHLAMYDIA?
Chlamydia is more common in young people, especially young women. You are more likely to get infected with chlamydia if you do not consistently use a condom or if you have multiple partners.

WHAT ARE THE SYMPTOMS OF CHLAMYDIA?
Chlamydia does not usually cause any symptoms. So you may not realize that you have it. But, even if you do not have symptoms, you can still pass the infection to others.

If you do have symptoms, they may not appear until several weeks after you have sex with someone who has chlamydia.

Symptoms in men include the following:
- discharge from the penis
- a burning sensation when urinating (peeing)
- pain and swelling in one or both testicles (although this is less common)

If the chlamydia infects the rectum, it can cause rectal pain, discharge, and bleeding.

HOW IS CHLAMYDIA DIAGNOSED?

There are lab tests to diagnose chlamydia. Your health-care provider may ask you to provide a urine sample.

WHO SHOULD BE TESTED FOR CHLAMYDIA?

You should go to your provider for a test if you have symptoms of chlamydia or if you have a partner who has an STD.

Men who have sex with men (MSM) should get checked for chlamydia every year.

WHAT OTHER PROBLEMS CAN CHLAMYDIA CAUSE?

Men often do not have health problems from chlamydia. Sometimes, it can infect the epididymis (the tube that carries sperm). This can cause pain, fever, and, rarely, infertility.

Men can also develop reactive arthritis because of a chlamydia infection. Reactive arthritis is a type of arthritis that happens as a "reaction" to an infection in the body.

Babies born to infected mothers can get eye infections and pneumonia from chlamydia. It may also make it more likely for your baby to be born too early.

Untreated chlamydia may also increase your chances of getting or giving HIV.

WHAT ARE THE TREATMENTS FOR CHLAMYDIA?

Antibiotics will cure the infection. You may get a one-time dose of the antibiotics, or you may need to take medicine every day for seven days. It is important to take all the medicine that your provider prescribed for you. Antibiotics cannot repair any permanent damage that the disease has caused.

To prevent spreading the disease to your partner, you should not have sex until the infection has cleared up. If you got a one-time dose of antibiotics, you should wait seven days after taking the medicine to have sex again. If you have to take medicine every day for seven days, you should not have sex again until you have finished taking all of the doses of your medicine.

It is common to get a repeat infection, so you need to get tested again about three months after treatment.

CAN CHLAMYDIA BE PREVENTED?

The only sure way to prevent chlamydia is to not have vaginal, anal, or oral sex.

Correct usage of latex condoms greatly reduces, but does not eliminate, the risk of catching or spreading chlamydia. If your or your partner is allergic to latex, you can use polyurethane condoms.[2]

Section 24.3 | Genital Herpes

WHAT IS GENITAL HERPES?

Genital herpes is a sexually transmitted disease (STD) caused by two types of viruses—herpes simplex virus type 1 (HSV-1) and herpes simplex virus type 2 (HSV-2). Genital herpes is common in the United States among people aged 14–49.

HOW IS GENITAL HERPES SPREAD?

You can get genital herpes by having vaginal, anal, or oral sex with someone who has the infection. You can get herpes if you have contact with:
- a herpes sore
- saliva from a partner with an oral herpes infection
- genital fluids from a partner with a genital herpes infection
- skin in the oral area of a partner with oral herpes
- skin in the genital area of a partner with genital herpes

You can also get genital herpes from a sex partner who does not have a visible sore or is unaware of their infection. It is also

---

[2] MedlinePlus, "Chlamydia Infections," National Institutes of Health (NIH), March 13, 2023. Available online. URL: https://medlineplus.gov/chlamydiainfections.html. Accessed June 20, 2023.

possible to get genital herpes if you receive oral sex from a partner with oral herpes.

You will not get herpes from toilet seats, bedding, or swimming pools. You will also not get it from touching objects, such as silverware, soap, or towels.

WHAT IS ORAL HERPES?

Herpes simplex virus type 1 often causes oral herpes, which can result in cold sores or fever blisters on or around the mouth. However, most people with oral herpes do not have any symptoms. Most people with oral herpes get it during childhood or young adulthood from nonsexual contact with saliva.

IS THERE A LINK BETWEEN GENITAL HERPES AND ORAL HERPES?

Yes. Oral herpes caused by HSV-1 can spread from the mouth to the genitals through oral sex. This is why some cases of genital herpes are due to HSV-1.

WHAT IS THE LINK BETWEEN GENITAL HERPES AND HUMAN IMMUNODEFICIENCY VIRUS?

Herpes infection can cause sores or breaks in the skin or lining of the mouth, vagina, and rectum. This provides a way for human immuno-deficiency virus (HIV) to enter the body. Even without visible sores, herpes increases the number of immune cells in the lining of the genitals. HIV targets immune cells for entry into the body. Having both HIV and genital herpes increases the chance of spreading HIV to an HIV-negative partner during oral, vaginal, or anal sex.

SYMPTOMS OF GENITAL HERPES

Most people with genital herpes have no symptoms or have very mild symptoms. Mild symptoms may go unnoticed or be mistaken for other skin conditions such as a pimple or ingrown hair. Because of this, most people do not know they have a herpes infection.

Herpes sores usually appear as one or more blisters on or around the genitals, rectum, or mouth. This is known as having an "outbreak." The blisters break and leave painful sores that may take a week or more to heal. Flu-like symptoms (e.g., fever, body aches, or swollen glands) may also occur during the first outbreak.

People who experience an initial outbreak of herpes can have repeated outbreaks, especially if they have HSV-2. However, repeat outbreaks are usually shorter and less severe than the first outbreak. Although genital herpes is a lifelong infection, the number of outbreaks may decrease over time.

Ask a health-care provider to examine you if:

- you notice any symptoms
- your partner has an STD or symptoms of an STD

STD symptoms can include an unusual sore, a smelly genital discharge, burning when peeing, or bleeding between periods (if you have a menstrual cycle).

HOW WOULD YOUR HEALTH-CARE PROVIDER KNOW IF YOU HAVE GENITAL HERPES?

Your health-care provider may diagnose genital herpes by simply looking at any sores that are present. Providers can also take a sample from the sore(s) and test it. If sores are not present, a blood test may be used to look for HSV antibodies.

Have an honest and open talk with your health-care provider about herpes testing and other STDs.

It is to be noted that a herpes blood test can help determine if you have herpes infection. It cannot tell you who gave you the infection or when you got the infection.

IS THERE A CURE FOR GENITAL HERPES?

There is no cure for genital herpes. However, there are medicines that can prevent or shorten outbreaks. A daily anti-herpes medicine can make it less likely to pass the infection on to your sex partner(s).

WHAT HAPPENS IF YOU DO NOT RECEIVE TREATMENT?

Genital herpes can cause painful genital sores and can be severe in people with suppressed immune systems.

If you touch your sores or fluids from the sores, you may transfer herpes to another body part such as your eyes. Do not touch the sores or fluids to avoid spreading herpes to another part of your body. If you do touch the sores or fluids, quickly wash your hands thoroughly to help avoid spreading the infection.

HOW COULD YOU PREVENT GENITAL HERPES?

The only way to completely avoid STDs is to not have vaginal, anal, or oral sex.

If you are sexually active, you can do the following things to lower your chances of getting genital herpes:
- being in a long-term mutually monogamous relationship with a partner who does not have herpes
- using condoms the right way every time you have sex

Be aware that not all herpes sores occur in areas that a condom can cover. Also, the skin can release the virus (shed) from areas that do not have a visible herpes sore. For these reasons, condoms may not fully protect you from getting herpes.

If your sex partner(s) has/have genital herpes, you can lower your risk of getting it if:
- your partner takes an anti-herpes medicine every day (This is something your partner should discuss with his or her health-care provider.)
- you avoid having vaginal, anal, or oral sex when your partner has herpes symptoms (i.e., during an "outbreak")

COULD YOU STILL HAVE SEX IF YOU HAVE HERPES?

If you have herpes, you should talk to your sex partner(s) about their risk. Using condoms may help lower this risk, but it will not get rid of the risk completely. Having sores or other symptoms of herpes can increase your risk of spreading the disease. Even if you do not have any symptoms, you can still infect your sex partners.

You may have concerns about how genital herpes will impact your health, sex life, and relationships. While herpes is not curable, it is important to know that it is manageable with medicine. Daily suppressive therapy (i.e., daily use of antiviral medication) can lower your risk of spreading the virus to others. Talk to a health-care provider about your concerns and treatment options.

A genital herpes diagnosis may affect how you will feel about current or future sexual relationships. Knowing how to talk to sexual partners about STDs is important.[3]

Section 24.4 | Gonorrhea

WHAT IS GONORRHEA?
Gonorrhea is a sexually transmitted disease (STD) that can cause infection in the genitals, rectum, and throat. It is very common, especially among young people aged 15–24.

HOW IS GONORRHEA SPREAD?
You can get gonorrhea by having vaginal, anal, or oral sex with someone who has gonorrhea.

ARE YOU AT RISK FOR GONORRHEA?
Sexually active people can get gonorrhea through vaginal, anal, or oral sex without a condom with a partner who has gonorrhea.

If you are sexually active, have an honest and open talk with your health-care provider. Ask them if you should get tested for gonorrhea or other STDs. If you are a sexually active gay or bisexual man, you should get tested for gonorrhea every year.

HOW COULD YOU REDUCE YOUR RISK OF GETTING GONORRHEA?
The only way to completely avoid STDs is to not have vaginal, anal, or oral sex.

---

[3] "Genital Herpes," Centers for Disease Control and Prevention (CDC), January 3, 2022. Available online. URL: www.cdc.gov/std/herpes/stdfact-herpes.htm. Accessed June 21, 2023.

If you are sexually active, the following things can lower your chances of getting gonorrhea:

- being in a long-term mutually monogamous relationship with a partner who has been tested and does not have gonorrhea
- using condoms the right way every time you have sex

HOW DO YOU KNOW IF YOU HAVE GONORRHEA?

Gonorrhea often has no symptoms, but it can cause serious health problems, even without symptoms.

Men who do have symptoms may have:

- a burning sensation when peeing
- a white, yellow, or green discharge from the penis
- painful or swollen testicles (although this is less common)

Rectal infections may either cause no symptoms or cause symptoms in men that may include the following:

- discharge
- anal itching
- soreness
- bleeding
- painful bowel movements

See your health-care provider if you notice any of these symptoms. You should also see a provider if your partner has an STD or symptoms of one. Symptoms can include an unusual sore, a smelly discharge, burning when peeing, or bleeding between periods.

HOW WOULD YOUR HEALTH-CARE PROVIDER KNOW IF YOU HAVE GONORRHEA?

Most of the time, a health-care provider will use a urine sample to diagnose gonorrhea. However, if you have had oral and/or anal sex, your health-care provider may use swabs to collect samples from your throat and/or rectum. In some cases, a health-care provider may also use a swab to collect a sample from a man's urethra (urine canal).

IS THERE A CURE FOR GONORRHEA?

Yes, the right treatment can cure gonorrhea. It is important that you take all of the medicine your health-care provider gives you to cure your infection. Do not share medicine for gonorrhea with anyone. Although medicine will stop the infection, it will not undo any permanent damage caused by the disease.

It is becoming harder to treat some gonorrhea, as drug-resistant strains of gonorrhea are increasing. Return to a health-care provider if your symptoms continue for more than a few days after receiving treatment.

WHAT HAPPENS IF YOU DO NOT RECEIVE TREATMENT?

Untreated gonorrhea can cause serious and permanent health problems.

In men, gonorrhea can cause a painful condition in the tubes attached to the testicles, which can, in rare cases, lead to infertility.

Rarely, untreated gonorrhea can also spread to your blood or joints. This condition can be life-threatening.

Untreated gonorrhea may also increase your chances of getting or giving HIV.

WHEN COULD YOU HAVE SEX AGAIN AFTER YOUR GONORRHEA TREATMENT?

Wait seven days after finishing all the medicine before having sex. You and your sex partner(s) should avoid having sex until you have each completed treatment and your symptoms are gone. This will help prevent you and your partner(s) from giving or getting gonorrhea again. Those with gonorrhea should be retested about three months after treatment of an initial infection, even if their partners received successful treatment.

If you have had gonorrhea and took medicine in the past, you can still get it again. This happens if you have sex without a condom with a person who has gonorrhea.[4]

---

[4] "Gonorrhea," Centers for Disease Control and Prevention (CDC), August 22, 2022. Available online. URL: www.cdc.gov/std/gonorrhea/stdfact-gonorrhea.htm. Accessed June 21, 2023.

Section 24.5 | **Hepatitis B**

WHAT IS HEPATITIS B?

Hepatitis B is a liver infection caused by the hepatitis B virus (HBV). HBV infection causes inflammation of the liver. When the liver is inflamed or damaged, its function can be affected. Hepatitis B is transmitted when blood, semen, or another body fluid from a person infected with HBV enters the body of someone who is not infected. This can happen through sexual contact; by sharing needles, syringes, or other drug injection equipment; or from the mother to the baby at birth. For some people, HBV infection is an acute, or short-term, illness; for others, it can become a long-term, chronic infection. Risk for chronic infection is related to age at infection: Approximately 90 percent of infected infants become chronically infected, compared with 2–6 percent of adults. Chronic hepatitis B can lead to cirrhosis, liver cancer, liver failure, and premature death.

HOW MANY PEOPLE HAVE HEPATITIS B?

In the United States, an estimated 880,000–1.89 million people are chronically infected with HBV. In 2020, 2,157 cases of acute hepatitis B were reported; however, because of low case detection and reporting, the Centers for Disease Control and Prevention (CDC) estimates that there were 14,000 acute hepatitis B infections. The rate of acute cases of HBV decreased by 32 percent after 2019 that may be related to the disruptions of the COVID-19 pandemic.

Globally, HBV is the most common blood-borne infection with an estimated 296 million people infected according to the World Health Organization (WHO).

WHO IS MOST AFFECTED BY HEPATITIS B?

In the United States, rates of new HBV infections are highest among adults aged 30–59, reflecting low hepatitis B vaccination coverage among adults at risk. The most common risk factor among people with new HBV infections is injecting drugs, related to the opioid crisis and other drug use.

The highest rates of chronic hepatitis B infection in the United States occur among foreign-born individuals, especially people born in Asia, the Pacific Islands, and Africa. Approximately 70 percent of cases in the United States are among people who were born outside of the United States. Other groups who have higher rates of chronic HBV infection include people who inject drugs and men who have sex with men.

HUMAN IMMUNODEFICIENCY VIRUS AND HEPATITIS B VIRUS COINFECTION

About 2 percent of people with human immunodeficiency virus (HIV) in the United States are coinfected with HBV; both infections have similar routes of transmission. People with HIV are at greater risk for complications and death from HBV infection. All people with HIV are recommended to be tested for HBV and, if susceptible, are further recommended to receive the hepatitis B vaccination or, if chronically infected, are evaluated for treatment to prevent liver disease and liver cancer.

HOW IS HEPATITIS B TRANSMITTED?

Hepatitis B is spread in several distinct ways: sexual contact; sharing needles, syringes, or other drug injection equipment; or from the mother to the child at birth.

In the United States, injection drug use was the most common risk factor reported among people with an acute HBV infection, followed by having multiple sex partners. Less commonly reported risk factors included accidental needle sticks, surgery, transfusions, and household contact with a person with HBV infection. Healthcare-related transmission of HBV is rare.

SCREENING AND TESTING FOR HEPATITIS B

The CDC estimates that 68 percent of people with chronic hepatitis B are unaware of their infection. The only way to find out if you have hepatitis B is to get tested. Hepatitis B testing is a covered preventive service under many health plans.

Being aware of your hepatitis B status is important because treatments are available that reduce the chance of developing liver disease and liver cancer. If you are diagnosed with hepatitis B, you can also protect your family members by getting them vaccinated.

All adults aged 18 years and older are recommended to receive screening for hepatitis B at least once in their lifetime using a triple panel test. To ensure increased access to testing, anyone who requests HBV testing should receive it regardless of disclosure of risk. Many people might be reluctant to disclose stigmatizing risks.

The CDC recommends HBV screening for hepatitis B surface antigen (HBsAg) for all pregnant people during each pregnancy, preferably in the first trimester, regardless of vaccination status or history of testing. Pregnant people with a history of appropriately timed triple panel screening without subsequent risk for exposure to HBV (i.e., no new HBV exposures since triple panel screening) only need HBsAg screening.

Persons at increased risk for HBV exposure or with symptoms for hepatitis B should receive HBV testing. Persons at increased risk, regardless of age, should receive periodic testing while risk for exposure is ongoing.

The following are the people at increased risk:
- people with a history of sexually transmitted infection (STI) or multiple sex partners
- people with hepatitis C infection or a history of hepatitis C virus infection
- people incarcerated or formerly incarcerated in a jail, prison, or other detention setting
- people born in countries with an HBV prevalence of 2 percent and greater
- people born in the United States not vaccinated as infants whose parents were born in regions with high rates of HBV infections (an HBsAg prevalence of 8% and greater)
- men who have sex with men
- people who inject drugs or have a history with injection drug use
- needle sharing or sexual contacts of people with known HBV infection

- people with HIV
- household and sexual contacts of HBV-infected people
- people requiring immunosuppressive therapy
- people with end-stage renal disease (including hemodialysis patients)
- blood and tissue donors
- people with elevated alanine aminotransferase levels (30 IU/L or greater for men)
- infants born to HBV-infected mothers

TREATMENT FOR HEPATITIS B

There are several antiviral treatments available for chronic hepatitis B. Everyone with chronic hepatitis B should be linked to care, considered for treatment, and regularly checked for liver damage and liver cancer. Hepatitis B treatments reduce the amount of virus in the body and reduce the chance of developing serious liver disease and liver cancer. There is no cure for hepatitis B, and treatment is recommended to continue for years if not for life. Research is ongoing for more effective treatments and a cure for HBV.

HEPATITIS B PREVENTION

Hepatitis B is a vaccine-preventable disease. The best way to prevent hepatitis B is to get vaccinated. The hepatitis B vaccine is safe and effective.

The hepatitis B vaccine is recommended for the following people:

- **Infants.** To receive protection against hepatitis B, universal hepatitis B vaccination within 24 hours of birth for all medically stable infants weighing 2,000 grams and more, followed by completion of the series is recommended.
- **Unvaccinated children aged younger than 19 years.** Three doses are required to complete the vaccine series.
- **Adults aged 19–60 and older with or without known risk factors for hepatitis B.** Two, three, or four doses are required. The two-dose vaccine is given over 30

days, which increases protection among adults more rapidly with fewer medical visits. There is also a combination vaccine that protects people from both hepatitis A and hepatitis B. The combined vaccine is usually given as three shots over a six-month period. These tools may support increased vaccination in settings such as jails, prisons, substance use disorder (SUD) prevention and treatment facilities, sexually transmitted disease (STD) treatment facilities, and HIV testing and treatment facilities.

The CDC and the Advisory Committee on Immunization Practices (ACIP) published additional guidance on the hepatitis B vaccine for adults aged 19–59 in 2022.

Hepatitis B can also be prevented by avoiding contact with contaminated blood and unprotected sexual exposure. Using condoms has also been shown to reduce the chance of STIs.[5]

Section 24.6 | HIV and AIDS

WHAT ARE HIV AND AIDS?

HIV stands for human immunodeficiency virus, which is the virus that causes HIV infection. The abbreviation "HIV" can refer to the virus or to HIV infection.

AIDS stands for acquired immunodeficiency syndrome. AIDS is the most advanced stage of HIV infection.

HIV attacks and destroys the infection-fighting CD4 cells (CD4 T lymphocyte) of the immune system. The loss of CD4 cells makes it difficult for the body to fight off infections and certain cancers. Without treatment, HIV can gradually destroy the immune system, and HIV infection advances to AIDS.

---

[5] "Hepatitis B Basics," U.S. Department of Health and Human Services (HHS), March 31, 2023. Available online. URL: www.hhs.gov/hepatitis/learn-about-viral-hepatitis/hepatitis-b-basics/index.html. Accessed June 21, 2023.

HOW DOES HIV SPREAD?

The spread of HIV from person to person is called "HIV transmission." HIV is spread only through certain body fluids from a person who has HIV. These body fluids include the following:

- blood
- semen
- pre-seminal fluid
- vaginal fluids
- rectal fluids
- breast milk

HIV transmission is only possible through contact with HIV-infected body fluids. In the United States, HIV is spread mainly by:

- having anal or vaginal sex with someone who has HIV without using a condom or taking medicines to prevent or treat HIV
- sharing injection drug equipment (works), such as needles or syringes, with someone who has HIV

The spread of HIV from a woman with HIV to her child during pregnancy, childbirth, or breastfeeding is called "perinatal transmission of HIV."

You cannot get HIV by shaking hands or hugging a person who has HIV. You also cannot get HIV from contact with objects, such as dishes, toilet seats, or doorknobs, used by a person with HIV. HIV is not spread through the air or water or by mosquitoes, ticks, or other blood-sucking insects.

HOW CAN A PERSON REDUCE THE RISK OF GETTING HIV?

To reduce your risk of HIV infection, use condoms correctly every time you have sex, limit your number of sexual partners, and never share injection drug equipment.

Also, talk to your health-care provider about pre-exposure prophylaxis (PrEP). PrEP is an HIV prevention option for people who do not have HIV but who are at high risk of becoming infected with HIV. PrEP involves taking a specific HIV medicine every day.

WHAT ARE THE SYMPTOMS OF HIV AND AIDS?

Within two to four weeks after infection with HIV, some people may have flu-like symptoms, such as fever, chills, or rash. The symptoms may last for a few days to several weeks.

Other possible symptoms of HIV include night sweats, muscle aches, sore throat, fatigue, swollen lymph nodes, and mouth ulcers. Having these symptoms does not mean you have HIV. Other illnesses can cause the same symptoms. Some people may not feel sick during early HIV infection (called "acute HIV infection"). During this earliest stage of HIV infection, the virus multiplies rapidly. After the initial stage of infection, HIV continues to multiply but at very low levels.

More severe symptoms of HIV infection, such as a badly damaged immune system and signs of opportunistic infections, generally do not appear for many years until HIV has advanced to AIDS. People with AIDS have badly damaged immune systems that make them prone to opportunistic infections. (Opportunistic infections are infections and infection-related cancers that occur more frequently or are more severe in people with weakened immune systems than in people with healthy immune systems.)

Without treatment with HIV medicines, HIV infection usually advances to AIDS in 10 years or longer though it may advance faster in some people.

HIV transmission is possible at any stage of HIV infection—even if a person with HIV has no symptoms of HIV.

HOW IS AIDS DIAGNOSED?

Symptoms such as fever, weakness, and weight loss may be a sign that a person's HIV has advanced to AIDS. However, a diagnosis of AIDS is based on one of the following criteria:

- a drop in CD4 count to less than 200 cells/mm^3 (A CD4 count measures the number of CD4 cells in a sample of blood.)
- the presence of certain opportunistic infections

Although an AIDS diagnosis indicates severe damage to the immune system, HIV medicines can still help people at this stage of HIV infection.

WHAT IS THE TREATMENT FOR HIV?

Antiretroviral therapy (ART) is the use of HIV medicines to treat HIV infection. People on ART take a combination of HIV medicines (called an "HIV treatment regimen") every day.

ART is recommended for everyone who has HIV. ART prevents HIV from multiplying, which reduces the amount of HIV in the body (called the "viral load"). Having less HIV in the body protects the immune system and prevents HIV infection from advancing to AIDS. ART cannot cure HIV, but HIV medicines help people with HIV live longer, healthier lives.

ART also reduces the risk of HIV transmission. The main goal of ART is to reduce a person's viral load to an undetectable level. An undetectable viral load means that the level of HIV in the blood is too low to be detected by a viral load test. People with HIV who maintain an undetectable viral load have effectively no risk of transmitting HIV to their HIV-negative partner through sex.[6]

Section 24.7 | Human Papillomavirus

Human papillomavirus (HPV) is the most common sexually transmitted infection (STI) in the United States. There are many different types of HPV. Some types can cause health problems, including genital warts and cancers. But there are vaccines that can stop these health problems from happening. HPV is a different virus than human immunodeficiency virus (HIV) and HSV (herpes).

HOW IS HUMAN PAPILLOMAVIRUS SPREAD?

You can get HPV by having vaginal, anal, or oral sex with someone who has the virus. It is most commonly spread during vaginal or

---

[6] HIVinfo, "HIV and AIDS: The Basics," U.S. Department of Health and Human Services (HHS), January 31, 2023. Available online. URL: https://hivinfo.nih.gov/understanding-hiv/fact-sheets/hiv-and-aids-basics. Accessed June 21, 2023.

anal sex. It also spreads through close skin-to-skin touching during sex. A person with HPV can pass the infection to someone even when they have no signs or symptoms.

If you are sexually active, you can get HPV, even if you have had sex with only one person. You can also develop symptoms years after having sex with someone who has the infection. This makes it hard to know when you first got it.

DOES HUMAN PAPILLOMAVIRUS CAUSE HEALTH PROBLEMS?

In most cases (9 out of 10), HPV goes away on its own within two years without health problems. But, when HPV does not go away, it can cause health problems such as genital warts and cancer.

Genital warts usually appear as a small bump or group of bumps in the genital area. They can be small or large, raised or flat, or shaped like a cauliflower. A health-care provider can usually diagnose warts by looking at the genital area.

DOES HUMAN PAPILLOMAVIRUS CAUSE CANCER?

Human papillomavirus can cause cancers, including cancer of the penis or anus. It can also cause cancer in the back of the throat (called "oropharyngeal cancer"). This can include the base of the tongue and tonsils.

Cancer often takes years, even decades, to develop after a person gets HPV. Genital warts and cancers result from different types of HPV.

There is no way to know who will develop cancer or other health problems from HPV. People with weak immune systems (including those with HIV) may be less able to fight off HPV. They may also be more likely to develop health problems from HPV.

HOW COULD YOU AVOID HUMAN PAPILLOMAVIRUS AND THE HEALTH PROBLEMS IT CAN CAUSE?

You can do several things to lower your chances of getting HPV:
- **Get vaccinated**. The HPV vaccine is safe and effective. It can protect against diseases (including cancers) caused by HPV when given in the recommended age groups.

444

If you are sexually active, do the following:

- **Use condoms the right way every time you have sex**. This can lower your chances of getting HPV. But HPV can infect areas the condom does not cover. So condoms may not fully protect against getting HPV.
- **Be in a mutually monogamous relationship**. Have sex only with someone who only has sex with you.

HOW DO YOU KNOW IF YOU HAVE HUMAN PAPILLOMAVIRUS?

There is no test to find out a person's "HPV status." Also, there is no approved HPV test to find HPV in the mouth or throat.

Most people with HPV do not know they have the infection. They never develop symptoms or health problems from it. Some people find out they have HPV when they get genital warts. Others may only find out once they have developed more serious problems from HPV, such as cancers.

IS THERE TREATMENT FOR HUMAN PAPILLOMAVIRUS OR HEALTH PROBLEMS THAT DEVELOP FROM HUMAN PAPILLOMAVIRUS?

There is no treatment for the virus itself. However, there are treatments for the health problems that HPV can cause:

- Genital warts can go away with treatment from your health-care provider or with prescription medicine. If left untreated, genital warts may go away, stay the same, or grow in size or number.
- Other HPV-related cancers are also more treatable when found and treated early.

WHO SHOULD GET THE HUMAN PAPILLOMAVIRUS VACCINE?

The Centers for Disease Control and Prevention (CDC) recommends HPV vaccination for:

- all preteens (including boys and girls) at the age of 11 or 12 years (or can start at the age of 9)
- everyone through the age of 26, if not vaccinated already

Vaccination is not recommended for everyone older than the age of 26 years. However, some adults aged 27–45 who are not already vaccinated may decide to get the HPV vaccine after speaking with their health-care provider about their risk for new HPV infections and the possible benefits of vaccination. HPV vaccination in this age range provides less benefit. Most sexually active adults have already been exposed to HPV although not necessarily all of the HPV types targeted by vaccination.

At any age, having a new sex partner is a risk factor for getting a new HPV infection. People who are already in a long-term, mutually monogamous relationship are not likely to get a new HPV infection.[7]

Section 24.8 | Pubic Lice

WHAT ARE PUBIC LICE?

Pubic lice (also called "crabs") are tiny insects that usually live in the pubic or genital area of humans. They are also sometimes found on other coarse body hair, such as hair on the legs, armpits, mustache, beard, eyebrows, or eyelashes. Pubic lice on the eyebrows or eyelashes of children or teens may be a sign of sexual exposure or abuse.

Pubic lice are parasites, and they need to feed on human blood to survive. They are one of the three types of lice that live on humans. The other two types are head lice and body lice. Each type of lice is different, and getting one type does not mean that you will get another type.

HOW DO PUBIC LICE SPREAD?

Pubic lice move by crawling because they cannot hop or fly. They usually spread through sexual contact. Occasionally, they may spread through physical contact with a person who has pubic lice or through

---

[7] "Genital HPV Infection—Basic Fact Sheet," Centers for Disease Control and Prevention (CDC), April 12, 2022. Available online. URL: www.cdc.gov/std/hpv/stdfact-hpv.htm. Accessed June 21, 2023.

contact with clothing, beds, bed linens, or towels that were used by a person with pubic lice. You cannot get pubic lice from animals.

WHO IS AT RISK FOR PUBIC LICE?

Since they spread mainly through sexual contact, pubic lice are most common in adults.

WHAT ARE THE SYMPTOMS OF PUBIC LICE?

The most common symptom of pubic lice is intense itching in the genital area. You may also see nits (lice eggs) or crawling lice.

HOW DO YOU KNOW IF YOU HAVE PUBIC LICE?

A diagnosis of pubic lice usually comes from seeing a louse or nit. But lice and nits can be difficult to find because there may be only a few present. Also, they often attach themselves to more than one hair, and they do not crawl as quickly as head and body lice. Sometimes, it takes a magnifying lens to see the lice or nits.

People who have pubic lice should also be checked for other sexually transmitted diseases (STDs), and their sexual partners should also be checked for pubic lice.

WHAT ARE THE TREATMENTS FOR PUBIC LICE?

The main treatment for pubic lice is a lice-killing lotion. Options include a lotion that contains permethrin or a mousse containing pyrethrins and piperonyl butoxide. These products are available over-the-counter (OTC) without a prescription. They are safe and effective when you use them according to the instructions. Usually, treatment will get rid of the lice. If not, you may need another treatment after 9–10 days.

There are other lice-killing medicines that are available with a prescription from your health-care provider.

You should also wash your clothes, bedding, and towels with hot water and dry them using the hot cycle of the dryer.[8]

---

[8] MedlinePlus, "Pubic Lice," National Institutes of Health (NIH), April 18, 2018. Available online. URL: https://medlineplus.gov/pubiclice.html. Accessed July 12, 2023.

Section 24.9 | **Scabies**

WHAT IS SCABIES?

Scabies is an infestation of the skin by the human itch mite (*Sarcoptes scabiei* var. *hominis*). The microscopic scabies mite burrows into the upper layer of the skin where it lives and lays its eggs. The most common symptoms of scabies are intense itching and a pimple-like skin rash. The scabies mite is usually spread by direct, prolonged, skin-to-skin contact with a person who has scabies.

Scabies is found worldwide and affects people of all races and social classes. Scabies can spread rapidly under crowded conditions where close body and skin contact is frequent. Institutions, such as nursing homes, extended-care facilities, and prisons, are often sites of scabies outbreaks. Childcare facilities are also a common site of scabies infestations.

HOW SOON AFTER INFESTATION DO SYMPTOMS OF SCABIES BEGIN?

If a person has never had scabies before, symptoms may take as long as four to six weeks to begin. It is important to remember that an infected person can spread scabies during this time, even if he does not have symptoms yet.

In a person who has had scabies before, symptoms usually appear much sooner (one to four days) after exposure.

HOW DO YOU GET SCABIES?

Scabies is usually spread by direct, prolonged, skin-to-skin contact with a person who has scabies. Contact generally must be prolonged; a quick handshake or hug usually will not spread scabies. Scabies is spread easily to sexual partners and household members. Scabies in adults is frequently sexually acquired. Scabies is sometimes spread indirectly by sharing articles, such as clothing, towels, or bedding used by an infected person; however, such indirect spread can occur much more easily when the infected person has crusted scabies.

WHAT IS CRUSTED (NORWEGIAN) SCABIES?

Crusted scabies is a severe form of scabies that can occur in some persons who are immunocompromised (have a weak immune system), are elderly, have a disability, or are debilitated. It is also called "Norwegian scabies." Persons with crusted scabies have thick crusts of skin that contain large numbers of scabies mites and eggs. Persons with crusted scabies are very contagious to other persons and can spread the infestation easily, both by direct skin-to-skin contact and by contamination of items, such as their clothing, bedding, and furniture. Persons with crusted scabies may not show the usual signs and symptoms of scabies, such as the characteristic rash or itching (pruritus). Persons with crusted scabies should receive quick and aggressive medical treatment for their infestation to prevent outbreaks of scabies.

WHAT ARE THE SIGNS AND SYMPTOMS OF SCABIES INFESTATION?

The most common signs and symptoms of scabies are intense itching (pruritus), especially at night, and a pimple-like (papular) itchy rash. The itching and rash each may affect much of the body or be limited to common sites, such as the wrist, elbow, armpit, webbing between the fingers, nipple, penis, waist, beltline, and buttocks. The rash can also include tiny blisters (vesicles) and scales. Scratching the rash can cause skin sores; sometimes, these sores become infected by bacteria.

Tiny burrows sometimes are seen on the skin; these are caused by the female scabies mite tunneling just beneath the surface of the skin. These burrows appear as tiny raised and crooked (serpiginous) grayish-white or skin-colored lines on the skin surface. Because mites are often few in number (only 10–15 mites per person), these burrows may be difficult to find. They are found most often in the webbing between the fingers; in the skin folds on the wrist, elbow, or knee; and on the penis, breast, or shoulder blades.

The head, face, neck, palms, and soles are often involved in infants and very young children, but usually not adults and older children.

Persons with crusted scabies may not show the usual signs and symptoms of scabies, such as the characteristic rash or itching (pruritus).

449

HOW IS SCABIES INFESTATION DIAGNOSED?

Diagnosis of a scabies infestation is usually made based on the customary appearance and distribution of the rash and the presence of burrows. Whenever possible, the diagnosis of scabies should be confirmed by identifying the mite, mite eggs, or mite fecal matter (scybala). This can be done by carefully removing a mite from the end of its burrow using the tip of a needle or by obtaining skin scraping to examine under a microscope for mites, eggs, or mite fecal matter. It is important to remember that a person can still be infected even if mites, eggs, or fecal matter cannot be found; typically fewer than 10–15 mites can be present on the entire body of an infected person who is otherwise healthy. However, persons with crusted scabies can be infected with thousands of mites and should be considered highly contagious.

HOW LONG CAN SCABIES MITES LIVE?

On a person, scabies mites can live for as long as one to two months. Off a person, scabies mites usually do not survive more than 48–72 hours. Scabies mites will die if exposed to a temperature of 122 °F (50 °C) for 10 minutes.

CAN SCABIES BE TREATED?

Yes. Products used to treat scabies are called "scabicides" because they kill scabies mites; some also kill eggs. Scabicides to treat human scabies are available only with a doctor's prescription; no "over-the-counter" (OTC; nonprescription) products have been tested and approved for humans.

Always carefully follow the instructions provided by the doctor and pharmacist, as well as those contained in the box or printed on the label. When treating adults and older children, scabicide cream or lotion is applied to all areas of the body from the neck down to the feet and toes; when treating infants and young children, the cream or lotion is also applied to the head and neck. The medication should be left on the body for the recommended time before it is washed off. Clean clothes should be worn after treatment.

Never use a scabicide intended for veterinary or agricultural use to treat humans.

WHO SHOULD BE TREATED FOR SCABIES?

Anyone who is diagnosed with scabies, as well as his sexual partners and other contacts who have had prolonged skin-to-skin contact with the infected person, should be treated. Treatment is recommended for members of the same household as the person with scabies, particularly those persons who have had prolonged skin-to-skin contact with the infected person. All persons should be treated at the same time to prevent reinfestation.

Re-treatment may be necessary if itching continues more than two to four weeks after treatment or if new burrows or rash continue to appear.

HOW SOON AFTER TREATMENT WOULD YOU FEEL BETTER?

If itching continues more than two to four weeks after initial treatment or if new burrows or rash continue to appear (if initial treatment includes more than one application or dose, then the two- to four-week time period begins after the last application or dose), re-treatment with scabicide may be necessary; seek the advice of a physician.

DO YOU GET SCABIES FROM YOUR PET?

No. Animals do not spread human scabies. Pets can become infected with a different kind of scabies mite that does not survive or reproduce on humans but causes "mange" in animals. If an animal with "mange" has close contact with a person, the animal mite can get under the person's skin and cause temporary itching and skin irritation. However, the animal mite cannot reproduce on a person and will die on its own in a couple of days. Although the person does not need to be treated, the animal should be treated because its mites can continue to burrow into the person's skin and cause symptoms until the animal has been treated successfully.

CAN SCABIES BE SPREAD BY SWIMMING IN A PUBLIC POOL?

Scabies is spread by prolonged skin-to-skin contact with a person who has scabies. Scabies sometimes can also be spread by contact with items, such as clothing, bedding, or towels that have been used by a person with scabies, but such spread is very uncommon unless the infected person has crusted scabies.

Scabies is very unlikely to be spread by water in a swimming pool. Except for a person with crusted scabies, only about 10–15 scabies mites are present on an infected person; it is extremely unlikely that any would emerge from under wet skin.

Although uncommon, scabies can be spread by sharing a towel or item of clothing that has been used by a person with scabies.

HOW COULD YOU REMOVE SCABIES MITES FROM YOUR HOUSE OR CARPET?

Scabies mites do not survive more than two to three days away from human skin. Items, such as bedding, clothing, and towels, used by a person with scabies can be decontaminated by machine-washing in hot water and drying using the hot cycle or by dry-cleaning. Items that cannot be washed or dry-cleaned can be decontaminated by removing from any body contact for at least 72 hours.

Because persons with crusted scabies are considered very infectious, careful vacuuming of furniture and carpets in rooms used by these persons is recommended.

Fumigation of living areas is unnecessary.

IF YOU COME IN CONTACT WITH A PERSON WHO HAS SCABIES, SHOULD YOU TREAT YOURSELF?

No. If a person thinks he might have scabies, he should contact a doctor. The doctor can examine the person, confirm the diagnosis of scabies, and prescribe an appropriate treatment. Products used to treat scabies in humans are available only with a doctor's prescription.

Sleeping with or having sex with any scabies-infected person presents a high risk for transmission. The longer a person has skin-to-skin exposure, the greater the likelihood for transmission to occur. Although briefly shaking hands with a person who has non-crusted scabies could be considered as presenting a relatively low risk, holding the hand of a person with scabies for 5–10 minutes could be considered to present a relatively high risk of transmission. However, transmission can occur even after brief skin-to-skin contact, such as a handshake, with a person who has crusted scabies. In general, a person who has skin-to-skin contact with a person who has crusted scabies would be considered a good candidate for treatment.

To determine when prophylactic treatment should be given to reduce the risk of transmission, early consultation should be sought with a health-care provider who understands:

- the type of scabies (i.e., noncrusted versus crusted) to which a person has been exposed
- the degree and duration of skin exposure that a person has had to the infected patient
- whether the exposure occurred before or after the patient was treated for scabies
- whether the exposed person works in an environment where he would be likely to expose other people during the asymptomatic incubation period (e.g., a nurse or caretaker who works in a nursing home or hospital would often be treated prophylactically to reduce the risk of further scabies transmission in the facility)[9]

Section 24.10 | Syphilis

WHAT IS SYPHILIS?

Syphilis is a sexually transmitted infection (STI) that can cause serious health problems without treatment. Infection develops in stages (primary, secondary, latent, and tertiary). Each stage can have different signs and symptoms.

---

[9] "Scabies Frequently Asked Questions (FAQs)," Centers for Disease Control and Prevention (CDC), October 24, 2018. Available online. URL: www.cdc.gov/parasites/scabies/gen_info/faqs.html. Accessed July 12, 2023.

HOW DOES SYPHILIS SPREAD?

You can get syphilis by direct contact with a syphilis sore during vaginal, anal, or oral sex.

You cannot get syphilis through casual contact with objects, such as:

- toilet seats
- doorknobs
- swimming pools
- hot tubs
- bathtubs
- sharing clothing or eating utensils

ARE YOU AT RISK FOR SYPHILIS?

Sexually active people can get syphilis through vaginal, anal, or oral sex without a condom with a partner who has syphilis. If you are sexually active, have an honest and open talk with your health-care provider. Ask them if you should get tested for syphilis or other sexually transmitted diseases (STDs).

You should get tested regularly for syphilis if you are sexually active and:

- are a gay or bisexual man
- have human immunodeficiency virus (HIV)
- are taking pre-exposure prophylaxis (PrEP) for HIV prevention
- have partner(s) who have tested positive for syphilis

HOW COULD YOU REDUCE YOUR RISK OF GETTING SYPHILIS?

The only way to completely avoid STDs is to not have vaginal, anal, or oral sex.

If you are sexually active, you can do the following things to lower your chances of getting syphilis:

- being in a long-term mutually monogamous relationship with a partner who has been tested and does not have syphilis
- using condoms the right way every time you have sex

Condoms prevent the spread of syphilis by preventing contact with a sore. Sometimes, sores occur in areas not covered by a condom. Contact with these sores can still transmit syphilis.

WHAT ARE THE SIGNS AND SYMPTOMS OF SYPHILIS?

There are four stages of syphilis: primary secondary, latent, and tertiary. Each stage has different signs and symptoms.

Primary Stage

During the first (primary) stage of syphilis, you may notice a single sore or multiple sores. The sore is the location where syphilis entered your body. These sores usually occur in, on, or around the:

- penis
- anus
- rectum
- lips or in the mouth

Sores are usually (but not always) firm, round, and painless. Because the sore is painless, you may not notice it. The sore usually lasts three to six weeks and heals regardless of whether you receive treatment. Even after the sore goes away, you must still receive treatment. This will stop your infection from moving to the secondary stage.

Secondary Stage

During the secondary stage, you may have skin rashes and/or sores in your mouth or anus. This stage usually starts with a rash on one or more areas of your body. The rash can show up when your primary sore is healing or several weeks after the sore has healed. The rash can be on the palms of your hands and/or the bottoms of your feet and look:

- rough
- red
- reddish-brown

The rash usually will not itch, and it is sometimes so faint that you would not notice it. Other symptoms may include the following:

- fever
- swollen lymph glands
- sore throat
- patchy hair loss
- headaches
- weight loss
- muscle aches
- fatigue (feeling very tired)

The symptoms from this stage will go away whether you receive treatment. Without the right treatment, your infection will move to the latent and possibly tertiary stages of syphilis.

Latent Stage

The latent stage of syphilis is a period when there are no visible signs or symptoms. Without treatment, you can continue to have syphilis in your body for years.

Tertiary Stage

Most people with untreated syphilis do not develop tertiary syphilis. However, when it does happen, it can affect many different organ systems. These include the heart and blood vessels and the brain and nervous system. Tertiary syphilis is very serious and would occur 10–30 years after your infection began. In tertiary syphilis, the disease damages your internal organs and can result in death. A health-care provider can usually diagnose tertiary syphilis with the help of multiple tests.

NEUROSYPHILIS, OCULAR SYPHILIS, AND OTOSYPHILIS

Without treatment, syphilis can spread to the brain and nervous system (neurosyphilis), the eye (ocular syphilis), or the ear (otosyphilis). This can happen during any of the stages described previously.

Signs and symptoms of neurosyphilis can include the following:
- severe headache
- muscle weakness and/or trouble with muscle movements
- changes to your mental state (trouble focusing, confusion, personality change) and/or dementia (problems with memory, thinking, and/or decision-making)

Signs and symptoms of ocular syphilis can include the following:
- eye pain and/or redness
- changes in your vision or even blindness

Signs and symptoms of otosyphilis may include the following:
- hearing loss
- ringing, buzzing, roaring, or hissing in the ears ("tinnitus")
- dizziness or vertigo (feeling like you or your surroundings are moving or spinning)

HOW WOULD YOU OR YOUR HEALTH-CARE PROVIDERS KNOW IF YOU HAVE SYPHILIS?

Most of the time, health-care providers will use a blood test to test for syphilis. Some will diagnose syphilis by testing fluid from a syphilis sore.

CAN YOU GET SYPHILIS AGAIN AFTER RECEIVING TREATMENT?

Having syphilis once does not protect you from getting it again. Even after successful treatment, you can get syphilis again. Only laboratory tests can confirm whether you have syphilis. Follow-up testing by your health-care provider is necessary to make sure your treatment was successful. It may not be obvious that a sex partner has syphilis. Syphilis sores in the anus, mouth, or under the foreskin of the penis can be hard to see. You may get syphilis again if your sex partner(s) does not receive testing and treatment.

IS THERE A CURE FOR SYPHILIS?

Yes, syphilis is curable with the right antibiotics from your health-care provider. However, treatment might not undo any damage the infection can cause.[10]

Section 24.11 | Trichomoniasis

WHAT IS TRICHOMONIASIS?

Trichomoniasis (or "trich") is a very common sexually transmitted disease (STD) caused by infection with *Trichomonas vaginalis* (a protozoan parasite). Although symptoms vary, most people who have trich cannot tell they have it.

HOW COMMON IS TRICHOMONIASIS?

Infection is more common in women than in men. Older women are more likely than younger women to have the infection.

HOW IS TRICHOMONIASIS SPREAD?

Sexually active people can get trich by having sex without a condom with a partner who has trich.

In men, the infection is most commonly found inside the penis (urethra). During sex, the parasite usually spreads from a penis to a vagina or from a vagina to a penis.

It is not common for the parasite to infect other body parts, such as the hands, mouth, or anus. It is unclear why some people with the infection get symptoms while others do not. It probably depends on factors such as a person's age and overall health. People with trich can pass the infection to others, even if they do not have symptoms.

---

[10] "Syphilis," Centers for Disease Control and Prevention (CDC), February 10, 2022. Available online. URL: www.cdc.gov/std/syphilis/stdfact-syphilis.htm. Accessed June 21, 2023.

WHAT ARE THE SIGNS AND SYMPTOMS OF TRICHOMONIASIS?

About 70 percent of people with the infection do not have any signs or symptoms. When trich does cause symptoms, they can range from mild irritation to severe inflammation. Some people get symptoms within 5–28 days after getting the infection. Others do not develop symptoms until much later. Symptoms can come and go.

Men with trich may notice:
- itching or irritation inside the penis
- burning after peeing or ejaculating
- discharge from the penis

Having trich can make sex feel unpleasant. Without treatment, the infection can last for months or even years.

WHAT ARE THE COMPLICATIONS OF TRICHOMONIASIS?

Trich can increase the risk of getting or spreading other sexually transmitted infections (STIs). For example, trich can cause genital inflammation, making it easier to get human immunodeficiency virus (HIV) or pass it to a sex partner.

HOW DO HEALTH-CARE PROVIDERS DIAGNOSE TRICHOMONIASIS?

It is not possible to diagnose trich based on symptoms alone. Your health-care provider can examine you, and a laboratory test will confirm the diagnosis.

WHAT IS THE TREATMENT FOR TRICHOMONIASIS?

Trich is the most common curable STD. A health-care provider can treat the infection with medication (pills) taken by mouth. This treatment is also safe for pregnant people. If you receive and complete treatment for trich, you can still get it again. Reinfection occurs in about one in five people within three months after receiving treatment. This can happen if you have sex without a condom with a person who has trich. To avoid reinfection, your sex partners should receive treatment at the same time.

You should not have sex again until you and your sex partner(s) complete treatment. You should receive testing again about three months after your treatment, even if your sex partner(s) received treatment.

HOW COULD YOU PREVENT TRICHOMONIASIS?

The only way to avoid STDs is to not have vaginal, anal, or oral sex.

If you are sexually active, you can do the following things to lower your chances of getting trich:

- being in a long-term mutually monogamous relationship with a partner who has been tested and does not have trich
- using condoms the right way every time you have sex

Also, talk about the potential risk of STDs before having sex with a new partner. This can help inform the choices you are comfortable taking with your sex life.

If you are sexually active, have an honest and open talk with your health-care provider. Ask them if you should get tested for trich or other STDs.[11]

---

[11] "Trichomoniasis," Centers for Disease Control and Prevention (CDC), April 25, 2022. Available online. URL: www.cdc.gov/std/trichomonas/stdfact-trichomoniasis.htm. Accessed June 21, 2023.

Chapter 25 | **Gynecomastia**

WHAT IS GYNECOMASTIA?

Gynecomastia is the enlargement of male breast tissue, most often due to an imbalance of estrogen and testosterone hormones. The condition can affect one or both breasts and can make the breast tender. It is usually not permanent or dangerous; however, affected males may experience social embarrassment and psychological distress. Pseudogynecomastia (false gynecomastia) can sometimes be confused with gynecomastia. The former is caused by excessive fat tissue on the chest, while the latter is an above-average growth of the breast tissue itself.

PREVALENCE

Gynecomastia can occur at any stage of a man's life, depending on the degree of hormonal change.

The following are the three peak stages of gynecomastia that occur in males:

- **Peak 1**. Almost 60–90 percent of newborn babies have this condition for roughly two to three weeks after birth when the mother's estrogen remains in their bloodstream.
- **Peak 2**. Around 50–60 percent of adolescents may develop the condition during puberty as a result of hormonal changes in them. The condition lasts a few months to two years.
- **Peak 3**. Men aged 50–69 experience no symptoms but may have the condition. One in every four men in this age group is affected; in these cases, other medical problems may be associated with the condition.

CAUSES AND RISK FACTORS

The male and female hormones are generally present in both sexes. However, when the production of the primary male hormone (testosterone) is less, and the primary female hormone (estrogen) is more in the male body, it causes gynecomastia.

Some other causes and risk factors of gynecomastia include:

- medication, such as antibiotics, antianxiety drugs, anabolic steroids, heart medications, antiandrogens, tricyclic antidepressants, gastric motility medications, and ulcer medications
- cancer and AIDS treatments
- consumption of alcohol, heroin, methadone, marijuana, and amphetamines
- various physical conditions, including hypogonadism, tumors, kidney failure, liver failure, cirrhosis, malnutrition, and starvation
- obesity or lack of proper diet and nutrition

DIAGNOSIS

To begin evaluating a patient for gynecomastia, a health-care provider will ask for a medical history, including such information as the symptoms being experienced, how long they have persisted, if tenderness is present around the breast area, type of medication being taken, general health condition, drug history, and family health history. The health-care provider will then carefully examine the breast tissue, genitals, and abdomen.

A doctor may order tests that include blood tests, hormone studies, computerized tomography (CT) scan, magnetic resonance imaging (MRI) scan, mammogram, and tissue biopsy to confirm gynecomastia.

TREATMENT

In young patients, treatment is often unnecessary since, in such cases, gynecomastia usually resolves on its own. For older individuals, several treatment methods can be recommended by health-care providers. For example, medications may be prescribed to help restore hormone balance. Certain medications, such as tamoxifen, aromatase inhibitors (Arimidex), and raloxifene (Evista), may help in some cases. If gynecomastia results from the usage of certain drugs, doctors may prescribe a different medication that may help improve other health conditions.

Surgery may be an option in rare cases if medication and other treatments prove ineffective. The surgical method has two options, namely liposuction and mastectomy. While liposuction involves the removal of breast fat and not the breast gland, mastectomy involves the removal of the breast gland.

To make good decisions and ensure the best possible outcome, before beginning any treatment, the patient should ask the health-care provider the following questions:

- Is the breast enlargement likely to resolve on its own?
- What types of treatments are available?
- How long will treatment last?
- Are there any health conditions that are triggering the gynecomastia?
- Should I avoid any particular substance or medication to improve the condition?
- Should I be tested for breast cancer?
- If breasts hurt, how can I stop the pain?

Treatment options also include getting psychological counseling and help and support from family. The condition can cause stress and embarrassment, so counseling, group therapy, and explaining the condition to family and friends can have a major impact on the recovery process.

References

Booth, Stephanie. "Enlarged Breasts in Men: Causes and Treatments," WebMD, December 13, 2015. Available online. URL: www.webmd.com/men/features/male-breast-enlargement-gynecomastia#12. Accessed August 11, 2023.

"Enlarged Breasts in Men (Gynecomastia)," Mayo Clinic, October 16, 2021. Available online. URL: www.mayoclinic.

org/diseases-conditions/gynecomastia/symptoms-causes/
syc-20351793. Accessed August 11, 2023.

"Gynecomastia," Cleveland Clinic, September 8, 2021.
Available online. URL: https://my.clevelandclinic.org/
health/articles/gynecomastia. Accessed August 11, 2023.

Lemaine, Valerie, et al., "Gynecomastia in Adolescent Males,"
National Library of Medicine (NLM), February 27, 2013.
Available online. URL: www.ncbi.nlm.nih.gov/pmc/
articles/PMC3706045. Accessed August 11, 2023.

Chapter 26 | Sexual Health Issues in Men with Cancer

Men being treated for cancer may experience changes that affect their sexual life during, and sometimes after, treatment. While you may not have the energy or interest in sexual activity that you did before treatment, being intimate with and feeling close to your spouse or partner is probably still important.

Your doctor or nurse may talk with you about how cancer treatment might affect your sexual life, or you may need to be proactive and ask questions such as "What sexual changes or problems are common among men receiving this type of treatment?" and "What methods of birth control or protection are recommended during treatment?"

Whether or not you will have problems that affect your sexual health depends on factors such as:

- the type of cancer
- the type of treatment(s)
- the amount (dose) of treatment
- the length (duration) of treatment
- your age at time of treatment
- the amount of time that has passed since treatment
- other personal health factors

CANCER TREATMENTS MAY CAUSE SEXUAL PROBLEMS IN MEN

Many problems that affect a man's sexual activity during treatment are temporary and improve once treatment has ended. Other side effects may be long term or may start after treatment.

Your doctor will talk with you about side effects you may have based on your treatment(s):

- **Chemotherapy.** This may lower your testosterone levels and libido during the treatment period. You may be advised to use a condom because semen may contain traces of chemotherapy for a period of time after treatment. Chemotherapy does not usually affect your ability to have an erection.

- **External beam radiation therapy and brachytherapy.** External beam radiation therapy to the pelvis (such as to the anus, bladder, penis, or prostate) and brachytherapy (also called "internal radiation therapy") can affect a man's sexual function. If blood vessels or nerves are damaged, it may be difficult to get or keep an erection; this is called "erectile dysfunction." If the prostate is damaged, you may have a dry orgasm.

- **Hormone therapy.** This can lower testosterone levels and decrease a man's sexual drive. It may be difficult to get or keep an erection.

- **Surgery.** Surgery for penile, rectal, prostate, testicular, and other pelvic cancers (such as the bladder, colon, and rectum) may affect the nerves, making it difficult to get and keep an erection. Sometimes, nerve-sparing surgery can be used to prevent these problems.

- **Medicines.** Medicines used to treat pain, some drugs used for depression, and medicines that affect the nerves and blood vessels may all affect your sex drive.

Health problems, such as heart disease, high blood pressure (HBP), diabetes, and smoking, can also contribute to changes in your sexual health.

WAYS TO MANAGE SEXUAL HEALTH ISSUES
People on your health-care team have helped others cope during this difficult time and can offer valuable suggestions. You may also want to talk with a sexual health expert to get answers to any questions or concerns.

Most men can be sexually active during treatment, but you will want to confirm this with your doctor. For example, there may be times during treatment when you are at increased risk of infection or bleeding and may be advised to abstain from sexual activity. Depending on the type of treatment you are receiving, condom use may be advised.

Your health-care team can help you with the following:

- **Learn about treatments**. Based on symptoms you are having, your oncologist or a urologist will advise you on treatment options. For example, there are medicines and devices that may be prescribed once a sexual health problem has been diagnosed. Medicines can be given to increase blood flow to the penis. There are also surgical procedures in which a firm rod or inflatable device (penile implant) is placed in the penis, making it possible to get and keep an erection.

- **Learn about condoms and/or contraceptives**. Condoms may be advised to prevent your partner's exposure to chemotherapy drugs that may remain in semen. Based on your partner's age, contraception may be advised to prevent pregnancy.

- **Manage related side effects**. Talk with your doctor or nurse about problems, such as pain, fatigue, hair loss, loss of interest in activities, sadness, or trouble sleeping, that may affect your sex life. Speaking up about side effects can help you get the treatment and support you need to feel better.

- **Get support and counseling**. During this time, sharing your feelings and concerns with people you are close to will help. You may also benefit from participating in a professionally moderated or led support group. Your nurse or social worker can recommend support groups and counselors in your area.

TALKING WITH YOUR HEALTH-CARE TEAM ABOUT SEXUAL HEALTH ISSUES

As you think about the changes that treatment has brought into your life, make a list of questions to ask your doctor, nurse, or social worker.

Consider adding these to your list:

- What sexual problems are common among men receiving this treatment?
- What sexual problems might I have during treatment?
- When might these changes occur?
- How long might these problems last? Will any of these problems be permanent?
- How can these problems be prevented, treated, or managed?
- What precautions do I need to take during treatment? For example, do I need to use a condom to protect my partner?
- Should my partners and I use contraception to avoid a pregnancy? What types of contraception (birth control) do you recommend?
- Is there a support group that you recommend?
- What specialist(s) would you suggest that I talk with to learn more?[1]

[1] "Sexual Health Issues in Men with Cancer," National Cancer Institute (NCI), December 29, 2022. Available online. URL: www.cancer.gov/about-cancer/treatment/side-effects/sexuality-men. Accessed June 16, 2023.

Chapter 27 | **Noncancerous Prostate Disorders**

Chapter Contents

WHAT IS THE PROSTATE?

The prostate is a walnut-shaped gland that is part of the male reproductive system. The main function of the prostate is to make a fluid that goes into semen. Prostate fluid is essential for a man's fertility. The gland surrounds the urethra at the neck of the bladder. The bladder neck is the area where the urethra joins the bladder. The bladder and urethra are parts of the lower urinary tract. The prostate has two or more lobes, or sections, enclosed by an outer layer of tissue, and it is in front of the rectum, just below the bladder. The urethra is the tube that carries urine from the bladder to the outside of the body. In men, the urethra also carries semen out through the penis (see Figure 27.1).

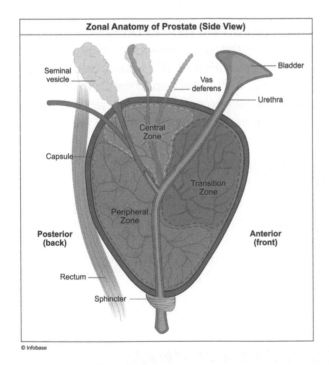

Figure 27.1. Prostate Anatomy

Infobase

WHAT IS BENIGN PROSTATIC HYPERPLASIA?

Benign prostatic hyperplasia (BPH) is a condition in men in which the prostate gland is enlarged and not cancerous. BPH is also called "benign prostatic hypertrophy" or "benign prostatic obstruction."

The prostate goes through two main growth periods as a man ages. The first occurs early in puberty when the prostate doubles in size. The second phase of growth begins around the age of 25 and continues during most of a man's life. BPH often occurs with the second growth phase.

As the prostate enlarges, the gland presses against and pinches the urethra. The bladder wall becomes thicker. Eventually, the bladder may weaken and lose the ability to empty completely, leaving some urine in the bladder. The narrowing of the urethra and urinary retention—the inability to empty the bladder completely—cause many of the problems associated with BPH.

HOW COMMON IS BENIGN PROSTATIC HYPERPLASIA?

Benign prostatic hyperplasia is the most common prostate problem for men older than the age of 50. Although BPH rarely causes symptoms before the age of 40, the occurrence and symptoms increase with age. BPH affects about 50 percent of men between the ages of 51 and 60 and up to 90 percent of men older than 80 years of age.

WHO IS MORE LIKELY TO DEVELOP BENIGN PROSTATIC HYPERPLASIA?

Men with the following factors are more likely to develop BPH:
- 40 years of age and older
- family history of BPH
- medical conditions, such as obesity, heart and circulatory disease, and type 2 diabetes
- lack of physical exercise
- erectile dysfunction (ED)

WHAT CAUSES BENIGN PROSTATIC HYPERPLASIA?

The cause of BPH is not well understood; however, it occurs mainly in older men. BPH does not develop in men whose testicles were removed before puberty. For this reason, some researchers believe that factors related to aging and the testicles may cause BPH.

Throughout their lives, men produce testosterone, a male hormone, and small amounts of estrogen, a female hormone. As men age, the amount of active testosterone in their blood decreases, which leaves a higher proportion of estrogen. Scientific studies have suggested that BPH may occur because the higher proportion of estrogen within the prostate increases the activity of substances that promote prostate cell growth.

Another theory focuses on dihydrotestosterone (DHT), a male hormone that plays a role in prostate development and growth. Some research has indicated that even with a drop in blood testosterone levels, older men continue to produce and accumulate high levels of DHT in the prostate. This accumulation of DHT may encourage prostate cells to continue to grow. Scientists have noted that men who do not produce DHT do not develop BPH.

WHAT ARE THE SYMPTOMS OF BENIGN PROSTATIC HYPERPLASIA?

Lower urinary tract symptoms suggestive of BPH may include the following:

- urinary frequency—urination eight or more times a day
- urinary urgency—the inability to delay urination
- trouble starting a urine stream
- a weak or an interrupted urine stream
- dribbling at the end of urination
- nocturia—frequent urination during periods of sleep
- urinary retention
- urinary incontinence—the accidental loss of urine
- pain after ejaculation or during urination
- urine that has an unusual color or smell

Symptoms of BPH most often come from:

- a blocked urethra
- a bladder that is overworked from trying to pass urine through the blockage

The size of the prostate does not always determine the severity of the blockage or symptoms. Some men with greatly enlarged prostates have little blockage and few symptoms, while other men who have minimally enlarged prostates have greater blockage and more symptoms. Less than half of all men with BPH have lower urinary tract symptoms.

Sometimes, men may not know they have a blockage until they cannot urinate. This condition, called "acute urinary retention" (AUR), can result from taking over-the-counter (OTC) cold or allergy medications that contain decongestants, such as pseudoephedrine and oxymetazoline. A potential side effect of these medications may prevent the bladder neck from relaxing and releasing urine. Medications that contain antihistamines, such as diphenhydramine, can weaken the contraction of bladder muscles and cause urinary retention, difficulty urinating, and painful urination. When men have partial urethra blockage, urinary retention can also occur as a result of alcohol consumption, cold temperatures, or a long period of inactivity.

WHAT ARE THE COMPLICATIONS OF BENIGN PROSTATIC HYPERPLASIA?

The complications of BPH may include the following:

- acute urinary retention
- chronic, or long-lasting, urinary retention
- blood in the urine
- urinary tract infections (UTIs)
- bladder damage
- kidney damage
- bladder stones

Most men with BPH do not develop these complications. However, kidney damage in particular can be a serious health threat when it occurs.

When to Seek Medical Care

A person may have urinary symptoms unrelated to BPH that are caused by bladder problems, UTIs, or prostatitis—inflammation of the prostate. Symptoms of BPH can also signal more serious conditions, including prostate cancer. Men with symptoms of BPH should see a health-care provider.

Men with the following symptoms should seek immediate medical care:

- complete inability to urinate
- painful, frequent, and urgent need to urinate, with fever and chills
- blood in the urine
- great discomfort or pain in the lower abdomen and urinary tract

HOW IS BENIGN PROSTATIC HYPERPLASIA DIAGNOSED?

A health-care provider diagnoses BPH based on the following.

Personal and Family Medical History

Taking a personal and family medical history is one of the first things a health-care provider may do to help diagnose BPH. A health-care provider may ask a man:

- what symptoms are present
- when the symptoms began and how often they occur
- whether he has a history of recurrent UTIs
- what medications he takes, both prescription and OTC
- how much liquid he typically drinks each day
- whether he consumes caffeine and alcohol
- about his general medical history, including any significant illnesses or surgeries

Physical Exam

A physical exam may help diagnose BPH. During a physical exam, a health-care provider most often:

- examines a patient's body, which can include checking for:
  - discharge from the urethra
  - enlarged or tender lymph nodes in the groin
  - a swollen or tender scrotum

- taps on specific areas of the patient's body
- performs a digital rectal exam (DRE)

A DRE, or rectal exam, is a physical exam of the prostate. To perform the exam, the health-care provider asks the man to bend over a table or lie on his side while holding his knees close to his chest. The health-care provider slides a gloved, lubricated finger into the rectum and feels the part of the prostate that lies next to the rectum. The man may feel slight, brief discomfort during the rectal exam. A health-care provider most often performs a rectal exam during an office visit, and men do not require anesthesia. The exam helps the health-care provider see if the prostate is enlarged or tender or has any abnormalities that require more testing.

Many health-care providers perform a rectal exam as part of a routine physical exam for men aged 40 or older, whether or not they have urinary problems.

Medical Tests

A health-care provider may refer men to a urologist—a doctor who specializes in urinary problems and the male reproductive system—though the health-care provider most often diagnoses BPH on the basis of symptoms and a DRE. A urologist uses medical tests to help diagnose lower urinary tract problems related to BPH and recommend treatment. Medical tests may include the following:

- **Urinalysis.** It involves testing a urine sample. The patient collects a urine sample in a special container in a health-care provider's office or a commercial facility. A health-care provider tests the sample during an office visit or sends it to a lab for analysis. For the test, a nurse or technician places a strip of chemically treated paper, called a "dipstick," into the urine. Patches on the dipstick change color to indicate signs of infection in urine.
- **Prostate-specific antigen (PSA) blood test**. A health-care provider may draw blood for a PSA test during an office visit or in a commercial facility and send the sample to a lab for analysis. Prostate cells create a

protein called PSA. Men who have prostate cancer may have a higher amount of PSA in their blood. However, a high PSA level does not necessarily indicate prostate cancer. In fact, BPH, prostate infections, inflammation, aging, and normal fluctuations often cause high PSA levels. Much remains unknown about how to interpret a PSA blood test; the test's ability to discriminate between cancer and prostate conditions, such as BPH; and the best course of action to take if the PSA level is high.

- **Urodynamic tests**. Urodynamic tests include a variety of procedures that look at how well the bladder and urethra store and release urine. A health-care provider performs urodynamic tests during an office visit or in an outpatient center or a hospital. Some urodynamic tests do not require anesthesia; others may require local anesthesia. Most urodynamic tests focus on the bladder's ability to hold urine and empty steadily and completely and may include the following:

  - **Uroflowmetry.** This test measures how rapidly the bladder releases urine.

  - **Postvoid residual measurement**. This measurement evaluates how much urine remains in the bladder after urination.

  - **Reduced urine flow or residual urine in the bladder.** This condition often suggests urine blockage due to BPH.

- **Cystoscopy**. It is a procedure that uses a tube-like instrument, called a "cystoscope," to look inside the urethra and bladder. A urologist inserts the cystoscope through the opening at the tip of the penis and into the lower urinary tract. A urologist performs cystoscopy during an office visit or in an outpatient center or a hospital. The urologist will give the patient local anesthesia; however, in some cases, the patient may require sedation and regional or general anesthesia. A urologist may use cystoscopy to look for blockage or stones in the urinary tract.

- **Transrectal ultrasound**. This procedure uses a device, called a "transducer," that bounces safe, painless sound waves off organs to create an image of their structure. The health-care provider can move the transducer to different angles to make it possible to examine different organs. A specially trained technician performs the procedure in a health-care provider's office, an outpatient center, or a hospital, and a radiologist—a doctor who specializes in medical imaging—interprets the images; the patient does not require anesthesia. Urologists most often use transrectal ultrasound to examine the prostate. In a transrectal ultrasound, the technician inserts a transducer slightly larger than a pen into the man's rectum, next to the prostate. The ultrasound image shows the size of the prostate and any abnormalities, such as tumors. Transrectal ultrasound cannot reliably diagnose prostate cancer.
- **Biopsy**. It is a procedure that involves taking a small piece of prostate tissue for examination with a microscope. A urologist performs the biopsy in an outpatient center or a hospital. The urologist will give the patient light sedation and local anesthetic; however, in some cases, the patient will require general anesthesia. The urologist uses imaging techniques, such as ultrasound, a computerized tomography (CT) scan, or magnetic resonance imaging (MRI), to guide the biopsy needle into the prostate. A pathologist—a doctor who specializes in examining tissues to diagnose diseases—examines the prostate tissue in a lab. The test can show whether prostate cancer is present.

HOW IS BENIGN PROSTATIC HYPERPLASIA TREATED?
Treatment options for BPH may include the following:
- lifestyle changes
- medications
- minimally invasive procedures
- surgery

A health-care provider treats BPH based on the severity of symptoms, how much the symptoms affect a man's daily life, and a man's preferences.

Men may not need treatment for a mildly enlarged prostate unless their symptoms are bothersome and affecting their quality of life (QOL). In these cases, instead of treatment, a urologist may recommend regular checkups. If BPH symptoms become bothersome or present a health risk, a urologist most often recommends treatment.

HOW CAN BENIGN PROSTATIC HYPERPLASIA BE PREVENTED?
Researchers have not found a way to prevent BPH. Men with risk factors for BPH should talk with a health-care provider about any lower urinary tract symptoms and the need for regular prostate exams. Men can get early treatment and minimize BPH effects by recognizing lower urinary tract symptoms and identifying an enlarged prostate.[1]

Section 27.2 | Prostatitis

WHAT IS PROSTATITIS?
Prostatitis is a frequently painful condition that involves inflammation of the prostate and sometimes the areas around the prostate.
Scientists have identified four types of prostatitis:
- chronic prostatitis or chronic pelvic pain syndrome
- acute bacterial prostatitis
- chronic bacterial prostatitis
- asymptomatic inflammatory prostatitis

Men with asymptomatic inflammatory prostatitis do not have symptoms. A health-care provider may diagnose asymptomatic

---

[1] "Prostate Enlargement (Benign Prostatic Hyperplasia)," National Institute of Diabetes and Digestive and Kidney Diseases (NIDDK), September 2014. Available online. URL: www.niddk.nih.gov/health-information/urologic-diseases/prostate-problems/prostate-enlargement-benign-prostatic-hyperplasia. Accessed July 5, 2023.

inflammatory prostatitis when testing for other urinary tract or reproductive tract disorders. This type of prostatitis does not cause complications and does not need treatment.

HOW COMMON IS PROSTATITIS?

Prostatitis is the most common urinary tract problem for men younger than the age of 50 and the third most common urinary tract problem for men older than the age of 50. Prostatitis accounts for about 2 million visits to health-care providers in the United States each year.

Chronic prostatitis or chronic pelvic pain syndrome:

- is the most common and least understood form of prostatitis
- can occur in men of any age group
- affects 10–15 percent of the U.S. male population

WHO IS MORE LIKELY TO DEVELOP PROSTATITIS?

The factors that affect a man's chances of developing prostatitis differ depending on the following types:

- **Chronic prostatitis/chronic pelvic pain syndrome.**
  Men with nerve damage in the lower urinary tract due to surgery or trauma may be more likely to develop chronic prostatitis/chronic pelvic pain syndrome. Psychological stress may also increase a man's chances of developing the condition.
- **Acute and chronic bacterial prostatitis.** Men with lower urinary tract infections (UTIs) may be more likely to develop bacterial prostatitis. UTIs that recur or are difficult to treat may lead to chronic bacterial prostatitis.

WHAT CAUSES PROSTATITIS?

The causes of prostatitis differ depending on the following types:

- **Chronic prostatitis or chronic pelvic pain syndrome.**
  The exact cause of chronic prostatitis/chronic pelvic pain syndrome is unknown. Researchers believe a

microorganism, though not a bacterial infection, may cause the condition. This type of prostatitis may relate to chemicals in the urine, the immune system's response to a previous UTI, or nerve damage in the pelvic area.

- **Acute and chronic bacterial prostatitis.** A bacterial infection of the prostate causes bacterial prostatitis. The acute type happens suddenly and lasts a short time, while the chronic type develops slowly and lasts a long time, often years. The infection may occur when bacteria travel from the urethra into the prostate.

WHAT ARE THE SYMPTOMS OF PROSTATITIS?

Each type of prostatitis has a range of symptoms that vary depending on the cause and may not be the same for every man. Many symptoms are similar to those of other conditions.

- **Chronic prostatitis/chronic pelvic pain syndrome.** The main symptoms of chronic prostatitis/chronic pelvic pain syndrome can include pain or discomfort lasting three or more months in one or more of the following areas:
  - between the scrotum and anus
  - the central lower abdomen
  - the penis
  - the scrotum
  - the lower back
- **Pain during or after ejaculation is another common symptom.** A man with chronic prostatitis/chronic pelvic pain syndrome may have pain spread out around the pelvic area or may have pain in one or more areas at the same time. The pain may come and go and appear suddenly or gradually. Other symptoms may include the following:
  - pain in the urethra during or after urination
  - pain in the penis during or after urination
  - urinary frequency—urination eight or more times a day (The bladder begins to contract even when

it contains small amounts of urine, causing more frequent urination.)

- urinary urgency—the inability to delay urination
- a weak or an interrupted urine stream

- **Acute bacterial prostatitis.** The symptoms of acute bacterial prostatitis come on suddenly and are severe. Men should seek immediate medical care. Symptoms of acute bacterial prostatitis may include the following:
  - urinary frequency
  - urinary urgency
  - fever
  - chills
  - a burning feeling or pain during urination
  - pain in the genital area, groin, lower abdomen, or lower back
  - nocturia—frequent urination during periods of sleep
  - nausea and vomiting
  - body aches
  - urinary retention—the inability to empty the bladder completely
  - trouble starting a urine stream
  - a weak or an interrupted urine stream
  - urinary blockage—the complete inability to urinate
  - a UTI—as shown by bacteria and infection-fighting cells in the urine

- **Chronic bacterial prostatitis.** The symptoms of chronic bacterial prostatitis are similar to those of acute bacterial prostatitis, though not as severe. This type of prostatitis often develops slowly and can last three or more months. The symptoms may come and go, or they may be mild all the time. Chronic bacterial prostatitis may occur after previous treatment of acute bacterial prostatitis or a UTI. The symptoms of chronic bacterial prostatitis may include the following:
  - urinary frequency
  - urinary urgency

- a burning feeling or pain during urination
- pain in the genital area, groin, lower abdomen, or lower back
- nocturia
- painful ejaculation
- urinary retention
- trouble starting a urine stream
- a weak or an interrupted urine stream
- urinary blockage
- a UTI

WHAT ARE THE COMPLICATIONS OF PROSTATITIS?
The complications of prostatitis may include the following:
- bacterial infection in the bloodstream
- prostatic abscess—a pus-filled cavity in the prostate
- sexual dysfunction
- inflammation of reproductive organs near the prostate

WHEN TO SEEK MEDICAL CARE
A person may have urinary symptoms unrelated to prostatitis that are caused by bladder problems, UTIs, or benign prostatic hyperplasia. Symptoms of prostatitis can also signal more serious conditions, including prostate cancer.

Men with symptoms of prostatitis should see a health-care provider.

Men with the following symptoms should seek immediate medical care:
- complete inability to urinate
- painful, frequent, and urgent need to urinate, with fever and chills
- blood in the urine
- great discomfort or pain in the lower abdomen and urinary tract

HOW IS PROSTATITIS DIAGNOSED?
A health-care provider diagnoses prostatitis based on:
- a personal and family medical history
- a physical exam
- medical tests

A health-care provider may have to rule out other conditions that cause similar signs and symptoms before diagnosing prostatitis.

Personal and Family Medical History
Taking a personal and family medical history is one of the first things a health-care provider may do to help diagnose prostatitis.

Physical Exam
A physical exam may help diagnose prostatitis. During a physical exam, a health-care provider usually:
- examines a patient's body, which can include checking for
  - discharge from the urethra
  - enlarged or tender lymph nodes in the groin
  - a swollen or tender scrotum
- performs a digital rectal exam

Many health-care providers perform a rectal exam as part of a routine physical exam for men aged 40 or older, whether or not they have urinary problems.

Medical Tests
A health-care provider may refer men to a urologist—a doctor who specializes in the urinary tract and male reproductive system. A urologist uses medical tests to help diagnose lower urinary tract problems related to prostatitis and recommend treatment. Medical tests may include the following:
- urinalysis
- blood tests
- urodynamic tests

- cystoscopy
- transrectal ultrasound
- biopsy
- semen analysis

HOW IS PROSTATITIS TREATED?
Treatment depends on the following types of prostatitis.

Chronic Prostatitis/Chronic Pelvic Pain Syndrome
Treatment for chronic prostatitis/chronic pelvic pain syndrome aims to decrease pain, discomfort, and inflammation. A wide range of symptoms exists, and no single treatment works for every man. Although antibiotics will not help treat nonbacterial prostatitis, a urologist may prescribe them, at least initially, until the urologist can rule out a bacterial infection. A urologist may prescribe other medications:

- silodosin (Rapaflo)
- 5-alpha reductase inhibitors, such as finasteride (Proscar) and dutasteride (Avodart)
- nonsteroidal anti-inflammatory drugs (NSAIDs), such as aspirin, ibuprofen, and naproxen sodium
- glycosaminoglycans, such as chondroitin sulfate
- muscle relaxants, such as cyclobenzaprine (Amrix, Flexeril) and clonazepam (Klonopin)
- neuromodulators, such as amitriptyline, nortriptyline (Aventyl, Pamelor), and pregabalin (Lyrica)

Alternative treatments may include the following:
- warm baths, called "sitz baths"
- local heat therapy with hot water bottles or heating pads
- physical therapy, such as
  - Kegel exercises—tightening and relaxing the muscles that hold urine in the bladder and hold the bladder in its proper position (also called "pelvic muscle exercises")

- myofascial release—pressing and stretching, sometimes with cooling and warming, of the muscles and soft tissues in the lower back, pelvic region, and upper legs (also known as "myofascial trigger point release")
- relaxation exercises
- biofeedback
- phytotherapy with plant extracts such as quercetin, bee pollen, and saw palmetto
- acupuncture

To help ensure coordinated and safe care, people should discuss their use of complementary and alternative medical practices, including their use of dietary supplements, with their health-care provider.

For men whose chronic prostatitis/chronic pelvic pain syndrome symptoms are affected by psychological stress, appropriate psychiatric treatment and stress reduction may reduce the recurrence of symptoms.

To help measure the effectiveness of treatment, a urologist may ask a series of questions from a standard questionnaire called the "National Institutes of Health (NIH) Chronic Prostatitis Symptom Index." The questionnaire helps a urologist assess the severity of symptoms and how they affect the man's quality of life (QOL). A urologist may ask questions several times, such as before, during, and after treatment.

Acute Bacterial Prostatitis

A urologist treats acute bacterial prostatitis with antibiotics. The antibiotic prescribed may depend on the type of bacteria causing the infection. Urologists usually prescribe oral antibiotics for at least two weeks. The infection may come back; therefore, some urologists recommend taking oral antibiotics for six to eight weeks. Severe cases of acute prostatitis may require a short hospital stay so that men can receive fluids and antibiotics through an intravenous (IV) tube. After the IV treatment, the man will need to take oral antibiotics for two to four weeks. Most cases of acute bacterial prostatitis clear up completely with medication and slight changes to diet. The urologist may recommend:

- avoiding or reducing intake of substances that irritate the bladder, such as alcohol, caffeinated beverages, and acidic and spicy foods
- increasing intake of liquids—64–128 ounces per day—to urinate often and help flush bacteria from the bladder

Chronic Bacterial Prostatitis

A urologist treats chronic bacterial prostatitis with antibiotics; however, treatment requires a longer course of therapy. The urologist may prescribe a low dose of antibiotics for up to six months to prevent recurrent infection. The urologist may also prescribe a different antibiotic or use a combination of antibiotics if the infection keeps coming back. The urologist may recommend increasing intake of liquids and avoiding or reducing intake of substances that irritate the bladder.

A urologist may use alpha blockers that treat chronic prostatitis/chronic pelvic pain syndrome to treat urinary retention caused by chronic bacterial prostatitis. These medications help relax the bladder muscles near the prostate and lessen symptoms such as painful urination. Men may require surgery to treat urinary retention caused by chronic bacterial prostatitis. Surgically removing scar tissue in the urethra often improves urine flow and reduces urinary retention.

HOW CAN PROSTATITIS BE PREVENTED?

Men cannot prevent prostatitis. Researchers are currently seeking to better understand what causes prostatitis and develop prevention strategies.[2]

[2] "Prostatitis: Inflammation of the Prostate," National Institute of Diabetes and Digestive and Kidney Diseases (NIDDK), July 2014. Available online. URL: www.niddk.nih.gov/health-information/urologic-diseases/prostate-problems/prostatitis-inflammation-prostate. Accessed June 19, 2023.

Chapter 28 | Birth Control, Infertility, and Menopause in Men

Section 28.1 | Condoms

WHAT ARE CONDOMS?

A male condom is a thin film cover that is placed over the penis and keeps sperm from entering a partner's body. Using a male condom consistently and correctly reduces the risk for human immuno-deficiency virus (HIV) infection and other sexually transmitted infections (STIs).[1]

Condoms provide less protection against sexually transmitted diseases (STDs) that can be transmitted through sores or cuts on the skin, such as human papillomavirus (HPV), genital herpes, and syphilis.

Condoms help prevent HIV for higher-risk sexual activities, such as anal or vaginal sex, and for lower-risk activities, such as oral sex and sharing sex toys.

You can buy condoms at many stores or online, and you can sometimes get them for free from clinics or health departments.

WHAT ARE THE MAIN TYPES OF CONDOMS?

There are two main types of condoms: condoms used externally and condoms used internally.

An external condom (sometimes called a "male condom" or just a "condom") is worn over the penis during sex. It is a thin layer of latex, plastic, synthetic rubber, or natural membrane.

- Latex condoms provide the best protection against HIV.
- Plastic (polyurethane) or synthetic rubber condoms are good for people with latex allergies. Plastic condoms break more often than latex condoms.
- Natural membrane (such as lambskin) condoms have small holes in them and do not block HIV and other STDs. These should not be used for HIV or STD prevention.

---

[1] Office of Population Affairs (OPA), "Contraception and Preventing Pregnancy," U.S. Department of Health and Human Services (HHS), August 17, 2020. Available online. URL: https://opa.hhs.gov/reproductive-health/preventing-pregnancy-contraception. Accessed July 24, 2023.

491

An internal condom (sometimes called a "female condom") is used in the vagina or anus during sex. It is a thin pouch made of a synthetic latex product called "nitrile." HIV cannot travel through the nitrile barrier.[2]

SOME RISKS OF USING A CONDOM
- irritation
- allergic reactions (If you are allergic to latex, you can try condoms made of polyurethane.)[3]

HOW DO YOU USE AN EXTERNAL CONDOM?
To use an external condom, do the following:
- Carefully open and remove the condom from the wrapper.
- Place the condom on the tip of the hard penis. If uncircumcised, pull back the foreskin first.
- Pinch the air out of the tip of the condom. While holding the tip, unroll the condom all the way down the penis.
- After sex but before pulling out, hold the bottom of the condom and carefully pull out the penis.
- Carefully remove the condom and throw it in the trash.

If you feel the condom break any time during sex, stop immediately, pull out the penis, take off the broken condom, and put on a new condom.

Use water-based or silicone-based lubricants during sex to help keep the condom from tearing. Do not use oil-based lubricants because they can weaken the condom and cause it to break.[4]

---

[2] "Condoms," Centers for Disease Control and Prevention (CDC), May 13, 2021. Available online. URL: www.cdc.gov/hiv/basics/hiv-prevention/condoms.html. Accessed June 20, 2023.
[3] "Birth Control," U.S. Food and Drug Administration (FDA), December 23, 2022. Available online. URL: www.fda.gov/consumers/free-publications-women/birth-control#EC. Accessed June 20, 2023.
[4] See footnote [2].

Chance of Getting Pregnant with Typical Use (Number of Pregnancies Expected per 100 Women Who Use This Method for One Year)

- Out of 100 women whose partners' use this method, 18 may get pregnant.
- The most important thing is that you use a condom every time you have sex.
- It can be used with other barrier methods to decrease your chances of becoming pregnant.

DOES IT PROTECT FROM SEXUALLY TRANSMITTED INFECTIONS?

- Yes. Consistent and correct use of the male latex condom reduces the risk of STIs. The condom cannot provide absolute protection against STIs.[5]

Section 28.2 | Withdrawal

WHAT IS WITHDRAWAL?

Withdrawal, or the pullout method, has been practiced for centuries to avoid the risk of unwanted pregnancy during sexual intercourse. Scientifically known as "coitus interruptus" (Latin for interrupted intercourse), withdrawal happens when a man removes his penis from the vagina before ejaculating (the moment when semen spurts out of the penis).

WHAT IS THE LOGIC BEHIND WITHDRAWAL?

Withdrawal prevents sperm from entering the woman's vagina, thereby preventing contact between the sperm and the egg.

---

[5] See footnote [3].

WHAT ARE THE RISKS OF WITHDRAWAL?

Even if the penis is pulled out of the vagina, there is still a risk of pregnancy from pre-ejaculate, or pre-cum—sperm that is still in the urinary tract from a previous ejaculation. It is advisable for a man to urinate to get rid of all the pre-cum from the urethra before intercourse and clean properly to get rid of any fluid before having intercourse again.

Even though the withdrawal method may prevent unwanted pregnancy if practiced correctly, it does not protect people from the risk of sexually transmitted diseases (STDs) and human immunodeficiency virus (HIV). It is always wiser to protect yourself from the risk of pregnancy, STDs, and the transmission of HIV by correctly and consistently using male latex condoms and/or other contraceptive methods.

WHY SHOULD YOU USE WITHDRAWAL?

Withdrawal continues to be a popular birth control method among younger couples. A number of factors that make this an attractive option are as follows:

- This can be used when no other method is available.
- It is absolutely free and available without any prescription.
- It does not have any side effects.
- This can be used with other birth control methods.

IS WITHDRAWAL FAIL PROOF?

No. For a number of reasons withdrawal is an unreliable form of birth control.

The practice of withdrawal requires a lot of trust, self-control, and experience and requires the male partner to know the sexual responses of his own body to know when to pull out. It is generally not recommended for teens and sexually inexperienced men. If done incorrectly and a man is unable to predict and unable to control the exact moment of his ejaculation, this method could be very ineffective.

References

David, Delvin. "Coitus Interruptus (Withdrawal Method)," netdoctor, December 22, 2014. Available online. URL: www.netdoctor.co.uk/conditions/sexual-health/a2208/ coitus-interruptus-withdrawal-method. Accessed August 7, 2023.

Mayo Clinic Staff, "Withdrawal Method (Coitus Interruptus)," Mayo Clinic, May 7, 2022. Available online. URL: www.mayoclinic.org/tests-procedures/ withdrawal-method/about/pac-20395283. Accessed August 7, 2023.

"Withdrawal (Pull Out Method)," Planned Parenthood, February 22, 2017. Available online. URL: www. plannedparenthood.org/learn/birth-control/withdrawal-pull-out-method. Accessed August 7, 2023.

Section 28.3 | Vasectomy

A vasectomy is a surgical procedure performed as a method of birth control. It involves cutting the vas deferens to close off the tubes that carry sperm from the testicles (there is one vas deferens per testicle; see Figure 28.1). If a man has a successful vasectomy, he can no longer get a woman pregnant.

Sperm are made in the two testicles, which are inside the scrotum. They are stored in a tube attached to each testicle called the "epididymis." When a man ejaculates, the sperm travel from the epididymis, through the vas deferens, and then mix with seminal fluid to form semen. The semen then travels through the urethra and out the penis.

Before a vasectomy, semen contains sperm and seminal fluid. After a vasectomy, sperm are no longer in the semen. The man's testicles will make less sperm over time, and his body will harmlessly absorb any sperm that are made.

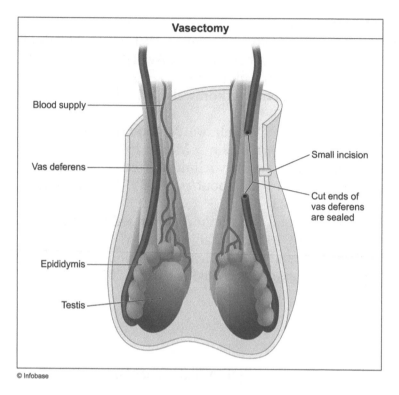

Vasectomy

Blood supply

Vas deferens

Epididymis

Testis

Small incision

Cut ends of
vas deferens
are sealed

© Infobase

Figure 28.1. Vasectomy

HOW IS A VASECTOMY DONE?

A vasectomy is usually performed in the office of a urologist, a doctor who specializes in the male urinary tract and reproductive system. In some cases, the urologist may decide to do a vasectomy in an outpatient surgery center or a hospital. This could be because of patient anxiety or because other procedures will be done at the same time.

There are two ways to perform a vasectomy. In either case, the patient is awake during the procedure, but the urologist uses a local anesthetic to numb the scrotum.

- **Conventional method**. With the conventional method, the doctor makes one or two small cuts in the scrotum to access the vas deferens. A small section of the vas deferens is cut out and then removed. The urologist may cauterize (seal with heat) the ends and then tie the ends with stitches. The doctor will then perform the same procedure on the other testicle, either through the same opening or through a second scrotal incision. For both testicles, when the vas deferens has been tied off, the doctor will use a few stitches or skin "glue" to close the opening(s) in the scrotum.

- **"No-scalpel" method**. With the "no-scalpel" method, a small puncture hole is made on one side of the scrotum. The health-care provider will find the vas deferens under the skin and pull it through the hole. The vas deferens is then cut, and a small section is removed. The ends are either cauterized or tied off and then put back in place. The procedure is then performed on the other testicle. No stitches are needed with this method because the puncture holes are so small.

After a vasectomy, most men go home the same day and fully recover in less than a week.

HOW EFFECTIVE IS VASECTOMY?

Vasectomy is one of the most effective forms of birth control. In the first year after a man has a vasectomy, a few couples will still get pregnant. But the number is far lower than the rates of pregnancy among couples using condoms or oral contraceptive pills.

However, a vasectomy is not effective right away. Men still need to use other birth control until the remaining sperm are cleared out of the semen. This takes 15–20 ejaculations, or about three months. Even then, one of every five men will still have sperm in his semen and will need to wait longer for the sperm to clear.

A health-care provider will check a man's semen for sperm at least once after the surgery. Once the sperm count has dropped to zero, it is safe to assume that the vasectomy is now an effective form of birth control. Until that time, men need to use another form of birth control to make sure their partner does not become pregnant.

WHAT ARE THE RISKS OF VASECTOMY?

Although vasectomy is safe and highly effective, men should be aware of problems that could occur after surgery and over time.

Surgical Risks

After surgery, most men have discomfort, bruising, and some swelling, all of which usually go away within two weeks. Problems that can occur after surgery and need to be checked by a health-care provider include the following:

- **Hematoma.** Bleeding under the skin that can lead to painful swelling.
- **Infection.** Fever and scrotal redness and tenderness are signs of infection.

Other Risks

The risk of other problems is small, but they do occur. These include the following:

- **A lump in the scrotum, called a "granuloma."** This is formed from sperm that leak out of the vas deferens into the tissue.
- **Postvasectomy pain syndrome.** This condition occurs in some men after a vasectomy procedure. It may affect their quality of life (QOL).
- **Vasectomy failure.** There is a small risk that the vasectomy will fail. This can lead to unintended pregnancy. Among 1,000 vasectomies, 11 will likely fail over two years, and half of these failures will occur within the first three months after surgery. The risk of failure depends on a number of factors. For example, some surgical techniques are more likely to fail than others. Additionally, there is a very small risk that the two ends of the vas deferens will grow back together. If this happens, sperm may be able to enter the semen and make pregnancy possible.
- **Risk of regret.** Vasectomy may be a good choice for men and/or couples who are certain that they do not want more or any children. Most men who

have vasectomy, as well as spouses of men who have vasectomy, do not regret the decision. Men who have vasectomy before the age of 30 are the group most likely to want a vasectomy reversal in the future.

WILL VASECTOMY AFFECT YOUR SEX LIFE?

Vasectomy will not affect your sex life. It does not decrease your sex drive because it does not affect the production of the male hormone testosterone. It also does not affect your ability to get an erection or ejaculate semen. Because the sperm make up a very small amount of the semen, you will not notice a difference in the amount of semen you ejaculate.[6]

Section 28.4 | Male Infertility

WHAT IS INFERTILITY?

In general, infertility is defined as not being able to get pregnant (conceive) after one year (or longer) of unprotected sex. Because fertility in women is known to decline steadily with age, some providers evaluate and treat women aged 35 or older after six months of unprotected sex. Individuals and couples who are unable to conceive a child should consider making an appointment with a reproductive endocrinologist—a doctor who specializes in managing infertility. Reproductive endocrinologists may also be able to help women with recurrent pregnancy loss, defined as having two or more spontaneous miscarriages.

Pregnancy is the result of a process that has many steps. To get pregnant,

- a woman's body must release an egg from one of her ovaries

---

[6] "About Vasectomy," *Eunice Kennedy Shriver* National Institute of Child Health and Human Development (NICHD), February 18, 2022. Available online. URL: www.nichd.nih.gov/health/topics/vasectomy/conditioninfo. Accessed June 19, 2023.

- a man's sperm must join with the egg along the way (fertilize)
- the fertilized egg must go through a fallopian toward the uterus (womb)
- the embryo must attach to the inside of the uterus (implantation)

Infertility may result from a problem with any or several of these steps.

IS INFERTILITY JUST A WOMAN'S PROBLEM?
No, infertility is not always a woman's problem. Both men and women can contribute to infertility.

WHAT CAUSES INFERTILITY IN MEN?
Infertility in men can be caused by different factors and is typically evaluated by a semen analysis. When a semen analysis is performed, the number of sperm (concentration), motility (movement), and morphology (shape) are assessed by a specialist. A slightly abnormal semen analysis does not mean that a man is necessarily infertile. Instead, a semen analysis helps determine if and how male factors are contributing to infertility.

Disruption of Testicular or Ejaculatory Function
- varicocele, a condition in which the veins within a man's testicle are enlarged (Although there are often no symptoms, varicoceles may affect the number or shape of the sperm.)
- trauma to the testes (It may affect sperm production and result in a lower number of sperm.)
- heavy alcohol use, smoking, anabolic steroid use, and illicit drug use
- cancer treatment involving certain types of chemotherapy, radiation, or surgery to remove one or both testicles
- medical conditions such as diabetes, cystic fibrosis, certain types of autoimmune disorders, and certain types of infections (These conditions may cause testicular failure.)

Hormonal Disorders
IMPROPER FUNCTION OF THE HYPOTHALAMUS OR PITUITARY GLANDS
The hypothalamus and pituitary glands in the brain produce hormones that maintain normal testicular function. Production of too much prolactin, a hormone made by the pituitary gland (often due to the presence of a benign pituitary gland tumor), or other conditions that damage or impair the function of the hypothalamus or the pituitary gland may result in low or no sperm production.

These conditions may include benign and malignant (cancerous) pituitary tumors, congenital adrenal hyperplasia, exposure to too much estrogen, exposure to too much testosterone, Cushing syndrome, and chronic use of medications called "glucocorticoids."

Genetic Disorders
Genetic conditions such as Klinefelter syndrome (KS), Y-chromosome microdeletion, myotonic dystrophy, and other less common genetic disorders may cause no sperm or low numbers of sperm to be produced.

WHAT INCREASES A MAN'S RISK OF INFERTILITY?
- age (Although advanced age plays a much more important role in predicting female infertility, couples in which the male partner is 40 years old or older are more likely to report difficulty conceiving.)
- being overweight or obese
- smoking
- excessive alcohol and drug use (opioids and marijuana)
- exposure to testosterone (This may occur when a doctor prescribes testosterone injections, implants, or topical gel for low testosterone or when a man takes testosterone or similar medications illicitly for the purposes of increasing their muscle mass.)
- exposure to radiation
- frequent exposure of the testes to high temperatures, such as that which may occur in men confined to a wheelchair or through frequent sauna or hot tub use

- exposure to certain medications such as flutamide, cyproterone, bicalutamide, spironolactone, ketoconazole, or cimetidine
- exposure to environmental toxins, including exposure to pesticides, lead, cadmium, or mercury

WHAT ARE SOME OF THE SPECIFIC TREATMENTS FOR MALE INFERTILITY?

Male infertility may be treated with medical, surgical, or assisted reproductive therapies (ARTs) depending on the underlying cause. Medical and surgical therapies are usually managed by a urologist who specializes in infertility. A reproductive endocrinologist may offer intrauterine insemination (IUI) or in vitro fertilization (IVF) to help overcome male factor infertility.[7]

Section 28.5 | Reproductive Health Problems Associated with Workplace Exposures

A number of workplace substances have been identified as reproductive hazards for men. Reproductive hazards are substances that affect the ability to have healthy children.

Some examples of reproductive hazards include the following:
- radiation
- pesticides
- various chemicals and solvents
- legal and illegal drugs
- cigarettes
- heat

Scientists are just beginning to understand how reproductive hazards affect the male reproductive system.

---

[7] "Infertility FAQs," Centers for Disease Control and Prevention (CDC), April 26, 2023. Available online. URL: www.cdc.gov/reproductivehealth/infertility/index.htm. Accessed June 19, 2023.

Birth Control, Infertility, and Menopause in Men

Although more than 1,000 workplace chemicals have been shown to have reproductive effects on animals, most have not been studied in humans. There are over 72 million unique chemicals registered by the American Chemical Society (ACS), with about 15,000 new substances added every day, most of which are not tested for reproductive health effects.

Table 28.1 shows examples of reproductive hazards for men in the workplace. Although studies have found that workplace exposures may affect the reproductive system in some men, these effects do not necessarily occur in every worker. Some of the agents listed in the table are well-known reproductive hazards (such as lead), while the scientific evidence for the others may not be as definitive.

Table 28.1. Potential Reproductive Hazards

Reproductive Problem	Examples
Low hormone levels Some reproductive hazards can change the level of hormones in a man's body. This could affect how sperm are made or the man's sexual performance.	insecticides, lead, organophosphates, dichlorodiphenyldichloroethylene (DDE), manganese, phthalates
Low number of sperm Some reproductive hazards can stop or slow the actual production of sperm. This means that there will be fewer sperm present to fertilize an egg; if no sperm are produced, the man is sterile.	lead, diesel exhaust, pesticides, bisphenol A, organophosphates, chromium, paraquat/malathion
Irregular sperm shape Reproductive hazards may cause the shape of sperm cells to be different. These sperm often have trouble swimming or are unable to fertilize the egg.	insecticides, lead, carbon disulfide, pesticides, bisphenol A, petrochemical, carbofuran, nickel
Irregular sperm genetics Some reproductive hazards can affect the genetics (DNA) found in sperm. The sperm and egg each contribute 23 chromosomes at fertilization. The genetic information, or DNA, stored in these chromosomes determines what we will look like and how our bodies will function. Radiation or chemicals may cause changes or breaks in the DNA. If a sperm's DNA is damaged, it may not be able to fertilize an egg, or if it does fertilize an egg, it may affect the development of the unborn baby.	phthalates, styrene, organophosphates, carbaryl, fenvalerate, lead, benzene

Table 28.1. Continued

Reproductive Problem	Examples
Chemicals in semen Hazardous chemicals may collect in the epididymis, seminal vesicles, or prostate. These chemicals may kill the sperm, change the way in which they swim, or attach to the sperm and be carried to the egg.	lead, trichloroethylene, boron, cadmium
Low amount of semen On average, a man ejaculates about three-fourths of a teaspoon of semen. Some exposures may reduce this to less than half a teaspoon. This may result in the fluid not transporting the sperm to the cervix (opening to the womb).	lead, organophosphates, paraquat/malathion
Low number of swimming sperm Sperm have to swim through much of the woman's reproductive tract. Slow or not swimming sperm reduce the number of sperm available for fertilization.	insecticides, diesel exhaust, lead, carbon disulfide, phthalates, pesticides, bisphenol A, fenvalerate, petrochemical, welding, N, N-dimethylformamide, abamectin, paraquat/malathion
Lower sex drive Some exposures may reduce the man's sex drive or libido. This could result in not having intercourse during the women's fertile time.	carbon disulfide, bisphenol A
Erectile dysfunction (ED) Some exposures affect the ability for a man's penis to be hard enough for sex.	bisphenol A, bicycle saddles
Lower penis sensitivity If an exposure reduces the feeling in the penis, the man may not be stimulated enough to ejaculate.	bicycle saddles
Lower ejaculation quality If an exposure limits the ejaculation process, sperm cannot reach the cervix (womb opening) and cannot get to the egg.	bisphenol A

Whether or not an exposure will cause a reproductive problem depends on:

- the amount of time you are exposed
- the amount of the hazard you are exposed to

- how you were exposed
- how your body reacts to the hazard

These are only examples of hazards. Do not assume that a substance is safe if it is missing from the table.

CAN YOU EXPOSE YOUR FAMILY TO WORKPLACE HAZARDS?

Your family may never come to your workplace but could be exposed to hazards in your workplace that you may accidentally bring home. This could affect your partner's health, the health of a pregnancy, or your children. Many chemicals can be carried to your car or to your home on your skin, hair, clothes, shoes, or tool box and expose others in the family. Some infections, including Zika virus, can be passed to sexual partners.[8]

Section 28.6 | Male Menopause

WHAT IS MALE MENOPAUSE?

Male menopause refers to a decline in male hormone levels that occurs due to the aging process. Since men aged 50 or older often undergo a drop in testosterone production, this condition is also known as "androgen (testosterone) decline," "andropause," or simply "low testosterone."

Testosterone is a hormone that is found in both men and women. In men, it is produced in the testes and is responsible for the development of male sex organs before birth, brings about changes during puberty, plays a role in sex drive and sperm production, fuels physical and mental energy, and helps maintain muscle mass.

Although menopause affects men at about the same age as women, it is not the same as female menopause. In women, menopause occurs as ovulation ends and hormone production drops

---

[8] "Men's Reproductive Health in the Workplace," Centers for Disease Control and Prevention (CDC), May 1, 2023. Available online. URL: www.cdc.gov/niosh/topics/repro/mensworkplace.html. Accessed June 19, 2023.

off quickly. In men, however, hormone production declines at a slower rate, and this may lead to only slight changes in the way the testes function.

WHAT ARE ITS SYMPTOMS?

Male menopause can lead to physical, sexual, and psychological problems that may worsen as the person ages. These problems can include the following:

- lack of energy
- decreased muscle mass
- feelings of physical weakness
- insomnia or other sleep disorders
- increased body fat
- decreased libido
- erectile dysfunction (ED)
- infertility
- lowered self-confidence
- decreased motivation
- difficulty concentrating
- depression

Other less common symptoms may include reduced testicle size, tender or enlarged breasts, hot flashes, loss of body hair, and, in rare cases, osteoporosis.

HOW IS IT DIAGNOSED?

To diagnose male menopause, your health-care provider will perform a physical examination and order a blood test to check for testosterone levels in the blood. He or she will also discuss about your symptoms and order additional blood tests to rule out other conditions that may be causing the symptoms of this condition.

HOW IS IT TREATED?

Symptoms of male menopause are commonly treated through lifestyle changes, such as eating a healthier diet, getting more sleep and regular exercise, and reducing stress. Antidepressants and therapy may be prescribed if the individual is suffering from depression.

Testosterone replacement therapy may also be suggested to help alleviate symptoms such as fatigue, decreased libido, and depression.

References
Derrer, David T. "Male Menopause," *Web*MD, August 17, 2014. Available online. URL: www.webmd.com/men/guide/male-menopause. Accessed August 7, 2023.

Krans, Brian. "What Is Male Menopause?" Healthline Media, March 8, 2016. Available online. URL: www.healthline.com/health/menopause/male. Accessed August 7, 2023.

Chapter 29 | Safer Sex Guidelines

WHAT IS "SAFER SEX"?

Having safer sex means avoiding risky practices that involve the transmission of sexually transmitted diseases (STDs) such as human immunodeficiency virus (HIV).

There are two reasons to practice safer sex: to protect yourself and to protect others.

Protecting Yourself

If you have HIV, you need to protect your health. When it comes to sex, this means practicing safer sex (such as using condoms) to avoid STDs such as herpes and hepatitis. HIV makes it harder for your body to fight off diseases. What might be a small health problem for someone without HIV could be a big health problem for you. Your health-care provider can prescribe condoms for you if you need them.

Protecting Your Partner

Taking care of others means making sure that you do not pass HIV or any other STDs to them.

"Being safe" usually means protecting yourself and others by using condoms for the highest-risk sex activities, specifically for anal and vaginal sex. When done correctly, condom use is very effective at preventing HIV transmission. In recent years, "being safe" has come to include two other important strategies for reducing HIV infections:

- HIV treatment (antiretroviral therapy (ART) medications) for people with HIV
- pre-exposure prophylaxis (PrEP) for HIV-negative people

Both are very effective at reducing the risk of HIV infection. One or more of them is likely to be appropriate for your situation—be sure to ask your health-care provider for more information.

ANTIRETROVIRAL THERAPY FOR HUMAN IMMUNODEFICIENCY VIRUS PREVENTION

One of the most effective ways you can prevent HIV from passing to an HIV-negative sex partner is to take your ART (HIV medications) every day. If they are working well to suppress the HIV in your body, they will also prevent transmission of HIV to others.

PRE-EXPOSURE PROPHYLAXIS

HIV-negative individuals may, under the supervision of their health-care provider, take a pill every day to prevent HIV infection. It is called "pre-exposure prophylaxis." Usually, these are persons who are at relatively high risk of becoming infected with HIV (e.g., because they have a partner with HIV, they have risky sexual exposures, or they share injection drug equipment). The medications used for PrEP are Truvada and Descovy. PrEP appears to be extremely effective if it is taken every day and is not effective if it is taken irregularly.[1]

---

[1] "What Is 'Safer Sex'?" U.S. Department of Veterans Affairs (VA), May 28, 2019. Available online. URL: www.hiv.va.gov/patient/daily/sex/safer-sex.asp. Accessed June 20, 2023.

Part 4 | Accidents, Violence, and Other Health Concerns

Chapter 30 | Motor Vehicle Accidents

Chapter Contents

Section 30.1 | Statistics on Traffic Fatalities

The National Highway Traffic Safety Administration (NHTSA) is partnering with advocates and experts from across the country to launch its "Speeding Wrecks Lives" speeding prevention campaign. The launch comes as new data show that while there has been three-quarters of a slight dip in overall roadway deaths, speeding fatalities reached a 14-year high in 2021 and made up almost one-third of all traffic fatalities.

The campaign, which will run from July 10 to 31, is one of many ways in which the U.S. Department of Transportation (DOT) is working to address the crisis of deaths on our roadways through its National Roadway Safety Strategy (NRSS). The NHTSA campaign is supported by a $9.6 million national media by featuring English and Spanish-language ads running on television, radio, and digital platforms. The ads target drivers aged 18–44, who data show are most likely to be involved in speeding-related fatal crashes.

During the press event, NHTSA Acting Administrator Ann Carlson, together with Lorraine Martin, president and CEO of the National Safety Council, and Dr. Will Smith, emergency department physician at St. John's Health in Jackson, Wyoming, emphasized the dangers of speeding and the efforts made around the country to prevent crashes. Also, lending their voices were Captain Cory Carlisle of the Kansas City, Missouri, Police Department; Captain Christopher Vetter, Commander of the New Hampshire Office of Highway Safety; and Lieutenant Maurice Raines of the Georgia Governor's Office of Highway Safety, who participated via taped remarks.

"Speeding accounts for nearly one-third of all fatalities on our roads and puts everyone at risk, including people in other vehicles, pedestrians, cyclists, motorcyclists and people with disabilities," Carlson said. "NHTSA reminds everyone to slow down and arrive safely—it's better to arrive a few minutes late than not at all."

The NHTSA released new data on speeding, showing that speeding-related fatalities increased 8 percent from 2020 to 2021, with 12,330 people killed in 2021 speeding-related crashes. This represents 29 percent of all traffic fatalities in 2021. The estimated number of people injured in speeding-related crashes also increased by 7 percent. And 33 percent of motorcycle riders in fatal crashes were speeding, more than drivers of any other vehicle type.

Many drivers in speeding-related crashes also engaged in other risky driving behaviors. Drivers in fatal crashes who were speeding were also impaired by alcohol more frequently than drivers who were not speeding. Additionally, more than half of speeding passenger vehicle drivers were not wearing a seat belt, as compared to 23 percent of non-speeding passenger vehicle drivers.

The NHTSA also released a study of efforts used by law enforcement officers to reduce speeding. The study found that the number of speeders on the road was a statistically significant predictor of speeding-related crashes, and the number of non-speeders was not, indicating that the number of vehicles on the road can increase without leading to more crashes if the additional vehicles are driving at or below the speed limit. The study also found that decoy (unoccupied) law enforcement vehicles, issuing citations, and digital speed signs can continue to reduce speeding at deployment locations, even after they are no longer at those locations.

In January 2022, the DOT released the comprehensive National Roadway Safety Strategy (NRSS), a roadmap to address the national crisis in traffic fatalities and serious injuries. It adopts the safe system approach and builds multiple layers of protection with safer roads, safer people, safer vehicles, safer speeds, and better postcrash care.

The NRSS is complemented by unprecedented safety funding included in President Biden's Bipartisan Infrastructure Law, including the Safe Streets and Roads for All grant program. In February, the Department announced over $800 million in grant awards for more than 500 communities to help carry out projects that can address high-crash areas.

The U.S. DOT also launched the next phase of the NRSS, its Call-to-Action campaign, and released a one-year progress report and accompanying data visualizations that highlight the extent and magnitude of the U.S. roadway safety problem.

The NHTSA is also working closely with states to use a variety of tools to address their individual speed problems, including setting speeds at safe limits and engaging with communities to tailor public education and enforcement efforts. Many states are conducting speed campaigns during the month of July to educate the public and enforce safe speeds to drive down speed-related crashes.

The DOT's other roadway safety actions include:

- issuing a proposed rulemaking on advanced pedestrian automatic emergency braking (AEB)
- releasing proposals for upgrades and a "road map" for the New Car Assessment Program—including developing a proposal to add a pedestrian protection program to NCAP
- issuing a final rule on rear impact guards
- issuing a standing general order to collect more data about crashes that occur when automated driving systems and advanced driver assistance systems are engaged
- producing the Vulnerable Road User Safety Assessment to guide states on required 2023 assessments
- establishing a cross-agency working group to issue the Complete Streets Report to Congress, "Moving to a Complete Streets Design Model."
- advancing a revised Manual on Uniform Traffic Control Devices by analyzing and resolving the more than 25,000 public comments
- publishing an Advance Supplemental Notice of Proposed Rulemaking concerning speed limiters with a motor-carrier-based approach.[1]

Section 30.2 | Aggressive Driving

Speeding endangers everyone on the road: In 2021, speeding killed 12,330 people. We all know the frustrations of modern life and juggling a busy schedule, but speed limits are put in place to protect

---

[1] "Almost One-Third of Traffic Fatalities Are Speed-Related Crashes," National Highway Traffic Safety Administration (NHTSA), July 10, 2023. Available online. URL: www.nhtsa.gov/press-releases/speed-campaign-speeding-fatalities-14-year-high. Accessed August 14, 2023.

all road users. Learn about the dangers of speeding and why faster does not mean safer.

DANGERS OF SPEEDING

For more than two decades, speeding has been involved in approximately one-third of all motor vehicle fatalities. In 2021, speeding was a contributing factor in 29 percent of all traffic fatalities.

Speed also affects your safety even when you are driving at the speed limit but too fast for road conditions, such as during bad weather, when a road is under repair, or in an area at night that is not well-lit.

Speeding endangers not only the life of the speeder but also all the people on the road around them, including law enforcement officers. It is a problem we all need to help solve.

CONSEQUENCES OF SPEEDING

Speeding is more than just breaking the law. The consequences are far-ranging:

- greater potential for loss of vehicle control
- reduced effectiveness of occupant protection equipment
- increased stopping distance after the driver perceives a danger
- increased degree of crash severity leading to more severe injuries
- economic implications of a speed-related crash
- increased fuel consumption/cost

WHAT DRIVES SPEEDING?

Speeding is a type of aggressive driving behavior. Several factors have contributed to an overall rise in aggressive driving:

- **Traffic.** It is one of the most frequently mentioned contributing factors to aggressive driving, such as speeding. Drivers may respond by using aggressive driving behaviors, including speeding, changing lanes frequently, or becoming angry at anyone who they believe impedes their progress.

- **Running late.** Some people drive aggressively because they have too much to do and are "running late" for work, school, their next meeting, lesson, soccer game, or other appointments.
- **Anonymity.** A motor vehicle insulates the driver from the world. Shielded from the outside environment, a driver can develop a sense of detachment, as if an observer of their surroundings, rather than a participant. This can lead to some people feeling less constrained in their behavior when they cannot be seen by others and/or when it is unlikely that they will ever again see those who witness their behavior.
- **Disregard for others and for the law.** Most motorists rarely drive aggressively, and some never do. For others, episodes of aggressive driving are frequent, and for a small proportion of motorists, it is their usual driving behavior. Occasional episodes of aggressive driving— such as speeding and changing lanes abruptly—might occur in response to specific situations, such as when the driver is late for an important appointment, but it is not the driver's normal driving behavior.

If it seems that there are more cases of rude and outrageous behavior on the road now than in the past, the observation is correct—if for no other reason than there are more drivers driving more miles on the same roads than ever before.

DEALING WITH SPEEDING AND AGGRESSIVE DRIVERS

Speeding behavior and aggressive drivers may not only affect the speeder but can also affect other drivers, pedestrians, and bicyclists. Here are some tips for encountering speeders on the road:

- If you are in the left lane and someone wants to pass, move over and let them by.
- Give speeding drivers plenty of space. Speeding drivers may lose control of their vehicles more easily.

- Adjust your driving accordingly. Speeding is tied to aggressive driving. If a speeding driver is tailgating you or trying to engage you in risky driving, use judgment to safely steer your vehicle out of the way.
- Call the police if you believe a driver is following you or harassing you.[2]

Section 30.3 | Distracted Driving

Distracted driving is dangerous, claiming 3,522 lives in 2021. The National Highway Traffic Safety Administration (NHTSA) leads the national effort to save lives by preventing this dangerous behavior.

WHAT IS DISTRACTED DRIVING?

Distracted driving is any activity that diverts attention from driving, including talking or texting on your phone, eating and drinking, talking to people in your vehicle, and fiddling with the stereo, entertainment, or navigation system—anything that takes your attention away from the task of safe driving.

Texting is the most alarming distraction. Sending or reading a text takes your eyes off the road for five seconds. At 55 mph, that is like driving the length of an entire football field with your eyes closed.

You cannot drive safely unless the task of driving has your full attention. Any nondriving activity you engage in is a potential distraction and increases your risk of crashing.

CONSEQUENCES OF DISTRACTED DRIVING

Using a cell phone while driving creates enormous potential for deaths and injuries on U.S. roads. In 2020, 3,142 people were killed in motor vehicle crashes involving distracted drivers.

[2] "Speeding," National Highway Traffic Safety Administration (NHTSA), December 16, 2016. Available online. URL: www.nhtsa.gov/risky-driving/speeding. Accessed June 20, 2023.

GET INVOLVED

We can all play a part in the fight to save lives by ending distracted driving.

- **Teens**. They can be the best messengers with their peers, so they are encouraged to speak up when they see a friend driving while distracted, to have their friends sign a pledge to never drive distracted, to become involved in their local Students Against Destructive Decisions chapter, and to share messages on social media that remind their friends, family, and neighbors not to make the deadly choice to drive distracted.
- **Parents**. They are the first people who should lead by example—by never driving distracted—as well as have a talk with their young driver about distraction and all of the responsibilities that come with driving. Have everyone in the family sign the pledge to commit to distraction-free driving. Remind your teen driver that in states with graduated driver licensing (GDL), a violation of distracted-driving laws could mean a delayed or suspended license.
- **Educators and employers**. They can play a part, too. Spread the word at your school or workplace about the dangers of distracted driving. Ask your students to commit to distraction-free driving or set a company policy on distracted driving.

Make your voice heard. If you feel strongly about distracted driving, be a voice in your community by supporting local laws, speaking out at community meetings, and highlighting the dangers of distracted driving on social media and in your local op-ed pages.[3]

---

[3] "Distracted Driving," National Highway Traffic Safety Administration (NHTSA), March 31, 2017. Available online. URL: www.nhtsa.gov/risky-driving/distracted-driving. Accessed July 13, 2023.

Section 30.4 | **Drowsy Driving**

Drowsy driving is a dangerous combination of driving when sleepy. This usually happens when a driver has not slept enough, but it can also happen because of untreated sleep disorders or shift work. Prescription and over-the-counter (OTC) medications can also cause drowsiness, and alcohol can interact with sleepiness to increase both impairment and drowsiness.

No one knows the exact moment when sleep will come over their body. Falling asleep at the wheel is clearly dangerous, but being sleepy also affects your ability to drive safely, even if you do not fall asleep. Drowsiness:

- makes you less able to pay attention to the road
- slows your reaction time if you must brake or steer suddenly
- affects your ability to make good decisions

DID YOU KNOW?

- In a Centers for Disease Control and Prevention (CDC) survey, an estimated 1 in 25 adult drivers (aged 18 or older) reported having fallen asleep while driving in the previous 30 days.
- In the same CDC survey, adult drivers who snore or usually sleep six or fewer hours per day were more likely to report falling asleep while driving than drivers who do not snore or usually sleep seven or more hours per day, respectively.
- In 2020, there were 633 deaths based on police reports. However, these numbers are underestimated, and over 6,000 fatal crashes each year may involve a drowsy driver.

WHO IS AT GREATER RISK OF DROWSY DRIVING AND RELATED CRASHES AND DEATHS?

- teen and young adult drivers
- drivers on the road between midnight and 6 a.m. or in the late afternoon

- drivers who do not get enough sleep
- commercial truck drivers
- drivers who work the night shift or long shifts
- drivers with untreated sleep disorders—such as sleep apnea, where breathing repeatedly stops and starts
- drivers who use medicines that make them sleepy

WARNING SIGNS OF DROWSY DRIVING
- yawning or blinking frequently
- trouble remembering the past few miles driven
- missing your exit
- drifting from your lane
- hitting a rumble strip on the side of the road[4]

TIPS TO DRIVE ALERT
How to Avoid Driving Drowsy
- Getting adequate sleep on a daily basis is the only true way to protect yourself against the risks of driving when you are drowsy. Experts urge consumers to make it a priority to get seven to eight hours of sleep per night.
- Before the start of a long family car trip, get a good night's sleep, or you could put your entire family and others at risk.
- Many teens do not get enough sleep at a stage in life when their biological need for sleep increases, which makes them vulnerable to the risk of drowsy-driving crashes, especially on longer trips. Advise your teens to delay driving until they are well-rested.
- Avoid drinking any alcohol before driving. Consumption of alcohol interacts with sleepiness to increase drowsiness and impairment.
- Always check your prescription and OTC medication labels to see if drowsiness could result from their use.

---

[4] "Drowsy Driving: Asleep at the Wheel," Centers for Disease Control and Prevention (CDC), November 21, 2022. Available online. URL: www.cdc.gov/sleep/features/drowsy-driving.html. Accessed June 21, 2023.

- If you take medications that could cause drowsiness as a side effect, use public transportation when possible.
- If you drive, avoid driving during the peak sleepiness periods (midnight to 6 a.m. and late afternoon). If you must drive during the peak sleepiness periods, stay vigilant for signs of drowsiness, such as crossing over roadway lines or hitting a rumble strip, especially if you are driving alone.

Short-Term Interventions

- Drinking coffee or energy drinks alone is not always enough. They might help you feel more alert, but the effects last only a short time, and you might not be as alert as you think you are. If you drink coffee and are seriously sleep-deprived, you still may have "micro sleep" or brief losses of consciousness that can last for four or five seconds. This means that at 55 miles per hour, you have traveled more than 100 yards down the road while asleep. That is plenty of time to cause a crash.
- If you start to get sleepy while you are driving, drink one to two cups of coffee and pull over for a short 20-minute nap in a safe place, such as a lighted, designated rest stop. This has been shown to increase alertness in scientific studies but only for short time periods.[5]

Section 30.5 | Drug-Impaired Driving

You cannot drive safely if you are impaired. That is why it is illegal everywhere in America to drive under the influence of alcohol, marijuana, opioids, methamphetamines, or any potentially impairing drug—prescribed or over-the-counter (OTC). Driving while

[5] "Drowsy Driving," National Highway Traffic Safety Administration (NHTSA), October 7, 2016. Available online. URL: www.nhtsa.gov/risky-driving/drowsy-driving. Accessed June 21, 2023.

impaired by any substance—legal or illegal—puts you and others in harm's way. Learn the latest research on drug-impaired driving, misconceptions about marijuana use, and what you can do to make smarter choices to drive safely.

MANY SUBSTANCES CAN IMPAIR DRIVING

Many substances can impair driving, including alcohol, some OTC and prescription drugs, and illegal drugs.

- Alcohol, marijuana, and other drugs can impair the ability to drive because they slow coordination, judgment, and reaction times.
- Cocaine and methamphetamine can make drivers more aggressive and reckless.
- Using two or more drugs at the same time, including alcohol, can amplify the impairing effects of each drug a person has consumed.
- Some prescription and OTC medicines can cause extreme drowsiness, dizziness, and other side effects. Read and follow all warning labels before driving and note that warnings against "operating heavy machinery" include driving a vehicle.

Impaired drivers cannot accurately assess their own impairment—which is why no one should drive after using any impairing substances. Remember: If you feel different, you drive different.

MARIJUANA IMPAIRS

There are many misconceptions about marijuana use, including rumors that marijuana cannot impair you or that marijuana use can actually make you a safer driver.

The National Highway Traffic Safety Administration (NHTSA) continues to conduct research to better understand the relationship between marijuana impairment and increased crash risk. The NHTSA's Drug and Alcohol Crash Risk Study found that marijuana users are more likely to be involved in crashes. However, the increased risk may be due in part because marijuana users are more likely to be young men, who are generally at a higher risk of crashes.

Research indicates drug prevalence is on the rise among drivers. The NHTSA's 2020 study of seriously or fatally injured road users at studied trauma centers suggested that the overall prevalence of alcohol, cannabinoids, and opioids increased during the public health emergency compared to before.

While evidence shows that drug-impaired driving is dangerous, we still have more to learn about the extent of the problem and how best to address it.

IT IS ILLEGAL

Driving impaired by any substance—alcohol or other drugs, whether legal or illegal—is against the law in all 50 states and the District of Columbia. Law enforcement officers are trained to observe drivers' behavior and to identify impaired drivers. Even in states where marijuana laws have changed, it is still illegal to drive under the influence of the drug.

RESPONSIBLE BEHAVIOR

We can all save lives by making smarter choices.

- Plan ahead for a sober driver if you plan to use an impairing drug.
- Do not let friends get behind the wheel if they are under the influence of drugs.
- If you are hosting a party where alcohol or other substances will be used, it is your job to make sure all guests leave with a sober driver.
- Always wear your seat belt—it is your best defense against impaired drivers.[6]

---

[6] "Drug-Impaired Driving," National Highway Traffic Safety Administration (NHTSA), December 15, 2020. Available online. URL: www.nhtsa.gov/risky-driving/drug-impaired-driving. Accessed June 21, 2023.

Section 30.6 | Older Drivers

If you are an older driver or a caregiver, the National Highway Traffic Safety Administration (NHTSA) encourages you to talk about driving safety. It also helps you understand how aging can affect driving and what you can do to continue driving safely as you age, such as adapting a vehicle to meet specific needs.

WHAT YOU CAN DO
If You Are a Family Caregiver: Talking about Driving with an Older Driver

Talking with an older person about their driving is often difficult. Most of us delay that talk until the person's driving has become what we believe to be dangerous. At that point, conversations can be tense and awkward for everyone involved. But there are things you can say and do to make those conversations more productive and less tense.

Learning how to understand and influence older drivers (www. nhtsa.gov/node/33911) will help you support an older driver's needs, as well as find community resources that can help put your older driver plan into action. If you have decided to initiate a conversation with an older loved one about driving safely, take the following three steps:
- Collect information.
- Develop a plan of action.
- Follow through on the plan.

You might also want to consider learning how to adapt a motor vehicle to accommodate the unique needs of an older driver and discussing it with your loved one.

If You Are an Older Driver: Tips to Drive Safely While Aging Gracefully

Decisions about your ability to drive should never be based on age alone. However, changes in vision, physical fitness, and reflexes may cause safety concerns. By accurately assessing age-related changes, you can adjust your driving habits to remain safe on the road or choose other kinds of transportation.

If you have noticed changes in your vision, physical fitness, attention, and ability to quickly react to sudden changes, it is important to understand how these changes may be affecting your ability to drive safely. Driving Safely While Aging Gracefully (www.nhtsa.gov/node/33936) is a resource developed by the USAA Educational Foundation, AARP, and NHTSA to help you recognize warning signs and pick up useful tips on what you can do to remain a safe driver.

One way to stay safe while driving is by making sure you understand how medical conditions can impact your ability to drive safely. Another way is by adapting your motor vehicle to make sure it fits you properly, as well as choosing appropriate features, installing and knowing how to use adaptive devices, and practicing good vehicle maintenance.[7]

---

[7] "Older Drivers," National Highway Traffic Safety Administration (NHTSA), May 12, 2010. Available online. URL: www.nhtsa.gov/road-safety/older-drivers. Accessed June 21, 2023.

Chapter 31 | Occupational Accidents and Injuries

Chapter Contents

Section 31.1 | Traumatic Occupational Injuries

Work-related injuries have a human and economic impact on employers, workers, and communities.[1]

NATIONAL CENSUS OF FATAL OCCUPATIONAL INJURIES IN 2021

The U.S. Bureau of Labor Statistics reported that there were 5,190 fatal work injuries recorded in the United States in 2021, an 8.9-percent increase from 4,764 in 2020 (see Figure 31.1). The fatal work injury rate was 3.6 fatalities per 100,000 full-time equivalent (FTE) workers, up from 3.4 per 100,000 FTE in 2020 and up from the 2019 prepandemic rate of 3.5 (see Figure 31.2). These data are from the Census of Fatal Occupational Injuries (CFOI).

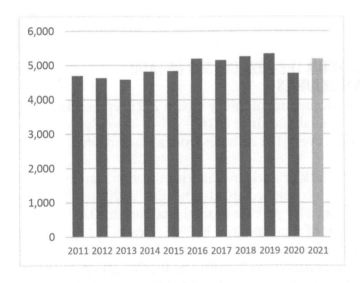

Figure 31.1. Number of Fatal Work Injuries, 2011–2021

U.S. Bureau of Labor Statistics (BLS)

---

[1] "Traumatic Occupational Injuries," Centers for Disease Control and Prevention (CDC), July 26, 2022. Available online. URL: www.cdc.gov/niosh/injury/default.html. Accessed June 22, 2023.

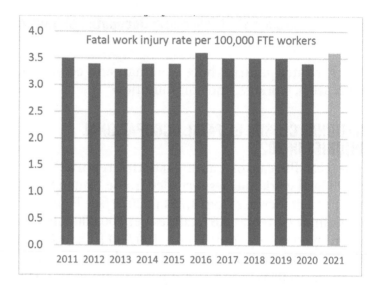

Figure 31.2. Fatal Work Injury Rate, 2011–2021

U.S. Bureau of Labor Statistics (BLS)

KEY FINDINGS FROM THE 2021 CENSUS OF FATAL OCCUPATIONAL INJURIES

- The 3.6 fatal occupational injury rate in 2021 represents the highest annual rate since 2016.
- A worker died every 101 minutes from a work-related injury in 2021.
- The share of Black or African-American workers fatally injured on the job reached an all-time high in 2021, increasing from 11.4 percent of total fatalities in 2020 to 12.6 percent of total fatalities in 2021. Deaths for this group climbed to 653 in 2021 from 541 in 2020, a 20.7-percent increase. The fatality rate for this group increased from 3.5 in 2020 to 4 per 100,000 FTE workers in 2021.
- Suicides continued to trend down, decreasing to 236 in 2021 from 259 in 2020, an 8.9-percent decrease.
- Workers in transportation and material moving occupations experienced a series high of 1,523 fatal work

injuries in 2021 and represented the occupational group with the highest number of fatalities. This is an increase of 18.8 percent from 2020.

- Transportation incidents remained the most frequent type of fatal event in 2021 with 1,982 fatal injuries, an increase of 11.5 percent from 2020. This major category accounted for 38.2 percent of all work-related fatalities in 2021.

WORKER CHARACTERISTICS

- Black or African-American workers, as well as Hispanic or Latinx workers, had fatality rates (4.0 and 4.5 per 100,000 FTE workers, respectively) in 2021 that were higher than the all-worker rate of 3.6. Transportation incidents were the highest cause of fatalities within both of these groups (267 for Black or African-American workers and 383 for Hispanic or Latino workers).
- The second highest cause of fatalities to Black or African-American workers was injuries due to violence and other injuries by persons or animals (155), whereas for Hispanic or Latinx workers it was falls, slips, or trips (272). Almost a quarter of Black or African-American workplace fatalities (23.7%) are a result of violence and other injuries by persons or animals as opposed to 14.7 percent for all workers.
- Women made up 8.6 percent of all workplace fatalities but represented 14.5 percent of intentional injuries by a person in 2021.
- In 2021, workers between the ages of 45 and 54 suffered 1,087 workplace fatalities, a 13.9-percent increase from 2020. This age group accounted for just over one-fifth of the total fatalities for the year (20.9%).

FATAL EVENT OR EXPOSURE

- Despite experiencing an increase from 2020 to 2021, transportation incidents are still down 6.6 percent from 2019 when there were 2,122 fatalities (see Figure 31.3).

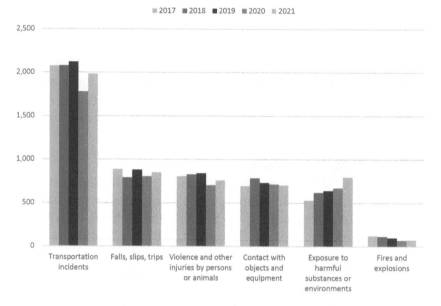

2017 ■ 2018 ■ 2019 ■ 2020 ■ 2021

Figure 31.3. Fatal Work Injuries by Major Event or Exposure, 2017–2021

U.S. Bureau of Labor Statistics (BLS)

- Fatalities due to violence and other injuries by persons or animals increased to 761 fatalities in 2021 from 705 fatalities in 2020 (7.9%). The largest subcategory, intentional injuries by person, increased 10.3 percent to 718 in 2021.
- Exposure to harmful substances or environments led to 798 worker fatalities in 2021, the highest figure since the series began in 2011. This major event category experienced the largest increase in fatalities in 2021, increasing 18.8 percent from 2020. Unintentional overdose from nonmedical use of drugs or alcohol accounted for 58.1 percent of these fatalities (464 deaths), up from 57.7 percent of this category's total in 2020.
- Work-related fatalities due to falls, slips, and trips increased by 5.6 percent in 2021, from 805 fatalities in 2020 to 850 in 2021. Falls, slips, and trips in construction and extraction occupations accounted for 370 of these

fatalities in 2021, an increase of 7.2 percent from 2020 when there were 345 fatalities. Despite the increase, this is still down 9.3 percent from 2019 when construction and extraction occupations experienced 408 fatalities due to this event.

OCCUPATION

- There was a 16.3 percent increase in deaths for driver/ sales workers and truck drivers that went up to 1,032 deaths in 2021 from 887 deaths in 2020 (see Figure 31.4). This was the primary factor behind the increase in fatalities of workers in transportation and material moving occupations, which reached a series high in 2021.
- Construction and extraction occupations had the second most occupational deaths (951) in 2021 despite experiencing a 2.6-percent decrease in fatalities from 2020. The fatality rate for this occupation also decreased from 13.5 deaths per 100,000 FTE workers in 2020 to 12.3 in 2021.
- Protective service occupations (such as firefighters, law enforcement workers, police and sheriff's patrol officers, and transit and railroad police) had a 31.9 percent increase in fatalities in 2021, increasing to 302 from 229 in 2020. Almost half (45.4%) of these fatalities are due to homicides (116) and suicides (21). About one-third (33.4%) are due to transportation incidents, representing the highest count since 2016.
- Installation, maintenance, and repair occupations had 475 fatalities in 2021, an increase of 20.9 percent. Almost one-third of these deaths (152) were to vehicle and mobile equipment mechanics, installers, and repairers.
- The fatal injury rate for fishing and hunting workers decreased from 132.1 per 100,000 FTEs in 2020 to 75.2 in 2021.

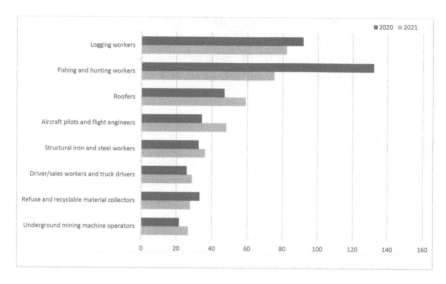

Figure 31.4. Fatal Work Injury Rates per 100,000 Full-Time Equivalent Workers by Selected Occupations, 2020–2021

U.S. Bureau of Labor Statistics (BLS)[2]

Section 31.2 | **Falls in the Workplace**

FALLS ARE SERIOUS AND COSTLY

- One out of five falls causes a serious injury, such as broken bones or a head injury.
- Each year, 3 million older people are treated in emergency departments (EDs) for fall injuries.
- Over 800,000 patients a year are hospitalized because of a fall injury, most often because of a head injury or hip fracture.
- Each year, at least 300,000 older people are hospitalized for hip fractures.

---

[2] "Census of Fatal Occupational Injuries Summary, 2021," U.S. Bureau of Labor Statistics (BLS), December 16, 2022. Available online. URL: www.bls.gov/news.release/pdf/cfoi.pdf. Accessed June 22, 2023.

- . More than 95 percent of hip fractures are caused by falling, usually by falling sideways.
- Falls are the most common cause of traumatic brain injuries (TBIs).

WHAT CAN HAPPEN AFTER A FALL?

Many falls do not cause injuries. But one out of five falls does cause a serious injury, such as a broken bone or a head injury. These injuries can make it hard for a person to get around, do everyday activities, or live on their own.

- Falls can cause broken bones, such as wrist, arm, ankle, and hip fractures.
- Falls can cause head injuries. These can be very serious, especially if the person is taking certain medicines (such as blood thinners). An older person who falls and hits their head should see their doctor right away to make sure they do not have a brain injury.
- Many people who fall, even if they are not injured, become afraid of falling. This fear may cause a person to cut down on their everyday activities. When a person is less active, they become weaker, and this increases their chances of falling.

WHAT CONDITIONS MAKE YOU MORE LIKELY TO FALL?

Research has identified many conditions that contribute to falling. These are called "risk factors." Many risk factors can be changed or modified to help prevent falls. They include the following:

- lower body weakness
- vitamin D deficiency (i.e., not enough vitamin D in your system)
- difficulties with walking and balance
- use of medicines, such as tranquilizers, sedatives, or antidepressants (Even some over-the-counter (OTC) medicines can affect balance and how steady you are on your feet.)
- vision problems

- foot pain or poor footwear
- home hazards or dangers, such as:
  - broken or uneven steps
  - throw rugs or clutter that can be tripped over

Most falls are caused by a combination of risk factors. The more risk factors a person has, the greater their chances of falling.

Health-care providers can help cut down a person's risk by reducing the fall risk factors listed above.

WHAT YOU CAN DO TO PREVENT FALLS

Falls can be prevented. These are some simple things you can do to keep yourself from falling.

Talk to Your Doctor

- Ask your doctor or health-care provider to evaluate your risk for falling and talk with them about specific things you can do.
- Ask your doctor or pharmacist to review your medicines to see if any might make you dizzy or sleepy. This should include prescription medicines and OTC medicines.
- Ask your doctor or health-care provider about taking vitamin D supplements.

Do Strength and Balance Exercises

Do exercises that make your legs stronger and improve your balance. Tai chi is a good example of this kind of exercise.

Have Your Eyes Checked

Have your eyes checked by an eye doctor at least once a year and be sure to update your eyeglasses if needed.

If you have bifocal or progressive lenses, you may want to get a pair of glasses with only your distance prescription for outdoor activities, such as walking. Sometimes, these types of lenses can make things seem closer or farther away than they really are.

Make Your Home Safer

- Get rid of things you could trip over.
- Add grab bars inside and outside your tub or shower and next to the toilet.
- Put railings on both sides of the stairs.
- Make sure your home has lots of light by adding more or brighter light bulbs.[3]

Section 31.3 | Falls Overboard

WHAT DO YOU KNOW ABOUT FALLS OVERBOARD?

Fall overboard events are the second leading contributor to fatalities among commercial fishermen nationwide. The following are a few data from 2000 to 2019:

- Two hundred and sixty-six fishermen died from falls overboard, representing 30 percent of all fatalities.
- None of the victims were wearing a functional personal flotation device (PFD) when they died.
- About 57 percent of falls overboard were not witnessed, usually due to the person working alone on deck or vessel.
- Fatal falls overboard most commonly occurred in the Gulf of Mexico shrimp, Alaska salmon, and East Coast lobster fisheries.

FALLING OVERBOARD IN COLD WATER

The most important step a person can take to survive a fall overboard is to wear a PFD. The ability to float provides a victim with more time to be rescued, even in cold water. A common misconception is that overboard victims die from hypothermia, but in reality, victims without flotation die from drowning after cold

---

[3] "Facts about Falls," Centers for Disease Control and Prevention (CDC), May 12, 2023. Available online. URL: www.cdc.gov/falls/facts.html. Accessed July 13, 2023.

incapacitation (the loss of ability to coordinate movement needed for swimming). The "1-10-1" principle can help you understand what happens when someone enters cold water:

- **1: Cold shock.** In the first minute following cold water immersion, you gasp and hyperventilate.
- **10: Cold incapacitation.** During the next 10 minutes, it becomes more difficult to use your hands, arms, and legs. Swimming failure and drowning can occur.
- **1: Hypothermia.** It can take about an hour before hypothermia sets in.

Wearing a PFD is the best way to make sure you buy yourself as much time as possible for recovery.

FALLS OVERBOARD RECOVERY PROCESS

Falls overboard incidents are survivable, but there are a number of actions that need to be taken by the victim and by rescuers to make survival more likely:

- **Float.** Wear a PFD on deck at all times!
- **Signal/notification.** Alert the skipper, crew, and/ or nearby vessels about the man overboard (MOB) incident.
- **Communication.** Maintain visual contact with the MOB.
- **Mark the MOB location.** Throw life rings, buoys, totes, or marker lights to mark the spot. Input the spot into your Global Positioning System (GPS) as well.
- **Turn the vessel.** Return to the location where the crewman went into the water.
- **Prepare a rescue swimmer.** They can assist the victim in getting back on board. Use an immersion suit and detachable tether.
- **Approach the MOB victim carefully.** Maintain visual contact and a safe distance depending on conditions.
- **Deploy a rescue device.** Throw a life ring or lower a sling, ladder, or other boarding devices to help them get back over the rail.

- **Mechanical advantage**. Use a hydraulic hauler or simple block and tackle to help lift the MOB out of the water more easily.

WHAT YOU CAN DO

Working on wet, pitching decks with moving lines and heavy gear poses fall overboard risks for fishermen. To reduce deaths from falls overboard, do the following:

- **Wear a PFD on deck**. Nationwide, none of the fishermen who died from falling overboard were wearing a properly working PFD when they died. PFDs can keep fishermen afloat, giving the crew time for rescue.
- **Use a man-overboard alarm system**. Many falls overboard are not witnessed, delaying recovery time and reducing chances of survival. A man-overboard system will alert the crew that a fall overboard occurred, and a device with GPS capabilities can signal the fisherman's location to assist in search and recovery efforts.
- **Add effective recovery devices and reboarding ladders**. A rescue sling or similar device is more effective than a life ring for bringing a crew member back on the vessel. If you fish alone, a plan should be in place for you to reboard your vessel unassisted after a fall.
- **Conduct man-overboard drills monthly**. Recovery procedures should be practiced regularly to ensure all crew members are prepared to respond to a fall overboard.[4]

---

[4] "Falls Overboard," Centers for Disease Control and Prevention (CDC), January 23, 2023. Available online. URL: www.cdc.gov/niosh/topics/fishing/fallsoverboard.html. Accessed June 22, 2023.

Section 31.4 | Fire-Related Injuries

Fires can occur anywhere—in structures, buildings, automobiles, and the outdoors. Fires that affect our homes are often the most tragic and the most preventable. While the loss of our possessions can be upsetting, the physical injuries and psychological impacts that fires can inflict on our lives are often far more devastating. It is a sad fact that each year, over 70 percent of all civilian fire injuries occur as a result of fires in residential buildings—our homes.

Annually, from 2017 to 2019, an estimated 11,650 civilian fire injuries resulted from 7,200 residential building fires resulting in injuries and an estimated 368,500 residential building fires. National estimates for 2017–2019 show that 75 percent of all civilian fire injuries occurred in residential buildings. On average, someone is injured in a residential building fire every 45 minutes.

By definition, civilian fire injuries involved people who were nonfatally injured as a result of a fire and were not on active duty with a firefighting organization. These injuries generally occurred from activities of fire control, escaping from the dangers of fire, or sleeping. Fires resulting in injuries were those where one or more injuries occurred. Although this section focuses on fire injuries and fires resulting in injuries, a fatal fire may be included if it also resulted in nonfatal civilian fire injuries.

CIVILIAN INJURY RATES FOR RESIDENTIAL BUILDING FIRES

Not all fires produce injuries. When civilian fire injuries were averaged over reported residential fires, the overall injury rate was nearly three civilian injuries per 100 residential fires (see Table 31.1). Residential fires that resulted in injuries, however, had 131 injuries for every 100 fires. Of the residential fires resulting in injuries, 82 percent resulted in one civilian injury; 12 percent resulted in two civilian injuries; and 6 percent resulted in three or more civilian injuries.

Table 31.1. Civilian Injury Rates for Residential Building Fires per 100 Fires (2017–2019)

Injuries per 100 Injury-Producing Residential Building Fires	Injuries per 100 Residential Building Fires
130.6	2.5

WHEN RESIDENTIAL BUILDING FIRES RESULTING IN INJURIES OCCUR

Residential fires resulting in injuries followed a daily pattern. In addition, unlike fatal residential fires, which occurred most frequently late at night or in the very early morning hours, residential fires resulting in civilian injuries followed a pattern similar to that of all residential fires with a less pronounced peak. As shown in Figure 31.5, residential fires resulting in injuries occurred most frequently in the late afternoon and early evening hours when many people are expected to be cooking dinner. The peak period from 5 to 8 p.m. accounted for 17 percent of the residential fires resulting in injuries. Cooking was the primary cause (31%) of residential fires that resulted in injuries. In general, residential fires resulting in injuries decreased to the lowest point of the day, between 5 and 8 a.m., and then steadily increased during the daytime hours until reaching the daily peak.

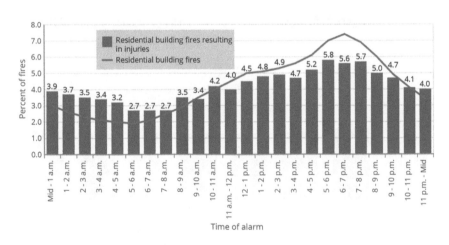

Figure 31.5. Residential Building Fires Resulting in Injuries by Time of Alarm (2017–2019)

Federal Emergency Management Agency (FEMA)

Residential fires resulting in injuries also follow a yearly pattern like that of all residential fires. In addition, residential fires resulting in injuries tend to follow a seasonal trend, with more fires taking place during the colder months than the warmer months (see Figure 31.6). January (10%) and March (10%) had the highest incidence of residential fires resulting in injuries. August and September resulted in the least amount of residential fires resulting in injuries. This drop may be explained by a decrease in residential heating fires and their associated injuries during the warmer months. Also, similar to all fires in residential buildings, residential fires resulting in injuries occurred most often on the weekend (see Figure 31.7).

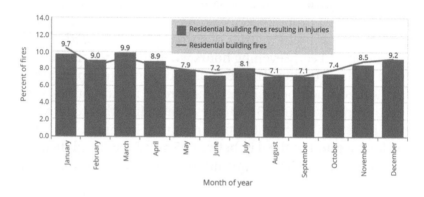

Figure 31.6. Residential Building Fires Resulting in Injuries by Month (2017–2019)

Federal Emergency Management Agency (FEMA)

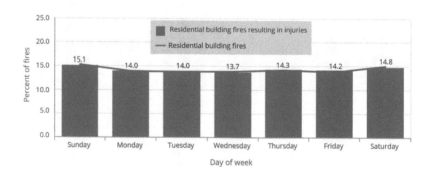

Figure 31.7. Residential Building Fires Resulting in Injuries by Day of Week (2017–2019)

Federal Emergency Management Agency (FEMA)

CAUSES OF RESIDENTIAL BUILDING FIRES RESULTING IN INJURIES

Cooking (31%) was the leading cause of residential fires that resulted in injuries. Other unintentional, careless actions (13%) and open flame (8%) were the next leading causes. Other unintentional, careless actions include misuse of materials or products, abandoned or discarded materials or products, and heat sources too close to combustibles. Open flame includes torches, candles, matches, lighters, embers, and the like.

CIVILIAN ACTIVITY WHEN INJURED

Most civilian fire injuries occurred when the victim was attempting to control the fire (33%), followed by attempting to escape (29%) and sleeping (11%). The U.S. Fire Administration (USFA) recommends leaving fighting a fire to trained firefighters and instead focusing efforts on following a preset escape plan. To escape a fire, many civilians make the mistake of trying to flee through the area where the fire is located. This area has tremendous heat, smoke, and a toxic atmosphere that can render a person unconscious. As a result, it is imperative that residents create and practice a home fire escape plan. A home fire escape plan includes multiple escape options and is created around the abilities of everyone in the home. In addition, studies show that people may not wake up from the smell of smoke while sleeping. Therefore, it is also vital to have smoke alarms inside and outside of each bedroom and on every level of the home. This will help alert sleeping people to the presence of fire.

CAUSE OF INJURY

The predominant cause of residential fire injuries, by far, involved exposure to fire products (80%), such as flame, heat, smoke, or gas (see Figure 31.8). The next two leading causes were exposure to toxic fumes other than smoke (8%) and other unspecified causes (4%).

PRIMARY SYMPTOMS OF CIVILIAN FIRE INJURIES

Smoke inhalation and thermal burns were the primary symptoms of reported injuries, accounting for 79 percent of all injuries resulting from residential fires (see Figure 31.9). Smoke inhalation alone accounted for 42 percent of residential fire injuries.

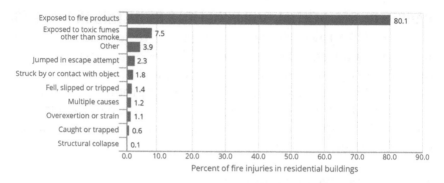

Figure 31.8. Civilian Fire Injuries in Residential Buildings by Cause of Injury (2017–2019)

Federal Emergency Management Agency (FEMA)

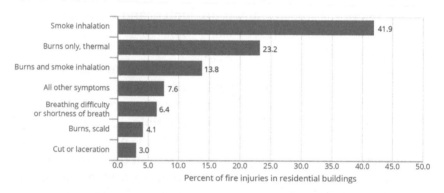

Figure 31.9. Civilian Fire Injuries in Residential Buildings by Primary Symptoms (2017–2019)

Federal Emergency Management Agency (FEMA)

Thermal burns (as opposed to scalds or chemical or electrical burns) accounted for another 23 percent and burns combined with smoke inhalation accounted for an additional 14 percent. Breathing difficulty or shortness of breath was reported for only 6 percent of injuries. Scalds (4%) and cuts or lacerations (3%) accounted for an even smaller proportion of the injuries. Thermal burns are caused by contact with flames, hot liquids, hot surfaces, and other sources of high heat. Of the thermal burns to the body, 70 percent were to the upper and lower extremities (56% and 14%, respectively).

Of the smoke inhalation injuries, 69 percent were internal injuries, which are particularly critical, as they can lead to lung damage. The inflammation and damage caused by smoke inhalation to delicate breathing sacs in the lungs actually grow worse in the hours after the incident. A chest x-ray can look clear, and oxygen levels in the blood may appear normal in the first few hours after a fire. A day or two later, however, the victim can suddenly take a turn for the worse as the lungs become unable to properly exchange oxygen.

Based on the severity of the injury, 55 percent of the civilian fire injuries in residential fires were deemed minor. Only 16 percent of the injuries were considered serious or life-threatening. The remaining 29 percent of civilian fire injuries in residential buildings were moderate.

AREAS OF THE BODY AFFECTED
The body parts affected most by residential fire injuries (see Figure 31.10) included internal parts (32%) and the upper extremities (25%). As discussed, the types of injuries that affected most areas of the body consisted of smoke inhalation, thermal burns, or a combination of both.

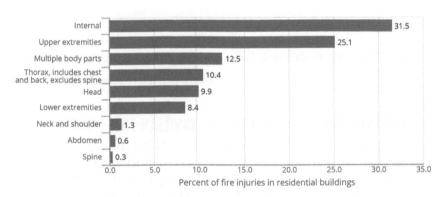

Figure 31.10. Civilian Fire Injuries in Residential Buildings by Part of Body Injured (2017–2019)

Federal Emergency Management Agency (FEMA)

FACTORS CONTRIBUTING TO CIVILIAN FIRE INJURIES

As shown in Figure 31.11, the most notable factors contributing to civilian fire injuries (outside of "other (unspecified) factor" at 24%) involved escape (27%), fire pattern (24%), and equipment-related factors (16%). Escape factors include unfamiliarity with exits, excessive travel distance to the nearest clear exit, a choice of an inappropriate exit route, reentering the building, and clothing catching fire while escaping. Fire pattern factors involve situations such as exits being blocked by smoke and flame, vision being blocked or impaired by smoke, and civilians being trapped above or below the fire. Equipment-related problems include factors such as the improper use of cooking or heating equipment and the use of unvented heating equipment.

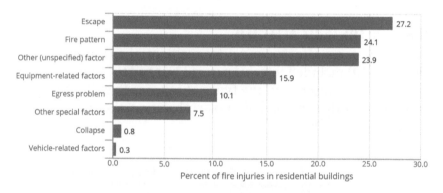

Figure 31.11. Factors Contributing to Civilian Fire Injuries in Residential Buildings (2017–2019)

Federal Emergency Management Agency (FEMA)

HUMAN FACTORS CONTRIBUTING TO CIVILIAN FIRE INJURIES

Human factors also contribute to residential fire injuries. Table 31.2 shows that the leading human factor contributing to injuries was being asleep (49%). This is not unexpected, as the largest number of injuries occurred in bedrooms (33%). Possibly impaired by alcohol (17%) was the second leading human factor contributing to injuries. This was followed by people with physical disabilities (14%) and unattended or unsupervised individuals (12%).

Occupational Accidents and Injuries

Table 31.2. Human Factors Contributing to Civilian Fire Injuries in Residential Buildings (2017–2019)

Human Factors Contributing to Injury	Percentage of Fire Injuries in Residential Buildings (Unknowns Apportioned; %)
Asleep	48.8
Possibly impaired by alcohol	16.5
Physical disabilities	13.9
Unattended or unsupervised	11.9
Possibly impaired by other drugs or chemicals	9.8
Possible intellectual disabilities	8.6
Unconscious	3.4
Physically restrained	0.6

GENDER, RACE, AND ETHNICITY OF CIVILIAN FIRE INJURIES

Males accounted for 54 percent, and females accounted for 46 percent of residential fire injuries. Figure 31.12 shows the percentage distribution of civilian fire injuries by race. Where racial information was provided, Whites constituted 63 percent of the injuries, followed by Blacks or African Americans (29%); other, including multiracial (6%); Asians (2%); American Indians or Alaska Natives (less than 1%); and Native Hawaiians or other Pacific Islanders (also less than 1%).

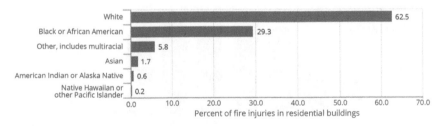

Figure 31.12. Civilian Fire Injuries in Residential Buildings by Race (2017–2019)

Federal Emergency Management Agency (FEMA)

The ethnicity element shows that 85 percent of the injuries occurred to non-Hispanics or non-Latinos, compared to Hispanics or Latinos (15%). Ethnicity was specified for 34 percent of reported injuries.

AGE OF CIVILIANS INJURED AND ACTIVITY WHEN INJURED

Civilians between the ages of 20 and 49 accounted for 44 percent of injuries in residential fires (see Figure 31.13). An additional 16 percent of those with injuries were less than 20 years old. Adults aged 50 and over accounted for 41 percent of those with injuries.

With the exception of children aged 9 or younger and adults aged 90 and over, the first reaction of civilians is either to try to control or to escape the fire (see Table 31.3). At the time of injury, for those aged 10–89, trying to control the fire and escaping were the two leading activities that resulted in injuries. Those aged 20–59 primarily got injured trying to control the fire (38%), followed by trying to escape the fire (25%). Those aged 10–19 and 60–89 primarily got injured trying to escape the fire (33%), followed by trying to control the fire (27%).

For children aged 0–9 and those aged 90 and over, escaping and sleeping were the two leading activities that resulted in injuries. Children aged 0–9 primarily got injured when trying to escape the fire (46%), followed by sleeping (24%). Older adults aged 90 and over primarily got injured when trying to escape (33%), followed by sleeping (18%).

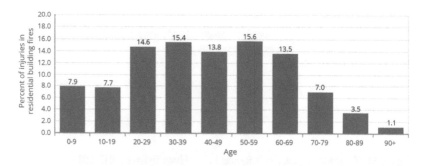

Figure 31.13. Civilian Fire Injuries in Residential Buildings by Age Group (2017–2019)

Federal Emergency Management Agency (FEMA)

Table 31.3. Leading Activities Resulting in Civilian Fire Injuries in Residential Buildings by Age Group (2017–2019)[5]

Percentage of Fire Injuries Where Age and Activity Reported (2017–2019)			
Age Group	Fire Control (%)	Escaping (%)	Sleeping (%)
0–9	6.9	45.6	24
10–19	29.5	37.9	8.5
20–29	39.6	24.8	7.6
30–39	40	25.4	7.3
40–49	39	23	7.6
50–59	34.2	25.2	12.7
60–69	27.2	28	12.5
70–79	24.5	35.1	11.5
80–89	22.2	37.1	9.7
90+	15.3	32.9	17.6
Overall	32.5	28.5	10.5

The young and the very old are less likely to be as mobile or ready to act in a fire situation. Of the reported injuries to children aged 0–9, 11 percent of the children were unable to act at the time of the fire. Of the reported injuries to those aged 90 and over, 15 percent of the older adults were unable to act at the time of the fire. Infants, young children, and older adults may require special provisions in a fire or emergency situation. Therefore, it is not surprising that these individuals are less likely to attempt to control the fire.

---

[5] "Civilian Fire Injuries in Residential Buildings (2017-2019)," U.S. Fire Administration (USFA), July 2021. Available online. URL: www.usfa.fema.gov/downloads/pdf/statistics/v21i4.pdf. Accessed July 13, 2023.

Chapter 32 | Violence against Men

Chapter Contents

Section 32.1 | Intimate Partner Violence and Stalking

Men and boys can be victims of sexual violence, stalking, and intimate partner violence (IPV). These forms of violence can happen in childhood, teen years, or adulthood.

- **Intimate partner violence.** Physical violence, sexual violence, stalking, psychological aggression, and control of reproductive or sexual health by a current or former intimate partner.
- **Sexual violence.** Sexual activity when consent is not obtained or given freely.
- **Contact sexual violence.** Including rape (penetration of the victim), being made to penetrate (MTP) someone else, sexual coercion, and/or unwanted sexual contact.
- **Stalking.** Occurring when someone repeatedly harasses or threatens someone else, causing fear or safety concerns.

UNDERSTANDING VIOLENCE AGAINST MEN

Male victimization is a significant public health problem, according to estimates in the National Intimate Partner and Sexual Violence Survey (NISVS).

Across U.S. states, nearly a quarter of men reported some form of contact sexual violence in their lifetime. Approximately 1 in 10 men in the United States experienced contact sexual violence, physical violence, and/or stalking by an intimate partner during their lifetime and reported some form of IPV-related impact. Commonly reported IPV-related impacts among male victims were fear, concern for safety, and symptoms of posttraumatic stress disorder (PTSD), among others.

FACTS ABOUT MALE VICTIMIZATION

Survey data have found that men experience a high prevalence of IPV, sexual violence, and stalking. Most first-time victimizations

555

occur before the age of 25, with many victims first experiencing violence before age 18.

Intimate Partner Violence

- About one in three men experienced contact sexual violence, physical violence, and/or stalking by an intimate partner during their lifetime.
- Nearly 56 percent of men who were victims of contact sexual violence, physical violence, and/or stalking by an intimate partner first experienced these or other forms of violence by that partner before age 25.

Sexual Violence

- Nearly 1 in 4 men in the United States experienced some form of contact sexual violence in their lifetime.
- About 1 in 14 men in the United States were MTP someone during their lifetime.
- More than 1 in 38 men in the United States experienced completed or attempted rape victimization in their lifetime.
- Among male victims of completed or attempted rape, about 71 percent first experienced such victimization prior to age 25.

Stalking

- About 1 in 17 men in the United States were victims of stalking at some point in their lifetime.
- Nearly 41 percent of male victims first experienced stalking before age 25.

RAPE VERSUS MADE TO PENETRATE

Made to penetrate is a form of sexual violence that some in the practice field consider similar to rape. The Centers for Disease Control and Prevention (CDC) measures rape and MTP as separate concepts and views the two as distinct types of violence with potentially different consequences. Given the burden of these forms of violence in the lives of Americans, it is important to understand the difference in order to raise awareness.

Rape entails any completed or attempted unwanted penetration of the victim through the use of physical force or when the victim was unable to consent due to being too drunk, high, or drugged (e.g., incapacitation, lack of consciousness, or lack of awareness) from their voluntary or involuntary use of alcohol or drugs.

Being MTP occurs when the victim was made to or there was an attempt to make them sexually penetrate someone without consent as a result of physical force or when the victim is unable to consent due to being too drunk, high, or drugged (e.g., incapacitation, lack of consciousness, or lack of awareness) from their voluntary or involuntary use of alcohol or drugs.

TYPE AND SEX OF PERPETRATORS OF INTIMATE PARTNER VIOLENCE, SEXUAL VIOLENCE, AND STALKING OF MALE VICTIMS

Perpetrators are usually known to their victims. Among male victims of stalking and sexual violence, perpetrators were most often a current or former intimate partner or an acquaintance.

The sex of the perpetrator depends on the type of violence. According to the NISVS, perpetrators of rape and unwanted sexual contact against male victims were mostly other men, while perpetrators of other forms of sexual violence such as MTP and sexual coercion against men were most often women. Both women and men perpetrate stalking of men. Women were mostly the perpetrators of IPV against men.

Sexual Violence
- Eighty-seven percent of male victims of (completed or attempted) rape reported only male perpetrators.
- Seventy-nine percent of male victims of being MTP reported only female perpetrators.
- Eighty-two percent of male victims of sexual coercion reported only female perpetrators.
- Fifty-three percent of male victims of unwanted sexual contact reported only female perpetrators.

- Forty-eight percent of male victims of lifetime noncontact unwanted sexual experiences reported only male perpetrators.

Stalking
- Forty-six percent of male victims reported being stalked by only female perpetrators.
- Forty-three percent of male victims reported being stalked by only male perpetrators.
- Eight percent of male victims reported being stalked by both male and female perpetrators.

Intimate Partner Violence
- Ninety-seven percent of men who experienced rape, physical violence, or stalking by an intimate partner had only female perpetrators.

PREVENTION IS KEY
By better understanding the specific experiences of male victims of violence, we can take action in our communities to stop violence before it starts.[1]

Section 32.2 | Sexual Assault of Men

At least 1 out of every 10 (or 10%) men in the United States has suffered from trauma as a result of sexual assault. Similar to women, men who experience sexual assault may suffer from depression, posttraumatic stress disorder (PTSD), and other emotional problems as a result. However, because women and men have different

[1] "Intimate Partner Violence, Sexual Violence, and Stalking among Men," Centers for Disease Control and Prevention (CDC), June 1, 2020. Available online. URL: www.cdc.gov/violenceprevention/intimatepartnerviolence/men-ipvsvandstalking.html. Accessed June 22, 2023.

life experiences due to their different gender roles, emotional symptoms following trauma can look different in men than they do in women.

WHO ARE THE PERPETRATORS OF MALE SEXUAL ASSAULT?

- Those who sexually assault men or boys differ in a number of ways from those who assault only females.
- Boys are more likely than girls to be sexually abused by strangers or by authority figures in organizations, such as schools, the church, or athletics programs.
- Those who sexually assault males usually choose young men and male adolescents (the average age is 17) as their victims and are more likely to assault many victims when compared to those who sexually assault females.
- Perpetrators often assault young males in isolated areas where help is not readily available. For instance, a perpetrator who assaults males may pick up a teenage hitchhiker on a remote road or find some other way to isolate his intended victim.
- As is true about those who assault and sexually abuse women and girls, most perpetrators of males are men. Specifically, men are perpetrators in about 86 out of every 100 (or 86%) male victimization cases.
- Despite popular belief that only gay men would sexually assault men or boys, most male perpetrators identify themselves as heterosexuals and often have consensual sexual relationships with women.

WHAT ARE SOME SYMPTOMS RELATED TO SEXUAL TRAUMA IN BOYS AND MEN?

Particularly when the assailant is a woman, the impact of sexual assault upon men may be downplayed by professionals and the public. However, men who have early sexual experiences with adults report problems in various areas at a much higher rate than those who do not.

Emotional Disorders

Men and boys who have been sexually assaulted are more likely to suffer from PTSD, anxiety disorders, and depression than those who have never been abused sexually.

Substance Abuse

Men who have been sexually assaulted have a high incidence of alcohol and drug use. For example, the probability of alcohol problems in adulthood is about 80 out of every 100 (or 80%) for men who have experienced sexual abuse, as compared to 11 out of every 100 (or 11%) for men who have never been sexually abused.

Risk-Taking Behavior

Exposure to sexual trauma can lead to risk-taking behavior during adolescence, such as running away and other delinquent behaviors. Having been sexually assaulted also makes boys more likely to engage in behaviors that put them at risk for contracting human immuno-deficiency virus (HIV), such as having sex without using condoms.

HELP FOR MEN WHO HAVE BEEN SEXUALLY ASSAULTED

Men who have been assaulted often feel stigmatized, which can be the most damaging aspect of the assault. It is important for men to discuss the assault with a caring and unbiased support person, whether that person is a friend, clergyman, or clinician. However, it is vital that this person be knowledgeable about sexual assault and men.

A local rape crisis center may be able to refer men to mental health practitioners who are well-informed about the needs of male sexual assault victims. If you are a man who has been assaulted and you suffer from any of these difficulties, please seek help from a mental health professional who has expertise working with men who have been sexually assaulted.[2]

---

[2] National Center for Posttraumatic Stress Disorder (NCPTSD), "Sexual Assault: Males," U.S. Department of Veterans Affairs (VA), September 22, 2022. URL: www.ptsd.va.gov/understand/types/sexual_trauma_male.asp. Accessed July 18, 2023.

Chapter 33 | **Suicide**

Suicide is death caused by injuring oneself with the intent to die. A suicide attempt is when someone harms themselves with any intent to end their life, but they do not die as a result of their actions.

Many factors can increase the risk of suicide or protect against it. Suicide is connected to other forms of injury and violence. For example, people who have experienced violence, including child abuse, bullying, or sexual violence, have a higher suicide risk. Being connected to family and community support and having easy access to health care can decrease suicidal thoughts and behaviors.

HOW BIG IS THE PROBLEM?

Suicide rates increased by approximately 36 percent between 2000 and 2021. Suicide was responsible for 48,183 deaths in 2021, which is about one death every 11 minutes. The number of people who think about or attempt suicide is even higher. In 2021, an estimated 12.3 million American adults seriously thought about suicide; 3.5 million planned a suicide attempt; and 1.7 million attempted suicide.

Suicide affects people of all ages. In 2021, suicide was among the top 9 leading causes of death for people aged 10–64. Suicide was the second leading cause of death for people aged 10–14 and 20–34.

Some groups have higher suicide rates than others. Suicide rates vary by race/ethnicity, age, and other factors, such as where someone lives. By race/ethnicity, the groups with the highest rates are non-Hispanic American-Indian/Alaska-Native people followed by non-Hispanic White people. Other Americans with higher-than-average rates of suicide are veterans, people who live in rural areas, and workers in certain industries and occupations such as mining and construction. Young people who identify as lesbian, gay, or bisexual have a higher prevalence of suicidal thoughts and behavior compared to their peers who identify as heterosexual.

FAR-REACHING EFFECTS OF SUICIDE

Suicide and suicide attempts cause serious emotional, physical, and economic impacts. People who attempt suicide and survive may experience serious injuries that can have long-term effects on their health. They may also experience depression and other mental health concerns.

Suicide and suicide attempts affect the health and well-being of friends, loved ones, coworkers, and the community. When people die by suicide, their surviving family and friends may experience prolonged grief, shock, anger, guilt, symptoms of depression or anxiety, and even thoughts of suicide themselves.

The financial toll of suicide on society is also costly. In 2020, suicide and nonfatal self-harm cost the nation over $500 billion in medical costs, work loss costs, value of statistical life, and quality of life (QOL) costs.

Suicidal behavior also has a far-reaching impact. There were 46,412 suicides among adults in 2021. But suicides are just the tip of the iceberg. For every suicide death, there were about:
- three hospitalizations for self-harm
- eight emergency department visits related to suicide
- thirty-eight self-reported suicide attempts in the past year
- two hundred sixty-five people who seriously considered suicide in the past year

HOW CAN YOU PREVENT SUICIDE?

Suicide is preventable, and everyone has a role to play to save lives and create healthy and strong individuals, families, and communities. Suicide prevention requires a comprehensive public health approach. The Centers for Disease Control and Prevention (CDC) developed the Suicide Prevention Resource for Action (Prevention Resource), which provides information on the best available evidence for suicide prevention. States and communities can use the

Prevention Resource to help make decisions about suicide prevention activities. Strategies range from those designed to support people at increased risk to a focus on the whole population, regardless of risk.

- strengthen economic supports
  - improve household financial security
  - stabilize housing
- create protective environments
  - reduce access to lethal means among persons at risk of suicide
  - create healthy organizational policies and culture
  - reduce substance use through community-based policies and practices
- improve access and delivery of suicide care
  - cover mental health conditions in health insurance policies
  - increase provider availability in underserved areas
  - provide rapid and remote access to help
  - create safer suicide care through systems change
- promote healthy connections
  - promote healthy peer norms
  - engage community members in shared activities
- teach coping and problem-solving skills
  - support social-emotional learning programs
  - teach parenting skills to improve family relationships
  - support resilience through education programs
- identify and support people at risk
  - train gatekeepers
  - respond to crises
  - plan for safety and follow-up after an attempt
  - provide therapeutic approaches
- lessen harm and prevent future risk
  - intervene after a suicide (postvention)
  - report and message about suicide safely

Need Help? Know Someone Who Does?

Contact the 988 Suicide and Crisis Lifeline if you are experiencing mental health-related distress or are worried about a loved one who may need crisis support.

- Call or text 988.
- Chat at 988lifeline.org.

Connect with a trained crisis counselor. 988 is confidential, free, and available 24/7/365.[1]

[1] "Facts about Suicide," Centers for Disease Control and Prevention (CDC), May 8, 2023. Available online. URL: www.cdc.gov/suicide/facts/index.html. Accessed June 29, 2023.

Chapter 34 | Alcohol, Tobacco, and Drug Use in Men

Chapter Contents

Section 34.1 | Alcohol, Tobacco, and Other Drugs

Misusing alcohol, tobacco, and other drugs can have both immediate and long-term health effects.

The misuse and abuse of alcohol, tobacco, illicit drugs, and prescription medications affect the health and well-being of millions of Americans. The National Survey on Drug Use and Health (NSDUH) estimates allow researchers, clinicians, policymakers, and the general public to better understand and improve the nation's behavioral health.

ALCOHOL

- Among the 133.1 million current alcohol users aged 12 or older in 2021, 60.0 million people (or 45.1%) were past month binge drinkers. The percentage of people who were past month binge drinkers was highest among young adults aged 18–25 (29.2% or 9.8 million people), followed by adults aged 26 or older (22.4% or 49.3 million people) and then by adolescents aged 12–17 (3.8% or 995,000 people).
- Among people aged 12–20 in 2021, 15.1 percent (or 5.9 million people) were past month alcohol users. Estimates of binge alcohol use and heavy alcohol use in the past month among underage people were 8.3 percent (or 3.2 million people) and 1.6 percent (or 613,000 people), respectively.
- In 2020, 50.0 percent of people aged 12 or older (or 138.5 million people) used alcohol in the past month (i.e., current alcohol users).
- Among the 138.5 million people who were current alcohol users, 61.6 million people (or 44.4%) were classified as binge drinkers, and 17.7 million people (28.8% of current binge drinkers and 12.8% of current alcohol users) were classified as heavy drinkers.
- The percentage of people who were past month binge alcohol users was highest among young adults

aged 18–25 (31.4%) compared with 22.9 percent of adults aged 26 or older and 4.1 percent of adolescents aged 12–17.

- Excessive alcohol use can increase a person's risk of stroke, liver cirrhosis, alcoholic hepatitis, cancer, and other serious health conditions.
- Excessive alcohol use can also lead to risk-taking behavior, including driving while impaired. The Centers for Disease Control and Prevention (CDC) reports that 29 people in the United States die in motor vehicle crashes that involve an alcohol-impaired driver daily.

TOBACCO

- In 2020, 20.7 percent of people aged 12 or older (or 57.3 million people) used nicotine products (i.e., used tobacco products or vaped nicotine) in the past month.
- Among past month users of nicotine products, nearly two-thirds of adolescents aged 12–17 (63.1%) vaped nicotine but did not use tobacco products. In contrast, 88.9 percent of past month nicotine product users aged 26 or older used only tobacco products.
- Tobacco use is the leading cause of preventable death, often leading to lung cancer, respiratory disorders, heart disease, stroke, and other serious illnesses. The CDC reports that cigarette smoking causes more than 480,000 deaths each year in the United States.
- The CDC's Office on Smoking and Health reports that more than 16 million Americans are living with a disease caused by smoking cigarettes.

Electronic Cigarette (E-cigarette)

- In 2021, 13.2 million people aged 12 or older (or 4.7%) used an e-cigarette or other vaping device to vape nicotine in the past month. The percentage of people who vaped nicotine was highest among young adults aged 18–25 (14.1% or 4.7 million people), followed by adolescents aged 12–17 (5.2% or 1.4 million people) and then by adults aged 26 or older (3.2% or 7.1 million people).

- Among people aged 12–20 in 2021, 11 percent (or 4.3 million people) used tobacco products or used an e-cigarette or other vaping device to vape nicotine in the past month. Among people in this age group, 8.1 percent (or 3.1 million people) vaped nicotine; 5.4 percent (or 2.1 million people) used tobacco products; and 3.4 percent (or 1.3 million people) smoked cigarettes in the past month.
- As per data from the CDC's 2020 National Youth Tobacco Survey, among both middle and high school students, current use of e-cigarettes declined from 2019 to 2020, reversing previous trends and returning current e-cigarette use to levels similar to those observed in 2018.
- E-cigarettes are not safe for youth or young adults, especially because they contain nicotine and other chemicals.

OPIOIDS

- Among people aged 12 or older in 2021, 3.3 percent (or 9.2 million people) misused opioids (heroin or prescription pain relievers) in the past year. Among the 9.2 million people who misused opioids in the past year, 8.7 million people misused prescription pain relievers compared with 1.1 million people who used heroin. These numbers include 574,000 people who both misused prescription pain relievers and used heroin in the past year.
- Among people aged 12 or older in 2020, 3.4 percent (or 9.5 million people) misused opioids in the past year. Among the 9.5 million people who misused opioids in the past year, 9.3 million people misused prescription pain relievers, and 902,000 people used heroin.
- According to the CDC's Understanding the Epidemic, an average of 128 Americans die every day from an opioid overdose.

MARIJUANA

- In 2021, marijuana was the most commonly used illicit drug, with 18.7 percent of people aged 12 or older (or 52.5 million people) using it in the past year. The percentage was highest among young adults aged 18–25 (35.4% or 11.8 million people), followed by adults aged 26 or older (17.2% or 37.9 million people) and then by adolescents aged 12–17 (10.5% or 2.7 million people).
- The percentage of people who used marijuana in the past year was highest among young adults aged 18 to 25 (34.5%) compared with 16.3 percent of adults aged 26 or older and 10.1 percent of adolescents aged 12–17.
- Marijuana can impair judgment and distort perception in the short term and can lead to memory impairment in the long term.
- Marijuana can have significant health effects on youth.

EMERGING TRENDS IN SUBSTANCE MISUSE

- **Methamphetamine.** In 2019, the NSDUH data show that approximately 2 million people used methamphetamine in the past year. Approximately 1 million people had a methamphetamine use disorder, which was higher than the percentage in 2016 but similar to the percentages in 2015 and 2018. The National Institute on Drug Abuse Data shows that overdose death rates involving methamphetamine have quadrupled from 2011 to 2017. Frequent meth use is associated with mood disturbances, hallucinations, and paranoia.
- **Cocaine.** In 2019, the NSDUH data show an estimated 5.5 million people aged 12 or older were past users of cocaine, including about 778,000 users of crack. The CDC reports that overdose deaths involving have increased by one-third from 2016 to 2017. In the short term, cocaine use can result in increased blood pressure, restlessness, and irritability. In the long term, severe medical complications of cocaine use include heart attacks, seizures, and abdominal pain.

- **Kratom.** In 2019, the NSDUH data show that about 825,000 people had used Kratom in the past month. Kratom is a tropical plant that grows naturally in Southeast Asia with leaves that can have psychotropic effects by affecting opioid brain receptors. It is currently unregulated and has a risk of abuse and dependence. The National Institute on Drug Abuse (NIDA) reports that the health effects of Kratom can include nausea, itching, seizures, and hallucinations.[1]

Section 34.2 | Men's Health and Smoking

CURRENT CIGARETTE SMOKING AMONG ADULTS IN THE UNITED STATES

In 2021, nearly 12 of every 100 U.S. adults aged 18 years or older (11.5%) smoked cigarettes. This means an estimated 28.3 million adults in the United States currently smoke cigarettes. More than 16 million Americans live with a smoking-related disease.

Smoking has declined from 20.9 percent (nearly 21 of every 100 adults) in 2005 to 11.5 percent (nearly 12 of every 100 adults) in 2021.

By Sex

- Current cigarette smoking was higher among men than women.
- About 13 of every 100 adult men (13.1%) smoked.
- About 10 of every 100 adult women (10.1%) smoked.

By Age

Cigarette smoking was highest among people aged 25–44 and 45–64. Cigarette smoking was lowest among people aged 18–24 years.

---

[1] "Alcohol, Tobacco, and Other Drugs," Substance Abuse and Mental Health Services Administration (SAMHSA), June 20, 2023. Available online. URL: www.samhsa.gov/find-help/atod. Accessed June 23, 2023.

- about 5 of every 100 adults aged 18–24 years (5.3%)
- nearly 13 of every 100 adults aged 25–44 years (12.6%)
- nearly 15 of every 100 adults aged 45–64 years (14.9%)
- about 8 of every 100 adults aged 65 years and older (8.3%)

By Race/Ethnicity

Cigarette smoking was highest among non-Hispanic adults from other racial groups and lowest among non-Hispanic Asian adults.

- nearly 15 of every 100 non-Hispanic adults from other racial groups* (14.9%)
- nearly 13 of every 100 non-Hispanic White adults (12.9%)
- nearly 12 of every 100 non-Hispanic Black adults (11.7%)
- nearly 8 of every 100 Hispanic adults (7.7%)
- about 5 of every 100 non-Hispanic Asian adults** (5.4%)

2021 tobacco product estimates for American-Indian/Alaska-Native adults were not statistically reliable.

The term "non-Hispanic adults" includes adults who were categorized as "non-Hispanic American Indian or Alaska Native and any other group" or "other single and multiple races."

**The term "non-Hispanic Asians" does not include Native Hawaiians or Other Pacific Islanders.*

By Education

Cigarette smoking was highest among people with a general education development (GED) certificate and lowest among those with a graduate degree.***

- nearly 31 of every 100 adults with a GED certificate (30.7%)

***Education estimates are limited to adults aged 25 or older.*

- about 20 of every 100 adults with some high school (no degree; 20.1%)
- about 17 of every 100 adults with a high school diploma (17.1%)
- about 16 of every 100 adults with some college (no degree; 16.1%)
- nearly 14 of every 100 adults with an associate degree (13.7%)
- about 5 of every 100 adults with an undergraduate degree (5.3%)
- about 3 of every 100 adults with a graduate degree (3.2%)

By Annual Household Income
Cigarette smoking was higher among people with a lower annual household income than those with higher annual household incomes.
- about 18 of every 100 adults with low income (18.3%)
- about 12 of every 100 adults with middle income (12.3%)
- nearly 7 of every 100 adults with high income (6.7%)

By U.S. Census Region
Cigarette smoking was highest in the Midwest and the South and lowest in the West.
- 14 of every 100 adults who live in the Midwest (14.0%)
- about 12 of every 100 adults who live in the South (12.4%)
- about 10 of every 100 adults who live in the Northeast (10.4%)
- nearly 9 of every 100 adults who live in the West (8.9%)

By Marital Status
Cigarette smoking was highest among persons who were divorced/separated or widowed and lowest among those who were married or living with a partner.

- nearly 17 of every 100 adults who were divorced/ separated or widowed (16.8%)
- nearly 11 of every 100 adults who were single/never married or not living with a partner (10.9%)
- about 10 of every 100 adults who were married or living with a partner (10.4%)

By Sexual Orientation

Cigarette smoking was higher among lesbian, gay, and bisexual adults than heterosexual/straight adults.

- about 15 of every 100 lesbian, gay, or bisexual adults (15.3%)
- about 11 of every 100 heterosexual/straight adults (11.4%)

By Health Insurance Coverage

Cigarette smoking was highest in adults and adults insured by Medicaid and uninsured adults and lowest in adults with Medicare only (aged 65 or over).

- nearly 22 of every 100 adults insured by Medicaid (21.5%)
- 20 of every 100 adults who were uninsured (20.0%)
- nearly 14 of every 100 adults who had other public insurance (13.9%)
- nearly 9 of every 100 adults with private insurance (8.6%)
- about 8 of every 100 adults insured by Medicare only (8.4%)

By Disability/Limitation

Cigarette smoking was higher among adults with a disability than those without.

- nearly 19 of every 100 adults with a disability (18.5%)
- nearly 11 of every 100 adults without a disability (10.9%)

By Mental Health Symptoms

Cigarette smoking was higher among adults who regularly had feelings of severe psychological distress than adults who did not.

- about 28 of every 100 adults who regularly had feelings of severe psychological distress (28.1%)
- nearly 11 of every 100 adults who did not regularly have feelings of severe psychological distress (10.9%)

Cigarette smoking was higher among adults who were ever told by a health-care provider that they had depression than adults who had not.

- about 19 of every 100 adults who were ever told by a health-care provider that they had depression (19.4%)
- nearly 10 of every 100 adults who were ever told by a health-care provider that they had depression (9.9%)[2]

SMOKING AND INCREASED HEALTH RISKS

Smokers are more likely than nonsmokers to develop heart disease, stroke, and lung cancer.

- Estimates show smoking increases the risk:
  - for coronary heart disease (CHD) by five to four times
  - for stroke by two to four times
  - of men developing lung cancer by 25 times
- Smoking causes diminished overall health, increased absenteeism from work, and increased health-care utilization and cost.

SMOKING AND CARDIOVASCULAR DISEASES

Smokers are at greater risk for diseases that affect the heart and blood vessels (cardiovascular diseases).

- Smoking causes stroke and CHD, which are among the leading causes of death in the United States.

[2] "Current Cigarette Smoking among Adults in the United States," Centers for Disease Control and Prevention (CDC), May 4, 2023. Available online. URL: www.cdc.gov/tobacco/data_statistics/fact_sheets/adult_data/cig_smoking/index.htm. Accessed June 23, 2023.

- Even people who smoke fewer than five cigarettes a day can have early signs of cardiovascular disease (CVD).
- Smoking damages blood vessels and can make them thicken and grow narrower. This makes your heart beat faster, and your blood pressure goes up. Clots can also form.
- A stroke occurs when:
  - a clot blocks the blood flow to part of your brain
  - a blood vessel in or around your brain bursts
- Blockages caused by smoking can also reduce blood flow to your legs and skin.

SMOKING AND RESPIRATORY DISEASES

Smoking can cause lung diseases by damaging your airways and the small air sacs (alveoli) found in your lungs.

- Lung diseases caused by smoking include chronic obstructive pulmonary disease (COPD), which includes emphysema and chronic bronchitis.
- Cigarette smoking causes most cases of lung cancer.
- If you have asthma, tobacco smoke can trigger an attack or make an attack worse.
- Smokers are 12–13 times more likely to die from COPD than nonsmokers.

SMOKING AND CANCER

Smoking can cause cancer almost anywhere in your body:

- bladder
- blood (acute myeloid leukemia)
- cervix
- colon and rectum (colorectal)
- esophagus
- kidney and ureter
- larynx
- liver
- oropharynx (which includes parts of the throat, tongue, soft palate, and the tonsils)
- pancreas

- stomach
- trachea, bronchus, and lung

Smoking also increases the risk of dying from cancer and other diseases in cancer patients and survivors.

If nobody smoked, one of every three cancer deaths in the United States would not happen.

SMOKING AND OTHER HEALTH RISKS

Smoking harms nearly every organ of the body and affects a person's overall health.

- Smoking affects men's sperm, which can reduce fertility and also increase risks of birth defects and miscarriage.
- Smoking affects the health of your teeth and gums and can cause tooth loss.
- Smoking can increase your risk for cataracts (clouding of the eye's lens that makes it hard for you to see). It can also cause age-related macular degeneration (AMD). AMD is damage to a small spot near the center of the retina, the part of the eye needed for central vision.
- Smoking is a cause of type 2 diabetes mellitus and can make it harder to control. The risk of developing diabetes is 30–40 percent higher for active smokers than nonsmokers.
- Smoking causes general adverse effects on the body, including inflammation and decreased immune function.
- Smoking is a cause of rheumatoid arthritis (RA).[3]

HOW SMOKING AFFECTS REPRODUCTIVE HEALTH IN MEN
Can Smoking Put You at Risk for Erectile Dysfunction?

Yes, smoking can increase your risk for erectile dysfunction (ED), a condition in which you are unable to get or keep an erection firm enough for satisfactory sexual intercourse.

---

[3] "Health Effects of Cigarette Smoking," Centers for Disease Control and Prevention (CDC), October 29, 2021. Available online. URL: www.cdc.gov/tobacco/data_statistics/fact_sheets/health_effects/effects_cig_smoking. Accessed June 23, 2023.

Can Smoking Increase Your Likelihood of Dying from Prostate Cancer?

Yes, smoking can increase your likelihood of dying from prostate cancer. The prostate is a gland in the male reproductive system and produces a fluid that forms part of the semen. Prostate cancer begins in the prostate.

If you have prostate cancer and smoke, you may be more likely to die from the disease than those with prostate cancer who do not smoke.[4]

Section 34.3 | Anabolic Steroid Use

WHAT ARE ANABOLIC STEROIDS?

Anabolic steroids are synthetically produced variants of the naturally occurring male hormone testosterone that are abused in an attempt to promote muscle growth, enhance athletic or other physical performance, and improve physical appearance.

Testosterone, trenbolone, oxymetholone, methandrostenolone, nandrolone, stanozolol, boldenone, and oxandrolone are some of the anabolic steroids that are most commonly encountered by U.S. law enforcement.

WHAT IS THEIR ORIGIN?

Most illicit steroids are smuggled into the United States from abroad. Steroids are also illegally diverted from legitimate sources (theft or inappropriate prescribing). The Internet is the most widely used means of buying and selling anabolic steroids. Steroids are also bought and sold at gyms, bodybuilding competitions, and schools by teammates, coaches, and trainers.

---

[4] "How Smoking Affects Reproductive Health," U.S. Food and Drug Administration (FDA), November 9, 2021. Available online. URL: www.fda.gov/tobacco-products/health-effects-tobacco-use/how-smoking-affects-reproductive-health#4. Accessed June 23, 2023.

WHAT ARE COMMON STREET NAMES?
Common street names include:
- Arnolds
- juice
- pumpers
- roids
- stackers
- weight gainers

WHAT DO THEY LOOK LIKE?
Steroids are available in tablets and capsules, sublingual tablets, liquid drops, gels, creams, transdermal patches, subdermal implant pellets, and water- and oil-based injectable solutions. The appearance of these products varies depending on the type and manufacturer.

HOW ARE THEY ABUSED?
Steroids are ingested orally, injected intramuscularly, or applied to the skin. The doses abused are often 10–100 times higher than the approved therapeutic and medical treatment dosages. Users typically take two or more anabolic steroids at the same time in a cyclic manner, believing that this will improve their effectiveness and minimize the adverse effects.

WHAT IS THEIR EFFECT ON THE MIND?
Case studies and scientific research indicate that high doses of anabolic steroids may cause mood and behavioral effects. In some individuals, anabolic steroid use can cause dramatic mood swings, increased feelings of hostility, impaired judgment, and increased levels of aggression (often referred to as "roid rage"). When users stop taking steroids, they may experience depression that may be severe enough to lead them to commit suicide. Anabolic steroid use may also cause psychological dependence and addiction.

WHAT IS THEIR EFFECT ON THE BODY?
A wide range of adverse effects is associated with the use or abuse of anabolic steroids. These effects depend on several factors, including

age, sex, and anabolic steroid used, amount used, and duration of use.

- In adolescents, anabolic steroid use can stunt the ultimate height that an individual might otherwise achieve.
- In boys, anabolic steroid use can cause early sexual development, acne, and stunted growth.
- In men, anabolic steroid use can cause shrinkage of the testicles, reduced sperm count, enlargement of the male breast tissue, sterility, and an increased risk of prostate cancer. In both men and women, anabolic steroid use can cause high cholesterol levels, which may increase the risk of coronary artery disease (CAD), strokes, and heart attacks. Anabolic steroid use can also cause acne and fluid retention. Oral preparations of anabolic steroids, in particular, can damage the liver.

Users who inject anabolic steroids run the risk of contracting various infections due to nonsterile injection techniques, sharing of contaminated needles, and the use of steroid preparations manufactured in nonsterile environments. All these factors put users at risk for contracting viral infections, such as human immunodeficiency virus infection and acquired immunodeficiency syndrome (HIV/AIDS) or hepatitis B or C, and bacterial infections at the sight of injection. Users may also develop endocarditis, a bacterial infection that causes a potentially fatal inflammation of the heart lining.

WHAT ARE THEIR OVERDOSE EFFECTS?

Anabolic steroids are not associated with overdoses. The adverse effects a user would experience develop from the use of steroids over time.

WHICH DRUGS CAUSE SIMILAR EFFECTS?

There are several substances that produce effects similar to those of anabolic steroids. These include human growth hormone (hHG), clenbuterol, gonadotropins, and erythropoietin.

WHAT IS THEIR LEGAL STATUS IN THE UNITED STATES?

Anabolic steroids are Schedule III substances under the Controlled Substances Act. Only a small number of anabolic steroids are approved for either human or veterinary use. Anabolic steroids may be prescribed by a licensed physician for the treatment of testosterone deficiency, delayed puberty, low red blood cell (RBC) count, breast cancer, and tissue wasting resulting from AIDS.[5]

---

[5] "Drug Fact Sheet: Steroids," U.S. Drug Enforcement Administration (DEA), April 20, 2020. Available online. URL: www.dea.gov/sites/default/files/2020-06/Steroids-2020_0.pdf. Accessed June 23, 2023.

Chapter 35 | **Body Image and Eating Disorders in Men**

Section 35.1 | Eating Disorders in Men

Eating disorders primarily affect girls and women, but boys and men also are vulnerable. Boys with eating disorders show the same types of emotional, physical, and behavioral signs and symptoms as girls, but for a variety of reasons, boys are less likely to be diagnosed with what is often considered a stereotypically "female" disorder. Males account for an estimated 5–15 percent of patients with anorexia or bulimia and an estimated 35 percent of those with binge-eating disorder.

Like females who have eating disorders, males with the illness have a distorted sense of body image and often have muscle dysmorphia, a type of disorder characterized by an extreme concern with becoming more muscular. Some boys with the disorder want to lose weight, while others want to gain weight or "bulk up." Boys who think they are too small are at a greater risk of using steroids or other dangerous drugs to increase muscle mass.[1]

Eating disorders involve extreme emotions, attitudes, and behaviors involving weight and food. Some types of eating disorders include anorexia nervosa, binge-eating disorder, and bulimia nervosa.

ANOREXIA NERVOSA

Anorexia nervosa is an eating disorder where people lose more weight than is considered healthy for their age and height. Persons with anorexia typically avoid or severely restrict food.

People with this disorder may have an intense fear of weight gain, even when they are underweight. They may diet or exercise too much or use other methods to lose weight.

Causes of Anorexia Nervosa

The exact causes of anorexia nervosa are not known. Many factors are involved, such as genes and hormones and social attitudes that promote very thin body types.

---

[1] MedlinePlus, "Preventing—NIH MedlinePlus Magazine," National Institutes of Health (NIH), 2008. Available online. URL: https://magazine.medlineplus.gov/pdf/spring2008.pdf. Accessed August 14, 2023.

Risk factors for anorexia include the following:

- being more worried about, or paying more attention to, weight and shape
- having an anxiety disorder as a child
- having a negative self-image
- having eating problems during infancy or early childhood
- having certain social or cultural ideas about health and beauty
- trying to be perfect or overly focused on rules

Anorexia usually begins during the teen years or young adulthood. Although more common among people who identify as women, anorexia affects all gender identities.

Symptoms of Anorexia Nervosa

Symptoms of anorexia nervosa include the following:

- have an intense fear of gaining weight or becoming fat, even when they are underweight
- refuse to keep weight at what is considered normal for their age, sex, height, and development
- have a distorted sense of body image, are very focused on body weight or shape, and are unable to understand the seriousness of weight loss

People with anorexia may severely limit the amount of food they eat, or they may eat and then make themselves throw up. Other behaviors include the following:

- cutting food into small pieces or moving them around the plate instead of eating
- exercising all the time, even if they are hurt
- going to the bathroom right after meals
- refusing to eat around other people
- using pills to make themselves urinate, have a bowel movement, or decrease their appetite

Other symptoms of anorexia may include the following:
- blotchy or yellow skin that is dry and covered with fine hair
- confused or slow thinking, along with poor memory or judgment
- depression
- dry mouth
- extreme sensitivity to cold (wearing several layers of clothing to stay warm)
- loss of bone strength, muscle, and body fat
- fatigue

BINGE-EATING DISORDER

Binge eating is when a person eats a much larger amount of food in a shorter period of time than they normally would. During binge eating, the person may feel a loss of control.

Causes of Binge-Eating Disorder

The cause of binge eating is unknown. However, binge eating sometimes begins during or after strict dieting. Binge eating may occur on its own or with another eating disorder, such as bulimia, and usually leads to becoming overweight.

Symptoms of Binge-Eating Disorder

A person who binge eats often:
- eats excessive numbers of calories in one sitting, often alone
- feeling unable to control their eating
- eating very quickly
- eating even when they are not hungry
- snacks, in addition to eating three meals a day
- overeats throughout the day
- feeling upset about their eating behaviors

BULIMIA NERVOSA

Bulimia is an illness in which a person binges on food or has regular episodes of overeating and feels a loss of control over their eating. The person then uses different methods to prevent weight gain, such as vomiting or abusing laxatives.

The affected person is usually aware that their eating pattern is abnormal and may feel fear or guilt when they binge and purge.

Causes of Bulimia Nervosa

The exact cause of bulimia is unknown. Genetics, psychological, trauma, family, society, or cultural factors may play a role. Bulimia is likely due to more than one factor.

Symptoms of Bulimia Nervosa

People with bulimia often eat large amounts of high-calorie foods, usually in secret. People can feel a lack of control over their eating during these episodes. Eating and binging episodes may occur as often as several times a day for many months or longer.

It is common that binge eating will lead to a feeling of self-disgust, which causes purging to prevent weight gain, bringing a sense of relief.

Bulimia may include the following:
- forcing oneself to vomit
- excessive exercise
- using laxatives, enemas, or diuretics (water pills)

People with bulimia are often at a normal weight or overweight, but they have a distorted view of their body image. Because the person's weight is often normal, other people may not notice this eating disorder.

Symptoms include the following:
- chronically inflamed and sore throat
- increasingly sensitive and decaying teeth (due to stomach acid when vomiting)
- severe dehydration (Electrolyte imbalances can lead to heart attack or stroke.)

- suddenly eating large amounts of food or buying large amounts of food that disappear right away
- regularly going to the bathroom right after meals
- throwing away packages of laxatives, diet pills, emetics (drugs that cause vomiting), or diuretics

GET HELP FOR EATING DISORDERS

Eating disorders can be fatal due to various medical complications and the high risk of associated suicide. Treatment plans can include psychotherapy, medical care, nutrition counseling, or medications.[2]

Section 35.2 | Muscle Dysmorphic Disorder

WHAT IS MUSCLE DYSMORPHIC DISORDER?

Muscle dysmorphic disorder (MDD) is a mental health condition in which a person becomes obsessed with their body physique and muscle mass. It is a type of body dysmorphic disorder (BDD) and is also called "reverse anorexia" or "bigorexia."

CAUSES OF MUSCLE DYSMORPHIC DISORDER

It is believed that psychological and environmental factors such as social media, bullying in schools, and childhood abuse can increase the risk of developing MDD. It has been found that some men develop this disorder because of their genetics. Also, people who are with low self-esteem have more of a tendency to develop MDD.

SIGNS AND SYMPTOMS OF MUSCLE DYSMORPHIC DISORDER

To determine the presence of this disorder, look for the following signs and symptoms:

- a strong belief that your body is not muscular enough
- comparing yourself with others' physiques

---

[2] "Eating Disorders," Substance Abuse and Mental Health Services Administration (SAMHSA), April 24, 2023. Available online. URL: www.samhsa.gov/mental-health/eating-disorders. Accessed July 23, 2023.

- compulsively and frequently looking at yourself in the mirror
- experiencing eagerness to check your weight often
- feeling a sense of disappointment in your physical appearance
- using steroids or other bodybuilding products, such as supplementary foods
- feeling anxious or depressed because of a missed workout
- experiencing distress in publicly exposing your body

Because of the tendency to panic over one's physique, a person with MDD often overtrains or overexercises their muscles, even after an injury.

CONSEQUENCES OF MUSCLE DYSMORPHIC DISORDER

Constant thinking about muscle insufficiency may interfere with your daily activities, and it can also affect friendships and other close relationships. Some of the risks involved in MDD are as follows:

- injuries due to overexercising
- damage to muscles and joints
- heart problems
- kidney damage
- liver damage
- mental problems

DIAGNOSIS OF MUSCLE DYSMORPHIC DISORDER

Muscle dysmorphic disorder is very difficult to diagnose, and it is likely underreported. The diagnosis of MDD primarily consists of:

- a psychological evaluation that assesses thoughts, risk factors, behaviors, and feelings related to negative self-esteem
- a medical history review, including personal, social, and family history

TREATMENT OF MUSCLE DYSMORPHIC DISORDER

Muscle dysmorphic disorder is curable, and individuals who are suffering from this disorder can overcome the illness with appropriate treatment. It can be done with the help of a psychiatrist, counselor, or experienced clinician. Cognitive-behavioral therapy (CBT) is one of the treatment methods that can be used to treat MDD. CBT involves eradicating negative and destructive behaviors and replacing them with good behaviors. Muscle dysmorphic disorder can also be treated with certain antidepressant medications, such as serotonin-reuptake inhibitors (SRIs). Both CBT and SRIs help prevent negative thoughts and behaviors. They also reduce anxiety or depression caused by MDD.

Living with MDD, without treating it, may affect your life and cause problems with your mental and physical health. When you begin to detect symptoms of MDD, consult your doctor.

References

"Body Dysmorphic Disorder," Mayo Clinic, April 28, 2016. Available online. URL: www.mayoclinic.org/diseases-conditions/body-dysmorphic-disorder/symptoms-causes/syc-20353938. Accessed August 7, 2023.

Muhlheim, Lauren. "Muscle Dysmorphia," Mirror-Mirror, June 30, 2014. Available online. URL: www.mirror-mirror.org/muscle-dysmorphia.htm. Accessed August 7, 2023.

"Muscle Dysmorphia," McCallum Place, March 10, 2011. Available online. URL: www.mccallumplace.com/muscle-dysmorphia. Accessed August 7, 2023.

"Muscle Dysmorphic Disorder (Bigorexia)," Anorexia Nervosa and Related Eating Disorders (ANRED), February 1, 2001. Available online. URL: www.anred.com/musdys.html. Accessed August 7, 2023.

Part 5 | Healthy Lifestyle Choices

Chapter 36 | Managing Common Disease Risk Factors

Chapter Contents

Section 36.1 | Controlling High Blood Pressure

More than one in three adults in the United States has high blood pressure (HBP), or hypertension. Many of those people do not know they have it because there are usually no warning signs. This can be dangerous because HBP can lead to life-threatening conditions, such as heart attack or stroke. The good news is that you can often prevent or treat HBP. Early diagnosis and heart-healthy lifestyle changes can keep HBP from seriously damaging your health.

WHAT IS BLOOD PRESSURE?

Blood pressure is the force of your blood pushing against the walls of your arteries. Each time your heart beats, it pumps blood into the arteries. Your blood pressure is highest when your heart beats, pumping the blood. This is called "systolic pressure." When your heart is at rest, between beats, your blood pressure falls. This is called "diastolic pressure." Table 36.1 shows the systolic and diastolic ranges for different blood pressure readings.

Your blood pressure reading uses these two numbers. Usually, the systolic number comes before or above the diastolic number. For example, 120/80 means a systolic of 120 and a diastolic of 80.

Table 36.1. Diagnosis of High Blood Pressure Readings

Blood Pressure Category	Systolic Blood Pressure		Diastolic Blood Pressure
Normal	Less than 120	and	Less than 80
High blood pressure (HBP; no other heart risk factors)	140 or higher	or	90 or higher
HBP (with other heart risk factors, according to some providers)	130 or higher	or	80 or higher
Dangerously HBP—seek medical care right away	180 or higher	and	120 or higher

HOW IS HIGH BLOOD PRESSURE DIAGNOSED?

High blood pressure usually has no symptoms. So the only way to find out if you have it is to get regular blood pressure checks from your health-care provider. Your provider will use a gauge, a stethoscope or electronic sensor, and a blood pressure cuff. He or she will take two or more readings at separate appointments before making a diagnosis.

For children and teens, the health-care provider compares the blood pressure reading to what is normal for other kids of the same age, height, and gender.

People with diabetes or chronic kidney disease (CKD) should keep their blood pressure below 130/80.

WHO IS AT RISK FOR HIGH BLOOD PRESSURE?

Anyone can develop HBP, but the following are a few factors that can increase your risk:

- **Age**. Blood pressure tends to rise with age.
- **Race/ethnicity**. HBP is more common in African-American adults.
- **Weight**. People who are overweight or have obesity are more likely to develop HBP.
- **Sex**. Before age 55, men are more likely than women to develop HBP. After age 55, women are more likely than men to develop it.
- **Lifestyle**. Certain lifestyle habits can raise your risk for HBP, such as eating too much sodium (salt) or not enough potassium, lack of exercise, drinking too much alcohol, and smoking.
- **Family history**. A family history of HBP raises the risk of developing HBP.

HOW COULD YOU PREVENT HIGH BLOOD PRESSURE?

You can help prevent HBP by having a healthy lifestyle in the following ways:

- **Eating a healthy diet**. To help manage your blood pressure, you should limit the amount of sodium (salt) that you eat and increase the amount of potassium in your diet. It is also important to eat foods that are lower in fat, as well as plenty of fruits, vegetables, and whole grains. The DASH eating plan is an example of an eating plan that can help you lower your blood pressure.

- **Getting regular exercise**. Exercise can help you maintain a healthy weight and lower your blood pressure. You should try to get moderate-intensity aerobic exercise for at least two and a half hours per week or vigorous-intensity aerobic exercise for one hour and fifteen minutes per week. Aerobic exercise, such as brisk walking, is any exercise in which your heart beats harder, and you use more oxygen than usual.
- **Being at a healthy weight**. Being overweight or having obesity increases your risk for HBP. Maintaining a healthy weight can help you control HBP and reduce your risk for other health problems.
- **Limiting alcohol**. Drinking too much alcohol can raise your blood pressure. It also adds extra calories, which may cause weight gain. Men should have no more than two drinks per day.
- **Not smoking**. Cigarette smoking raises your blood pressure and puts you at higher risk for heart attack and stroke. If you do not smoke, do not start. If you do smoke, talk to your health-care provider for help in finding the best way for you to quit.
- **Managing stress**. Learning how to relax and manage stress can improve your emotional and physical health and lower HBP. Stress management techniques include exercising, listening to music, focusing on something calm or peaceful, and meditating.

If you already have HBP, it is important to prevent it from getting worse or causing complications. You should get regular medical care and follow your prescribed treatment plan. Your plan will include healthy lifestyle habit recommendations and possibly medicines.[1]

Section 36.2 | Managing High Cholesterol

WHAT IS CHOLESTEROL?

Cholesterol is a waxy, fat-like substance that is found in all the cells in your body. Your liver makes cholesterol, and it is also in some foods, such as meat and dairy products. Your body needs some cholesterol to work properly. But, if you have too much cholesterol in your blood, you have a higher risk of coronary artery disease.

HOW DO YOU MEASURE CHOLESTEROL LEVELS?

A blood test called a "lipoprotein panel" can measure your cholesterol levels. Before the test, you will need to fast (not eat or drink anything but water) for 9–12 hours. The test gives the following information:

- **Total cholesterol.** A measure of the total amount of cholesterol in your blood. It includes both low-density lipoprotein (LDL) cholesterol and high-density lipoprotein (HDL) cholesterol.
- **LDL (bad) cholesterol.** The main source of cholesterol buildup and blockage in the arteries.
- **HDL (good) cholesterol.** HDL helps remove cholesterol from your arteries.
- **Non-HDL.** This number is your total cholesterol minus your HDL. Your non-HDL includes LDL and other types of cholesterol, such as very-low-density lipoprotein (VLDL).
- **Triglycerides.** Another form of fat in your blood that can raise your risk for heart disease, especially in women.

---

[1] MedlinePlus, "How to Prevent High Blood Pressure," National Institutes of Health (NIH), November 20, 2020. Available online. URL: https://medlineplus.gov/howtopreventhighbloodpressure.html. Accessed June 22, 2023.

WHAT DO YOUR CHOLESTEROL NUMBERS MEAN?

Cholesterol numbers are measured in milligrams per deciliter (mg/dL). Here are the healthy levels of cholesterol, based on your age and gender (see Table 36.2):

Table 36.2. Healthy Levels of Cholesterol

Type of Cholesterol	Healthy Level (mg/dL)
Anyone aged 19 or younger:	
Total cholesterol	Less than 170
Non-HDL	Less than 120
LDL	Less than 100
HDL	More than 45
Men aged 20 or older:	
Total cholesterol	125–200
Non-HDL	Less than 130
LDL	Less than 100
HDL	40 or higher
Triglycerides are not a type of cholesterol, but they are part of a lipoprotein panel (the test that measures cholesterol levels). A normal triglyceride level is below 150 mg/dL. You might need treatment if you have triglyceride levels that are borderline high (150–199 mg/dL) or high (200 mg/dL or more).	

HOW OFTEN SHOULD YOU GET A CHOLESTEROL TEST?

When and how often you should get a cholesterol test depends on your age, risk factors, and family history. The general recommendations are as follows:

- for people who are aged 19 or younger:
  - The first test should be between ages 9 and 11.
  - Children should have the test again every five years.
  - Some children may have this test starting at age two if there is a family history of high blood cholesterol, heart attack, or stroke.

- for people who are aged 20 or older:
  - Younger adults should have the test every five years.
  - Men aged 45–65 should have it every one to two years.

WHAT AFFECTS YOUR CHOLESTEROL LEVELS?

A variety of things can affect cholesterol levels. The following are a few things you can do to lower your cholesterol levels:

- **Diet**. Saturated fat and cholesterol in the food you eat make your blood cholesterol level rise. Saturated fat is the main problem, but cholesterol in foods also matters. Reducing the amount of saturated fat in your diet helps lower your blood cholesterol level. Foods that have high levels of saturated fats include some meats, dairy products, chocolate, baked goods, and deep-fried and processed foods.
- **Weight**. Being overweight is a risk factor for heart disease. It also tends to increase your cholesterol. Losing weight can help lower your LDL (bad) cholesterol, total cholesterol, and triglyceride levels. It also raises your HDL (good) cholesterol level.
- **Physical activity**. Not being physically active is a risk factor for heart disease. Regular physical activity can help lower LDL (bad) cholesterol and raise HDL (good) cholesterol levels. It also helps you lose weight. You should try to be physically active for 30 minutes on most, if not all, days.
- **Smoking**. Cigarette smoking lowers your HDL (good) cholesterol. HDL helps remove bad cholesterol from your arteries. So a lower HDL can contribute to a higher level of bad cholesterol.

The following are a few things that are outside your control that can also affect cholesterol levels:

- **Age and sex**. As men get older, their cholesterol levels rise.
- **Heredity**. Your genes partly determine how much cholesterol your body makes. High blood cholesterol can run in families.

- **Race**. Certain races may have an increased risk of high blood cholesterol. For example, African Americans typically have higher HDL and LDL cholesterol levels than Whites.

HOW CAN YOU LOWER YOUR CHOLESTEROL?

The following are the two main ways to lower your cholesterol:
- **Heart-healthy lifestyle changes**. Some lifestyle changes are as follows:
  - **Heart-healthy eating**. A heart-healthy eating plan limits the amount of saturated and trans fats that you eat.
  - **Weight management**. If you are overweight, losing weight can help lower your LDL (bad) cholesterol.
  - **Physical activity**. Everyone should get regular physical activity (30 minutes on most, if not all, days).
  - **Managing stress**. Research has shown that chronic stress can sometimes raise your LDL cholesterol and lower your HDL cholesterol.
  - **Quitting smoking**. Quitting smoking can raise your HDL cholesterol. Since HDL helps remove LDL cholesterol from your arteries, having more HDL can help lower your LDL cholesterol.
- **Drug treatment**. If lifestyle changes alone do not lower your cholesterol enough, you may also need to take medicines. There are several types of cholesterol medicines available, including statins. The medicines work in different ways and can have different side effects. Talk to your health-care provider about which one is right for you. While you are taking medicines to lower your cholesterol, you should continue with the lifestyle changes.[2]

---

[2] MedlinePlus, "Cholesterol Levels: What You Need to Know," National Institutes of Health (NIH), October 2, 2020. Available online. URL: https://medlineplus.gov/cholesterollevelswhatyouneedtoknow.html. Accessed August 1, 2023.

Section 36.3 | Promoting Healthy Sleep Habits

It is important to get enough sleep. Sleep helps keep your mind and body healthy.

HOW MUCH SLEEP DO YOU NEED?

Most adults need seven or more hours of good-quality sleep on a regular schedule each night.

Getting enough sleep is not only about total hours of sleep. It is also important to get good-quality sleep on a regular schedule, so you feel rested when you wake up.

If you often have trouble sleeping—or if you often still feel tired after sleeping—talk with your doctor.

WHY IS GETTING ENOUGH SLEEP IMPORTANT?

Getting enough sleep has many benefits. It can help you:

- get sick less often
- stay at a healthy weight
- lower your risk for serious health problems, such as diabetes and heart disease
- reduce stress and improve your mood
- think more clearly and do better in school and at work
- get along better with people
- make good decisions and avoid injuries—for example, drowsy drivers cause thousands of car accidents every year

DOES IT MATTER WHEN YOU SLEEP?

Yes. Your body sets your "biological clock" according to the pattern of daylight where you live. This helps you naturally get sleepy at night and stay alert during the day.

If you have to work at night and sleep during the day, you may have trouble getting enough sleep. It can also be hard to sleep when you travel to a different time zone.

Get sleep tips to help you:
- work the night shift
- deal with jet lag (trouble sleeping in a new time zone)

WHY CAN YOU NOT FALL ASLEEP?

Many things can make it harder for you to sleep, including the following:
- stress or anxiety
- pain
- certain health conditions, such as heartburn or asthma
- some medicines
- caffeine (usually from coffee, tea, and soda)
- alcohol and other drugs
- untreated sleep disorders, such as sleep apnea or insomnia

If you are having trouble sleeping, try making changes to your routine to get the sleep you need. You may want to:
- change what you do during the day—for example, get your physical activity in the morning instead of at night
- create a comfortable sleep environment—for example, make sure your bedroom is dark and quiet
- set a bedtime routine—for example, go to bed at the same time every night

HOW COULD YOU TELL IF YOU HAVE A SLEEP DISORDER?

Sleep disorders can cause many different problems. Keep in mind that it is normal to have trouble sleeping every now and then. People with sleep disorders generally experience these problems on a regular basis.

Common signs of sleep disorders include the following:
- trouble falling or staying asleep
- still feeling tired after a good night's sleep
- sleepiness during the day that makes it difficult to do everyday activities, such as driving or concentrating at work

605

- frequent loud snoring
- pauses in breathing or gasping while sleeping
- tingling or crawling feelings in your legs or arms at night that feel better when you move or massage the area
- feeling like it is hard to move when you first wake up

If you have any of these signs, talk to a doctor or nurse. You may need testing or treatment for a sleep disorder.[3]

Section 36.4 | Coping with Stress

Not all stress is bad. But long-term stress can lead to health problems.

Preventing and managing long-term stress can lower your risk for other conditions—such as heart disease, obesity, high blood pressure (HBP), and depression.

You can prevent or reduce stress by:
- planning ahead
- deciding which tasks to do first
- preparing for stressful events

Some stress is hard to avoid. You can find ways to manage stress by:
- noticing when you feel stressed
- taking time to relax
- getting active and eating healthy
- finding solutions to problems you are having
- talking to friends and family

---

[3] Office of Disease Prevention and Health Promotion (ODPHP), "Get Enough Sleep," U.S. Department of Health and Human Services (HHS), July 17, 2022. Available online. URL: https://health.gov/myhealthfinder/healthy-living/mental-health-and-relationships/get-enough-sleep. Accessed June 20, 2023.

WHAT CAUSES STRESS?

Stress is how the body reacts to a challenge or demand.

Change is often a cause of stress. Even positive changes, like having a baby or getting a job promotion, can be stressful.

Stress can be short- or long-term.

- Common causes of short-term stress are as follows:
  - needing to do a lot in a short amount of time
  - having a lot of small problems on the same day, such as getting stuck in a traffic jam or running late
  - getting ready for a work or school presentation
  - having an argument
- Common causes of long-term stress are as follows:
  - having problems at work or at home
  - having money problems
  - having a long-term illness
  - taking care of someone with an illness
  - dealing with the death of a loved one

WHAT ARE THE SIGNS OF STRESS?

When you are under stress, you may feel:
- worried
- angry
- irritable
- depressed
- unable to focus

Stress also affects your body. Physical signs of stress include the following:
- headaches
- trouble sleeping or sleeping too much
- upset stomach
- weight gain or loss
- tense muscles

Stress can also lead to a weakened immune system (the system in the body that fights infections), which could make you more likely to get sick.

BENEFITS OF LOWER STRESS
What Are the Benefits of Managing Stress?

Over time, long-term stress can lead to health problems. Managing stress can help you:

- sleep better
- control your weight
- have less muscle tension
- be in a better mood
- get along better with family and friends[4]

Section 36.5 | Adopting Healthier Habits

Are you thinking about being more active? Have you been trying to cut back on less healthy foods? Are you starting to eat better and move more but having a hard time sticking with these changes?

Old habits die hard. Changing your habits is a process that involves several stages. Sometimes, it takes a while before changes become new habits. And you may face roadblocks along the way.

Adopting new, healthier habits may protect you from serious health problems, such as obesity and diabetes. New habits, such as healthy eating and regular physical activity, may also help you manage your weight and have more energy. After a while, if you stick with these changes, they may become part of your daily routine.

The following information outlines four stages you may go through when changing your health habits or behavior. You will also find tips to help you improve your eating, physical activity

---

[4] Office of Disease Prevention and Health Promotion (ODPHP), "Manage Stress," U.S. Department of Health and Human Services (HHS), July 20, 2022. Available online. URL: https://health.gov/myhealthfinder/health-conditions/heart-health/manage-stress. Accessed July 21, 2023.

habits, and overall health. The four stages of changing a health behavior are as follows:

- contemplation
- preparation
- action
- maintenance

WHAT STAGE OF CHANGE ARE YOU IN?
Contemplation: "I'm Thinking about It."

In this first stage, you are thinking about change and becoming motivated to get started.

You might be in this stage if you:

- have been considering change but are not quite ready to start
- believe that your health, energy level, or overall well-being will improve if you develop new habits
- are not sure how you will overcome the roadblocks that may keep you from starting to change

Preparation: "I Have Made Up My Mind to Take Action."

In this next stage, you are making plans and thinking of specific ideas that will work for you.

You might be in this stage if you:

- have decided that you are going to change and are ready to take action
- have set some specific goals that you would like to meet
- are getting ready to put your plan into action

Action: "I Have Started to Make Changes."

In this third stage, you are acting on your plan and making the changes you set out to achieve.

You might be in this stage if you:

- have been making eating, physical activity, and other behavior changes in the past six months or so

- are adjusting to how it feels to eat healthier, be more active, and make other changes such as getting more sleep or reducing screen time
- have been trying to overcome things that sometimes block your success

Maintenance: "I Have a New Routine."

In this final stage, you have become used to your changes and have kept them up for more than six months.

You might be in this stage if:
- your changes have become a normal part of your routine
- you have found creative ways to stick with your routine
- you have had slipups and setbacks but have been able to get past them and make progress

Did you find your stage of change? Read on for ideas about what you can do next.

CONTEMPLATION: ARE YOU THINKING OF MAKING CHANGES?

Making the leap from thinking about change to taking action can be hard and may take time. Asking yourself about the pros (benefits) and cons (things that get in the way) of changing your habits may be helpful. How would life be better if you made some changes?

Think about how the benefits of healthy eating or regular physical activity might relate to your overall health. For example, suppose your blood glucose, also called "blood sugar," is a bit high, and you have a parent, brother, or sister who has type 2 diabetes. This means you also may develop type 2 diabetes. You may find that it is easier to be physically active and eat healthy knowing that it may help control blood glucose and protect you from a serious disease.

Table 36.1 lists the pros and cons of healthy eating. Find the items you believe are true for you. Think about factors that are important to you.

You may learn more about the benefits of changing your eating and physical activity habits from a health-care professional. Table 36.2 lists the pros and cons of physical activity. This knowledge may help you take action.

Managing Common Disease Risk Factors

Table 36.1. Pros and Cons of Healthy Eating

Pros	Cons
Having more energy	Spending more money and time on food
Improving health	Having to cook more often at home
Lowering risk for health problems	Having to eat less of foods you love
Maintaining a healthy weight	Having to buy different foods
Feeling proud of yourself	Having to convince your family that they all have to eat healthier foods
Setting an example for friends and family	

Table 36.2. Pros and Cons of Physical Activity

Pros	Cons
Improving health	Taking too much time and energy
Reducing risk for serious health problems	Being too hot or cold outside
Feeling better about yourself	Feeling self-conscious
Becoming stronger	Being nervous about your health
Having fun	Hurting yourself
Taking time to care for yourself	Being not good at being active
Meeting new people and spending time with them	Not knowing what to do
Having more energy	Having no one to be active with
Maintaining a healthy weight	Being not young or fit enough
Becoming a role model for others	Keeping you from family and friends

PREPARATION: HAVE YOU MADE UP YOUR MIND?

If you are in the preparation stage, you are about to take action. To get started, look at your list of pros and cons. How can you make a plan and act on it?

Table 36.3 lists the common roadblocks you may face and possible solutions to overcome roadblocks as you begin to change your habits. Think about these things as you make your plan.

Table 36.3. Lists Common Roadblocks and Possible Solutions to Overcome

Roadblock	Solution
Not having time	Make your new healthy habit a priority. Fit in physical activity whenever and wherever you can. Try taking the stairs or getting off the bus a stop early if it is safe to do so. Set aside one grocery shopping day a week and make healthy meals that you can freeze and eat later when you do not have time to cook.
Costing too much	You can walk around the mall, a school track, or a local park for free. Eat healthy on a budget by buying in bulk and when items are on sale and by choosing frozen or canned fruits and vegetables.
Not making this change alone	Recruit others to be active with you, which will help you stay motivated and safe. Consider signing up for a fun fitness class, such as salsa dancing. Get your family or coworkers on the healthy eating bandwagon. Plan healthy meals together with your family or start a healthy potluck once a week at work.
Not liking physical activity	Forget the old notion that being physically active means lifting weights in a gym. You can be active in many ways, including dancing, walking, or gardening. Make your own list of options that appeal to you. Explore options you never thought about and stick with what you enjoy.
Not liking healthy foods.	Try making your old favorite recipes in new healthier ways. For example, you can trim fat from meats and reduce the amount of butter, sugar, and salt you cook with. Use low-fat cheeses or milk rather than whole-milk foods. Add a cup or two of broccoli, carrots, or spinach to casseroles or pasta.

Once you have made up your mind to change your habits, make a plan and set goals for taking action. Here are some ideas for making your plan:
- Make lists of:
  - healthy foods that you like or may need to eat more of—or more often
  - foods you love that you may need to eat less often
  - things you could do to be more physically active

- fun activities you like and could do more often, such as dancing

After making your plan, start setting goals for putting your plan into action. Start with small changes. For example, "I'm going to walk for 10 minutes, three times a week." What is the one step you can take right away?

ACTION: HAVE YOU STARTED TO MAKE CHANGES?
You are making real changes to your lifestyle, which is fantastic. To stick with your new habits, do the following:
- review your plan
- look at the goals you set and how well you are meeting them
- overcome roadblocks by planning ahead for setbacks
- reward yourself for your hard work

Track Your Progress
- Tracking your progress helps you spot your strengths, find areas where you can improve, and stay on course. Record not only what you did, but how you felt while doing it—your feelings can play a role in making your new habits stick.
- Recording your progress may help you stay focused and catch setbacks in meeting your goals. Remember that a setback does not mean you have failed. All of us experience setbacks. The key is to get back on track as soon as you can.
- You can track your progress with online tools such as the NIH Body Weight Planner (www.niddk.nih.gov/bwp). The NIH Body Weight Planner lets you tailor your calorie and physical activity plans to reach your personal goals within a specific time period.

Overcome Roadblocks
- Remind yourself why you want to be healthier. Perhaps you want the energy to play with your nieces and nephews

or to be able to carry your own grocery bags. Recall your reasons for making changes when slipups occur. Decide to take the first step to get back on track.

- Problem solve to "outsmart" roadblocks. For example, plan to walk indoors, such as at a mall, on days when bad weather keeps you from walking outside.
- Ask a friend or family member for help when you need it and always try to plan ahead. For example, if you know that you will not have time to be physically active after work, go walking with a coworker at lunch or start your day with an exercise video.

Reward Yourself

- After reaching a goal or milestone, allow for a nonfood reward such as new workout gear or a new workout device. Also, consider posting a message on social media to share your success with friends and family.
- Choose rewards carefully. Although you should be proud of your progress, keep in mind that a high-calorie treat or a day off from your activity routine are not the best rewards to keep you healthy.
- Pat yourself on the back. When negative thoughts creep in, remind yourself how much good you are doing for your health by moving more and eating healthier.

MAINTENANCE: HAVE YOU CREATED A NEW ROUTINE?

Make your future a healthy one. Remember that eating healthy, getting regular physical activity, and other healthy habits are life-long behaviors, not one-time events. Always keep an eye on your efforts and seek ways to deal with the planned and unplanned changes in life.

Now that healthy eating and regular physical activity are part of your routine, keep things interesting, avoid slipups, and find ways to cope with what life throws at you.

Add Variety and Stay Motivated

- Mix up your routine with new physical activities and goals, physical activity buddies, foods, recipes, and rewards.

Deal with Unexpected Setbacks

- Plan ahead to avoid setbacks. For example, find other ways to be active in case of bad weather, injury, or other issues that arise. Think of ways to eat healthy when traveling or dining out, such as packing healthy snacks while on the road or sharing an entrée with a friend in a restaurant.
- If you do have a setback, do not give up. Setbacks happen to everyone. Regroup and focus on meeting your goals again as soon as you can.

Challenge Yourself

- Revisit your goals and think of ways to expand them. For example, if you are comfortable walking five days a week, consider adding strength training twice a week. If you have limited your saturated fat intake by eating less fried foods, try cutting back on added sugars, too. Small changes can lead to healthy habits worth keeping.[5]

---

[5] "Changing Your Habits for Better Health," National Institute of Diabetes and Digestive and Kidney Diseases (NIDDK), November 2020. Available online. URL: www.niddk.nih.gov/health-information/diet-nutrition/changing-habits-better-health. Accessed August 14, 2023.

Chapter 37 | Aiming for a Healthy Weight

Chapter Contents

Achieving and maintaining a healthy weight includes healthy eating, physical activity, optimal sleep, and stress reduction. Several other factors may also affect weight gain.

Healthy eating features a variety of healthy foods. Fad diets may promise fast results, but such diets limit your nutritional intake, can be unhealthy, and tend to fail in the long run.

How much physical activity you need depends partly on whether you are trying to maintain your weight or lose weight. Walking is often a good way to add more physical activity to your lifestyle.

Managing your weight contributes to good health now and as you age. In contrast, people who have obesity, compared to those with a healthy weight, are at increased risk for many serious diseases and health conditions.

ASSESSING YOUR WEIGHT

A high amount of body fat can lead to weight-related diseases and other health issues, and being underweight can also put one at risk for health issues. Body mass index (BMI) and waist circumference are two measures that can be used as screening tools to estimate weight status in relation to potential disease risk. However, BMI and waist circumference are not diagnostic tools for disease risks. A trained health-care provider should perform other health assessments in order to evaluate disease risk and diagnose disease status.

How to Measure and Interpret Weight Status
ADULT BODY MASS INDEX

Body mass index is a person's weight in kilograms divided by the square of height in meters. A high BMI can be an indicator of high body fatness, and having a low BMI can be an indicator of having too low body fatness. BMI can be used as a screening tool but is not diagnostic of the body fatness or health of an individual.

If your BMI is less than 18.5, it falls within the underweight range. If your BMI is 18.5–24.9, it falls within the normal or healthy weight range. If your BMI is 25–29.9, it falls within the overweight range. If your BMI is 30 or higher, it falls within the obese range.

Weight that is higher than what is considered a healthy weight for a given height is described as "overweight" or "obese." Weight that is lower than what is considered healthy for a given height is described as "underweight."

How to Measure Height and Weight for Body Mass Index

Height and weight must be measured in order to calculate BMI. It is most accurate to measure height in meters and weight in kilograms. However, the BMI formula has been adapted for height measured in inches and weight measured in pounds. These measurements can be taken in a health-care provider's office or at home using a tape measure and scale.

Waist Circumference

Another way to estimate your potential disease risk is to measure your waist circumference. Excessive abdominal fat may be serious because it places you at a greater risk for developing obesity-related conditions, such as type 2 diabetes, high blood pressure (HBP), and coronary artery disease (CAD). Your waistline may be telling you that you have a higher risk of developing obesity-related conditions if you are a man whose waist circumference is more than 40 inches.

Waist circumference can be used as a screening tool but is not diagnostic of the body fatness or health of an individual. A trained health-care provider should perform appropriate health assessments in order to evaluate an individual's health status and risks.[1]

---

[1] "Healthy Weight, Nutrition, and Physical Activity," U.S. Department of Health and Human Services (HHS), June 9, 2023. Available online. URL: www.cdc.gov/healthyweight/index.html. Accessed June 22, 2023.

Section 37.2 | Understanding Body Mass Index

WHAT IS BODY MASS INDEX?

Body mass index (BMI) is a person's weight in kilograms divided by the square of height in meters. BMI is an inexpensive and easy screening method for weight categories—underweight, healthy weight, overweight, and obesity.

BMI does not measure body fat directly, but BMI is moderately correlated with more direct measures of body fat. Furthermore, BMI appears to be as strongly correlated with various metabolic and disease outcomes as are these more direct measures of body fatness.

HOW IS BODY MASS INDEX USED?

Body mass index can be a screening tool, but it does not diagnose the body fatness or health of an individual. To determine if BMI is a health risk, a health-care provider performs further assessments. Such assessments include skinfold thickness measurements, evaluations of diet, physical activity, and family history.

WHAT ARE THE BODY MASS INDEX TRENDS FOR ADULTS IN THE UNITED STATES?

The prevalence of adult BMI greater than or equal to 30 kg/m^2 (obese status) has greatly increased since the 1970s. Recently, however, this trend has leveled off, except for older women.

WHAT ARE OTHER WAYS TO ASSESS EXCESS BODY FATNESS BESIDES BODY MASS INDEX?

Other methods to measure body fatness include skinfold thickness measurements (with calipers), underwater weighing, bioelectrical impedance, dual-energy x-ray absorptiometry (DXA), and isotope dilution. However, these methods are not always readily available, and they are either expensive or need to be conducted by highly trained personnel. Furthermore, many of these methods can be difficult to standardize across observers or machines, complicating comparisons across studies and time periods.

HOW IS BODY MASS INDEX CALCULATED?

Body mass index is calculated the same way for both adults and children. The calculation is based on the formulas in Table 37.1:

Table 37.1. Body Mass Index Calculation

Measurement Units	Formula and Calculation
Kilograms and meters (or centimeters)	Formula: weight (kg)/(height (m))^2 With the metric system, the formula for BMI is weight in kilograms divided by height in meters squared. Because height is commonly measured in centimeters, divide height in centimeters by 100 to obtain height in meters. Example: Weight = 68 kg, Height = 165 cm (1.65 m) Calculation: 68 ÷ (1.65)^2 = 24.98
Pounds and inches	Formula: weight (lb)/(height (in))^2 x 703 Calculate BMI by dividing weight in pounds (lbs) by height in inches (in) squared and multiplying by a conversion factor of 703. Example: Weight = 150 lbs, Height = 5'5" (65") Calculation: (150 ÷ (65)^2) x 703 = 24.96

HOW IS BODY MASS INDEX INTERPRETED FOR ADULTS?

For adults aged 20 and older, BMI is interpreted using standard weight status categories (see Table 37.2). These categories are the same for men and women of all body types and ages.

Table 37.2. Body Mass Index Weight Status for Adults

Body Mass Index	Weight Status
Below 18.5	Underweight
18.5–24.9	Healthy weight
25–29.9	Overweight
30 and above	Obesity

IS BODY MASS INDEX INTERPRETED THE SAME WAY FOR CHILDREN AND TEENS AS IT IS FOR ADULTS?

For children and teens, the interpretation of BMI depends upon age and sex even though it is calculated using the same formula as adult BMI. Children's and teen's BMI need to be age- and sex-specific because the amount of body fat changes with age and the amount of body fat differs between girls and boys. The BMI-for-age growth charts of the Centers for Disease Control and Prevention (CDC) take into account these differences and visually show BMI as a percentile ranking. These percentiles were determined using representative data of the U.S. population of 2- to 19-year-olds that was collected in various surveys.

Obesity among 2- to 19-year-olds is defined as a BMI at or above the 95th percentile of children of the same age and sex in this 1963–1994 reference population. For example, a 10-year-old boy of average height (56 inches) who weighs 102 pounds would have a BMI of 22.9 kg/m². This would place the boy in the 95th percentile for BMI—meaning that his BMI is greater than that of 95 percent of similarly aged boys in this reference population—and he would be considered to have obesity.

For adults, the interpretation of BMI does not depend on sex or age. Figure 37.1 shows the BMI calculation for boys aged 2–20.

HOW GOOD IS BODY MASS INDEX AS AN INDICATOR OF BODY FATNESS?

The correlation between BMI and body fatness is fairly strong, but even if two people have the same BMI, their level of body fatness may differ.

In general, at the same BMI:

- women tend to have more body fat than men
- the amount of body fat may be higher or lower depending on the racial/ethnic group
- older people, on average, tend to have more body fat than younger adults
- athletes have less body fat than do nonathletes

The accuracy of BMI as an indicator of body fatness also appears to be higher in persons with higher levels of BMI and body fatness. While a person with a very high BMI (e.g., 35 kg/m²) is very likely to have high body fat, a relatively high BMI can be the result of

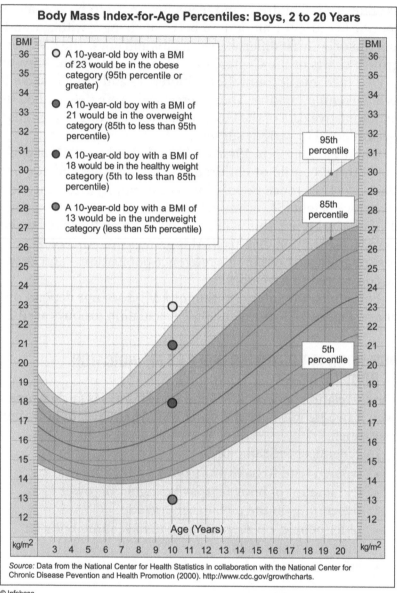

Body Mass Index-for-Age Percentiles: Boys, 2 to 20 Years

Source: Data from the National Center for Health Statistics in collaboration with the National Center for Chronic Disease Pevention and Health Promotion (2000). http://www.cdc.gov/growthcharts.

© Infobase

Figure 37.1. BMI for Age Percentiles

Infobase

either high body fat or high lean body mass (muscle and bone). A trained health-care provider should perform appropriate health assessments to evaluate an individual's health status and risks.

IF AN ATHLETE OR OTHER PERSON WITH A LOT OF MUSCLE HAS A BODY MASS INDEX OVER 25, IS THAT PERSON STILL CONSIDERED TO BE OVERWEIGHT?

According to the BMI weight status categories, anyone with a BMI between 25 and 29.9 would be classified as overweight, and anyone with a BMI over 30 would be classified as having obesity.

However, athletes may have a high BMI because of increased muscularity rather than increased body fat. In general, a person who has a high BMI is likely to have body fat and would be considered to be overweight or obese, but this may not apply to athletes. A trained health-care provider should perform appropriate health assessments to evaluate an individual's health status and risks.

WHAT ARE THE HEALTH CONSEQUENCES OF OBESITY FOR ADULTS?

People who have obesity are at increased risk for many diseases and health conditions, including the following:

- all causes of death (mortality)
- high blood pressure (HBP; hypertension)
- high LDL cholesterol, low HDL cholesterol, or high levels of triglycerides (dyslipidemia)
- type 2 diabetes
- coronary heart disease (CHD)
- stroke
- gallbladder disease
- osteoarthritis (a breakdown of cartilage and bone within a joint)
- sleep apnea and breathing problems
- chronic inflammation and increased oxidative stress
- some cancers (endometrial, breast, colon, kidney, gallbladder, and liver)
- low quality of life (QOL)

- mental illnesses, such as clinical depression, anxiety, and other mental disorders
- body pain and difficulty with physical functioning[2]

Section 37.3 | Addressing Overweight and Obesity

WHAT ARE OVERWEIGHT AND OBESITY?

Overweight and obesity are common conditions in the United States that are defined as the increase in size and amount of fat cells in the body. Overweight and obesity are caused by many factors including behaviors such as eating patterns, lack of sleep or physical activity, and some medicines, as well as genetics and family history. Obesity is a chronic health condition that raises the risk for heart disease—the leading cause of death in the United States—and is linked to many other health problems, including type 2 diabetes and cancer.

Nearly three in four adults aged 20 or older in the United States have either overweight or obesity. Nearly one in five children and teens aged 2–19 have obesity. Overweight and obesity can lead to serious health issues for people of all ages.

Health-care providers use a body mass index (BMI) chart to screen for overweight and obesity in adults (see Figure 37.2). BMI is a measure of body fat based on height and weight and is defined as the body mass (in kilograms) divided by the square of the body height (in meters) and expressed in units of kg/m². Your provider may talk to you about overweight and obesity if your BMI shows that your weight is above average for your height. But there is more to obesity than BMI.

Unhealthy lifestyle habits, such as not getting enough physical activity and eating high-calorie, low-nutrient foods, and beverages, can raise your risk of overweight and obesity. Some people find that their weight goes up when they start taking medicine for other health conditions, such as diabetes, depression, or high

---

[2] "About Adult BMI," Centers for Disease Control and Prevention (CDC), June 3, 2022. Available online. URL: www.cdc.gov/healthyweight/assessing/bmi/adult_bmi/index.html. Accessed June 22, 2023.

Body Mass Index (BMI)

Are you overweight or obese?

The Body Mass Index (BMI) is used to determine whether a person is at a healthy weight, overweight, or obese. BMI has some limitations, in that it can overestimate body fat in people who are very muscular and it can underestimate body fat in people who have lost muscle mass, such as many elderly.

Calculating your BMI

$$\text{Body Mass Index (BMI)} = \frac{\text{Weight (pounds)}}{\text{Height (inches)}^2} \times 703$$

Body Mass Index (BMI) Chart

Weight (pounds)

Height	120	130	140	150	160	170	180	180	200	210	220	230	240	250
4'6"	29	31	34	36	39	41	43	46	48	51	53	56	58	60
4'8"	27	29	31	34	36	38	40	43	45	47	49	52	54	56
4'10"	25	27	29	31	34	36	38	40	42	44	46	48	50	52
5'0"	23	25	27	29	31	33	35	37	39	41	43	45	47	49
5'2"	22	24	26	27	29	31	33	35	37	38	40	42	44	46
5'4"	21	22	24	26	28	29	31	33	34	36	38	40	41	43
5'6"	19	21	23	24	26	27	29	31	32	34	36	37	39	40
5'8"	18	20	21	23	24	26	27	29	30	32	34	35	37	38
5'10"	17	19	20	22	23	24	26	27	29	30	32	33	35	36
6'	16	18	19	20	22	23	24	26	27	28	30	31	33	34
6'2"	15	17	18	19	21	22	23	24	26	27	28	30	31	32
6'4"	15	16	17	18	20	21	22	23	24	26	27	28	29	30
6'6"	14	15	16	17	19	20	21	22	23	24	25	27	28	29
6'8"	13	14	15	17	18	19	20	21	22	23	24	25	26	28

Underweight (<18.5) Overweight (25–29.9)
Healthy weight (18.5–24.9) Obese (30+)

Note: Chart is for Adults aged 20 and older.
Source: Data from the Office of the Surgeon General.

© Infobase

Figure 37.2. BMI Chart

Infobase

blood pressure (HBP). Talk to your provider before you consider stopping any medicine you are taking for another condition that you think is also impacting your weight.

Lifestyle changes that can reduce weight include following a heart-healthy eating plan lower in calories and unhealthy saturated fats and increasing physical activity. The U.S. Food and Drug Administration (FDA) has also approved medicines and other treatments for weight loss. Surgery may also be a treatment option but is not available for everyone.

CAUSES AND RISK FACTORS OF OVERWEIGHT AND OBESITY
What Causes Overweight and Obesity?

Overweight and obesity can develop over time when you consume more calories than you use. This is also described as an energy imbalance: when your energy in (calories) does not equal your energy out (calories your body uses for things, such as breathing, digesting food, and being physically active).

Your body uses certain nutrients, such as carbohydrates or sugars, proteins, and fats, from the foods you eat to make and store energy.

Food is turned into energy for immediate use to power routine daily body functions and physical activity.

Food is stored as energy for future use by your body. Sugars are stored as glycogen in the liver and muscles. Fats are stored mainly as triglycerides in fatty tissue.

An energy imbalance causes your body to store more fat than can be used now or in the future. But your risk of developing overweight or obesity is determined by more than how much you eat. It also includes the types and amount of food and drinks you consume each day, your level of physical activity (such as whether you sit at an office desk or are on your feet all day), and how much good-quality sleep you get each night.

All of these factors, as well as many others, can contribute to weight gain.

What Raises the Risk of Overweight and Obesity?

There are many risk factors for overweight and obesity. Some are individual factors such as knowledge, skills, and behaviors.

Others are in your environment, such as school, workplace, and neighborhood. Additionally, food industry practices and marketing as well as social and cultural norms and values can also impact your risk.

You may not be able to change all of your risk factors for overweight or obesity. But knowing your risk is important to help you take steps to reach a healthy weight and lower your risk for obesity-related health problems, such as heart disease.

Lack of Physical Activity

Lack of physical activity, combined with high amounts of TV, computer, video game, or other screen time has been associated with a high BMI. Most adults need at least 150 minutes of aerobic activity a week. It is also recommended that adults do muscle-strengthening activities for major muscle groups on two or more days each week, as these activities give additional health benefits. Children should get 60 minutes of aerobic activity each day.

Unhealthy Eating Behaviors

Some unhealthy eating behaviors can increase your risk for overweight and obesity.

- **Eating more calories than you use.** The number of calories you need will vary based on your sex, age, and physical activity level. Find daily calorie needs or goals for adults as part of the Dietary Approaches to Stop Hypertension (DASH) eating plan (www.nhlbi.nih. gov/education/dash-eating-plan). You can also find Tip Sheets for Parents at www.nhlbi.nih.gov/health/ educational/wecan/tools-resources/parent-tip-sheets. htm for guidance on how many calories children need and ways to reduce screen time.
- **Eating too much saturated fat.** According to DASH, the amount of saturated fat in your daily diet should be no more than 10 percent of your total calories. For a 2,000-calorie diet, that is about 200 calories or about 22 grams of saturated fat.

- **Eating foods high in added sugar**. On a daily basis, try to limit the amount of added sugar in your diet to no more than 10 percent of your calories.

Not Getting Enough Good-Quality Sleep
Research has shown a link between poor sleep—not getting enough sleep or not getting enough good-quality sleep—and a high BMI. Regularly getting less than seven hours of sleep per night can affect the hormones that control hunger urges. In other words, not getting good-quality sleep can make us more likely to overeat or not recognize our body's signals that we are full.

High Amounts of Stress
Long-term and even short-term stress can affect the brain and trigger your body to make hormones, such as cortisol, that control energy balances and hunger urges. These hormone changes can make you eat more and store more fat.

Health Conditions
Some conditions, such as metabolic syndrome and polycystic ovary syndrome (PCOS), cause people to gain weight. These medical conditions must be treated for a person's weight to come close to or into the normal range.

GENETICS
Some people are predisposed to being heavier. Researchers have found at least 15 genes that influence obesity. Studies show that genetics may play a more important role in people with obesity than in people who are overweight. For people with a genetic high risk for obesity, making healthy lifestyle changes can help lower that risk.

MEDICINES
Some medicines cause weight gain by disrupting the chemical signals that tell your brain you are hungry. These include the following:
- antidepressants
- antipsychotics

- beta-blockers, which are used to treat HBP
- birth control
- glucocorticoids, which are often used to treat autoimmune disease
- insulin, which is a hormone taken to control blood sugar levels in people with diabetes

Talk to your provider if you notice weight gain while you are using one of these medicines. Ask whether there are other forms of the same medicine or other medicines that can treat your medical condition but have less of an effect on your weight.

Your Environment

Your environment can contribute to unhealthy eating and a lack of physical activity. Your environment includes all of the parts where you live and work—your home, buildings in which you work or shop, streets, and open spaces. The types of restaurants and the amount of green space you have can contribute to overweight and obesity.

Studies have shown that access to sidewalks and green spaces can help people be more physically active, and grocery stores and farmers' markets can help people eat healthier. On the other hand, people living in neighborhoods with more fast food restaurants and inaccessible or no sidewalks or bath paths are more likely to be overweight or obese.

SYMPTOMS AND DIAGNOSIS OF OVERWEIGHT AND OBESITY

There are no specific symptoms of overweight and obesity. Your health-care provider may diagnose overweight and obesity based on your medical history and high BMI. Your provider may also order tests to rule out other medical conditions.

Body Mass Index

Your BMI is a measure of body fat based on your weight and height. It is important to know that BMI is a screening tool and does not necessarily diagnose body fatness. Other related measures, such as waist circumference, are used to evaluate a person's health and risk of overweight and obesity.

Unhealthy Body Fat Distribution

To better understand the health risks that overweight and obesity may pose to a specific person providers can measure the person's distribution of body fat. You may have a normal BMI, but if you have a large waist circumference, you may have more fat in your abdomen than elsewhere. For men, an unhealthy waist circumference is greater than 40 inches.

Fatty tissue is found in different parts of your body. Fatty tissue produces hormones, cushions your joints, and stores energy.

However, depending on where the fatty tissue is found, it may do more harm than good. Fatty tissue found inside your abdomen is called "visceral" or "abdominal fat." We do not know what causes the body to create and store visceral fat. But we do know that this type of fat interferes with your body's endocrine and immune systems. It also promotes inflammation and contributes to obesity-related complications, including heart disease and diabetes.

Talk to your health-care provider about your BMI results and body fat distribution and what steps you may need to take to reach a healthy weight.

Testing for Causes of Overweight and Obesity

Sometimes, other medical conditions or medicines that you take may lead to overweight and obesity. These conditions or medicines may disrupt the delicate balance of hormones that control how we use and store energy. Your provider may order blood tests to rule out one of these conditions.

Cushing syndrome is a disorder that happens when your body makes too much of the stress hormone cortisol.

Hypothyroidism is a condition in which your body does not produce enough thyroid hormone. This slows down your body's use of energy (food), called "metabolism."

Polycystic ovary syndrome (PCOS) is a condition that affects the ovaries and results in hormone imbalance. PCOS can also be ruled out using ultrasound, a test where sound waves are used to create images of organs.

Talk with your provider if you start gaining or losing weight when you take prescribed medicines.

TREATMENT OF OVERWEIGHT AND OBESITY

If you are diagnosed with overweight or obesity, you and your health-care provider will work together to develop a treatment plan. Your plan will likely include reducing the number of calories you eat each day, getting more physical activity, and adopting lifelong healthy lifestyle changes.

The goal of your treatment plan is to reduce your risk of obesity-related complications and improve your quality of life (QOL). Depending on your BMI and other health conditions you have, your provider may also talk to you about dietary or nutritional counseling, behavioral weight-loss treatment programs, medicines, or surgery. The obesity screening, counseling, and weight-loss programs may be covered by your insurance.

Healthy Lifestyle Changes

To help you aim for and maintain a healthy weight, your provider may recommend that you adopt lifelong healthy lifestyle changes. A 5–10 percent weight loss can significantly improve your health and QOL.

- **Choose heart-healthy foods.** It is important to eat the right number of calories to maintain a healthy weight. If you need to lose weight, try to reduce your total daily calories gradually. Use the DASH eating plan to find out your daily calorie needs and to set goals. View healthy recipes and plan for success. Talk with your provider before beginning any diet or eating plan.
- **Get regular physical activity.** Many health benefits are associated with physical activity and getting the recommended amount of physical activity needed each week. Before starting any exercise program, ask your provider about what level of physical activity is right for you.

- **Get enough good-quality sleep.** The NHLBI research has shown a relationship between lack of sleep and obesity that begins as early as infancy. Experts recommend seven to eight hours of sleep per night for adults. Children need 12–16 hours of sleep (including naps).

Behavioral Weight-Loss Programs

Research has shown that there are areas of your brain that respond to pleasure. A chemical messenger is released whenever this part of the brain is stimulated by something we enjoy, such as eating food. The stimulation makes us feel good. Research shows that these connections may be stronger in some people than in others, which may explain why some people have a harder time losing weight.

Individual or group behavioral weight-loss programs are run by people who understand these brain connections. In these programs, one or more trained health-care professionals, such as a registered dietitian and nutritionist (RDN), psychologist, or exercise physiologist, will work with you to develop a customized weight-loss plan. The plan will likely include a reduced-calorie diet, physical activity goals, and behavioral strategies to help you make and maintain these lifestyle changes.

Your weight-loss specialist usually reviews or modifies your goals every six months, based on your progress and overall health.

When you are choosing a behavioral weight-loss program, you may want to consider whether the program:

- offers the service of multiple professionals, such as registered dietitians, doctors, nurses, psychologists, and exercise physiologists
- provides goals that have been customized for you and that consider things such as the types of food you like, your schedule, your physical fitness, and your overall health
- provides individual or group counseling to help you change your eating patterns and personal unhealthy habits

- teaches long-term strategies to deal with problems that can lead to future weight gain, such as stress or slipping back into unhealthy habits

Other things to consider when selecting a program include the following:
- the number of people who have successfully completed the program
- the average weight loss for people who finish the program
- possible side effects or risks
- fees or costs for additional items, such as dietary supplements

Medicine

When healthy lifestyle changes are not enough, your provider may treat overweight and obesity with medicines. The U.S. Food and Drug Administration (FDA) has approved several medicines for weight loss or management. These medicines target different parts of your body.
- **Brain.** Several medicines change the way the brain regulates the urge to eat, reducing your appetite. These include liraglutide, which is now approved for both children and adults aged 12 or older with obesity. Other medicines that work in a similar way are naltrexone/ bupropion, diethylpropion, and phendimetrazine. Setmelanotide is used to treat rare genetic conditions that cause obesity and increase resting metabolism.
- **Gastrointestinal (GI) tract.** Orlistat blocks your intestines from absorbing fat from foods in your diet.
- **Pancreas.** Semaglutide is an injectable medicine that works by helping the pancreas release the right amount of insulin when blood sugar levels are high. Insulin helps move sugar from the blood into other body tissues, where it is used for energy. The injections also work by slowing the movement of food through the stomach and may reduce appetite and cause weight loss.

Weight-loss medicines are not recommended as a single treatment for weight loss. These medicines can help you lose weight but should be combined with lifestyle changes for greater and longer-lasting weight loss.

Tell your provider about all the medicines you take because some of these medicines should not be used if you have certain conditions or are taking certain other medicines. Also, these medicines may have side effects. Talk to your provider if you are pregnant, are planning to get pregnant, are breastfeeding, or have a family history of cardiovascular conditions, such as HBP, heart attack, or stroke.

Weight-Loss Devices

The FDA has approved three weight-loss devices for adults. About half the people who undergo procedures to implant these devices lose at least 5 percent of their initial body weight as a result of the devices.

- Gastric balloons are placed in the stomach via a swallowable capsule attached to a thin catheter or via an endoscope (a long flexible tube with a small camera and a light at the end). Then, depending on the device, the balloons may be filled with gas or liquid (such as salt water) and sealed. Later, they are removed.

- Gastric bands are surgically implanted around the stomach, limiting the amount of food a person can eat at one time and increasing digestion time. This helps people eat less.

- Gastric emptying systems include a tube placed in the stomach via an endoscope and a port that lies against the skin of the abdomen. The tube drains a portion of the stomach contents into a container 20–30 minutes after meals. The device is removed when the patient reaches their goal weight.

Your doctor will monitor you for pain, vitamin deficiencies, anemia, persistent nausea and vomiting, intolerance to solid food, and failure to lose weight. These complications can be treated if they occur.

Surgery

Some people do not lose weight by making healthy lifestyle changes or taking medicines. If your BMI is 35 or greater and you are at risk for obesity-related complications, you may be eligible for surgery if you develop obesity-related complications.

The following are a few types of weight-loss (also called "bariatric") surgeries:

- **Gastrectomy.** A big portion of the stomach is removed to reduce the amount of food that you can eat.
- **Gastric banding.** The gastric band mentioned above is placed around the upper part of the stomach. This creates a smaller stomach.
- **Gastric bypass surgery.** A small part of the stomach is connected to the middle part of the intestine, bypassing the first part of the intestine. This reduces the amount of food that you can eat and the amount of fat your body can take in and store.

Talk to your doctor to learn more about the benefits and risks of each type of surgery. All surgeries carry some type of risk of possible complications, including bleeding, infection, or even death.

PREVENTION OF OVERWEIGHT AND OBESITY

You and your child should each see a health-care provider once a year to monitor changes in BMI. Your provider or your child's pediatrician may recommend lifestyle changes if BMI regularly increases. This is to prevent you or your child from developing overweight or obesity.[3]

---

[3] "Overweight and Obesity," National Heart, Lung, and Blood Institute (NHLBI), March 24, 2022. Available online. URL: www.nhlbi.nih.gov/health/overweight-and-obesity. Accessed June 22, 2023.

Section 37.4 | Tips for Healthy Weight Loss

Healthy weight is not about following a diet or program. Instead, it involves a lifestyle with healthy eating patterns, regular physical activity, and stress management.

People with gradual, steady weight loss (about 1–2 pounds per week) are more likely to keep the weight off than people who lose weight quickly.

Sleep, age, genetics, diseases, medications, and environments may also contribute to weight management. If you are concerned about your weight or have questions about your medications, talk with your health-care provider.

GETTING STARTED

Losing weight takes a well-thought-out plan. Here is how to get started.

Step 1: Make a Commitment

Whether you have a family history of heart disease, want to see your kids get married, or want to feel better in your clothes, write down why you want to lose weight. Writing it down can confirm your commitment. Post these reasons where they serve as a daily reminder of why you want to make this change.

Step 2: Take Stock of Where You Are

- **Write down everything you eat and drink for a few days in a food and beverage diary**. Being more aware of what you eat and drink will help you avoid mindless consumption. Tracking physical activity, sleep, and emotions can also help you understand current habits and stressors. This can also help identify areas where you can start making changes.
- **Next, examine your lifestyle**. Identify things that might pose challenges to your weight loss efforts. For example, does your work or travel schedule make it hard to get

enough physical activity? Do you find yourself eating sugary foods because that is what you buy for your kids? Do your coworkers often bring high-calorie items, such as doughnuts, to the workplace? Think through things you can do to help overcome these challenges.

- **If you have a chronic condition or a disability, ask your health-care provider for resources to support a healthy weight**. This may include referral to a registered dietitian and other clinical or community programs, federally approved medications or devices, or surgery. Ask for a follow-up appointment to monitor changes in your weight or any related health conditions.

Step 3: Set Realistic Goals

Set short-term goals and reward your efforts along the way. Maybe your long-term goal is to lose 40 pounds and to control your high blood pressure. Short-term goals might be to drink water instead of sugary beverages, take a 15-minute evening walk, or have a vegetable with supper.

Focus on two or three goals at a time. Effective goals are:

- specific
- realistic
- forgiving (less than perfect)

For example, "exercise more" is not specific. But "I will walk 15 minutes, 3 days a week for the first week" is specific and realistic.

Setting unrealistic goals, such as losing 20 pounds in two weeks, can leave you feeling defeated and frustrated.

Being realistic also means expecting occasional setbacks. When setbacks happen, get back on track as quickly as possible. Also, think about how to prevent setbacks in similar future situations.

Keep in mind everyone is different—what works for someone else might not be right for you. Try a variety of activities, such as walking, swimming, tennis, or group exercise classes. See what you enjoy most and can fit into your life. These activities will be easier to stick with over the long term.

Step 4: Identify Resources for Information and Support

Find family members or friends who will support your weight loss efforts. Coworkers or neighbors with similar goals might share healthy recipes and plan group physical activities. Joining a weight loss group or visiting a health-care professional, such as a registered dietitian, may also help.

Step 5: Continually Monitor Your Progress

Revisit the goals you set in step 3 and evaluate your progress regularly. Evaluate which parts of your plan are working well and which ones need tweaking. Then rewrite your goals and plan accordingly.

If you consistently achieve a particular goal, add a new goal to help you continue your pathway to success.

Reward yourself for your successes. Recognize when you are meeting your goals and be proud of your progress. Use nonfood rewards, such as a bouquet of fresh flowers, a sports outing with friends, or a relaxing bath. Rewards help keep you motivated on the path to better health.[4]

Section 37.5 | Choosing a Weight-Loss Program

Do you think you need to lose weight? Have you been thinking about trying a weight-loss program?

You are not alone. More than 70 percent of U.S. adults are overweight or have obesity—and many of them try to lose the extra pounds through different kinds of weight-loss programs. A number of these programs are advertised in magazines and newspapers, as well as on the radio, TV, and the Internet. But are they safe? And will they work for you?

This section provides tips on how to choose a program that may help you lose weight safely and keep it off over time. You will

---

[4] "Losing Weight," Centers for Disease Control and Prevention (CDC), June 15, 2023. Available online. URL: www.cdc.gov/healthyweight/losing_weight/index.html. Accessed June 22, 2023.

also learn how to talk with a health-care professional about your weight.

Your health-care professional may be able to help you make lifestyle changes to reach and maintain a healthy weight. However, if you are having trouble making these lifestyle changes—or if these changes are not enough to help you reach and stay at a healthy weight—you may want to consider a weight-loss program or other types of treatment.

WHERE DO YOU START?

Talking with a health-care professional about your weight is an important first step. Sometimes, health-care professionals may not address issues, such as healthy eating, physical activity, and weight during general office visits. You may need to raise these issues yourself. If you feel uneasy talking about your weight, bring your questions with you and practice talking about your concerns before your office visit. Aim to work with your health-care professional to improve your health.

Prepare for Your Visit

Before your visit with a health-care professional, think about the following questions:

- How can I change my eating habits, so I can be healthier and reach a healthy weight?
- How much and what type of physical activity do I think I need to be healthier and reach a healthy weight?
- Could I benefit from seeing a nutrition professional or weight-loss specialist or joining a weight-loss program?

You can be better prepared for a visit with a health-care professional if you:

- write down all of your questions ahead of time
- record all of the medicines and dietary supplements you take or bring them with you
- write down the types of diets or programs you have tried in the past to lose weight

- bring a pen and paper, smartphone, or other mobile
  device to read your questions and take notes

During your visit, a health-care professional may do the following:
- Review any medical problems you have and medicines
  you take to see whether they may be affecting your
  weight or your ability to lose weight.
- Ask you about your eating, drinking, and physical
  activity habits.
- Determine your body mass index (BMI) to see whether
  you are overweight or have obesity.

People who are overweight have a BMI between 25 and 29.9. People with obesity have a BMI of 30 or higher, and those with extreme obesity have a BMI of 40 or higher.

If a health-care professional says you should lose weight, you may want to ask for a referral to a weight-loss program, dietitian, or weight-loss specialist. If you decide to choose a weight-loss program on your own, consider talking with a health-care professional about the program before you sign up, especially if you have any health problems.

WHAT SHOULD YOU LOOK FOR IN A WEIGHT-LOSS PROGRAM?

To reach and stay at a healthy weight over the long term, you must focus on your overall health and lifestyle habits, not just on what you eat. Successful weight-loss programs should promote healthy behaviors that help you lose weight safely, that you can stick with every day, and that help you keep the weight off.

Safe and successful weight-loss programs should include the following:
- behavioral treatment, also called "lifestyle counseling,"
  that can teach you how to develop and stick with
  healthier eating and physical activity habits—for
  example, keeping food and activity records or journals
- information about getting enough sleep, managing stress,
  and the benefits and drawbacks of weight-loss medicines

- ongoing feedback, monitoring, and support throughout the program, in person, by phone, online, or through a combination of these approaches
- slow and steady weight-loss goals—usually one to two pounds per week (though weight loss may be faster at the start of a program)
- a plan for keeping the weight off, including goal setting, self-checks such as keeping a food journal, and counseling support

The most successful weight-loss programs provide 14 sessions or more of behavioral treatment over at least six months—and are led by trained staff.

Some commercial weight-loss programs have all of these components for a safe and successful weight-loss program.

Although these diets may help some people lose a lot of weight quickly—for example, 15 pounds in a month—they may not help people keep the weight off long-term. These diets may also have related health risks, the most common being gallstones.

For people who are overweight or have obesity, experts recommend a beginning weight-loss goal of 5–10 percent of your starting weight within six months. If you weigh 200 pounds, it would amount to a loss of 10 pounds, which is 5 percent of starting weight, to 20 pounds, which is 10 percent of starting weight, in six months.

Changing your lifestyle is not easy, but adopting healthy habits that you do not give up after a few weeks or months may help you maintain your weight loss.

WHAT IF THE PROGRAM IS OFFERED ONLINE?

Many weight-loss programs are now being offered partly or completely online and through apps for mobile devices. Researchers are studying how well these programs work on their own or together with in-person programs, especially long term. However, experts suggest that these weight-loss programs should provide the following:

- organized, weekly lessons, offered online or by podcast, and tailored to your personal goals

- support from a qualified staff person to meet your goals
- a plan to track your progress on changing your lifestyle habits, such as healthy eating and physical activity, using tools, such as cellphones, activity counters, and online journals
- regular feedback on your goals, progress, and results provided by a counselor through email, phone, or text messages
- the option of social support from a group through bulletin boards, chat rooms, or online meetings

Whether a program is online or in person, you should get as much background as you can before you decide to join.

Weight-Loss Programs to Avoid

Avoid weight-loss programs that make any of the following promises:
- Lose weight without diet or exercise!
- Lose weight while eating as much as you want of all your favorite foods!
- Lose 30 pounds in 30 days!
- Lose weight in specific problem areas of your body!

Other warning signs to look out for include:
- very small print, asterisks, and footnotes, which may make it easy to miss important information
- before-and-after photos that seem too good to be true
- personal endorsements that may be made up

WHAT QUESTIONS SHOULD YOU ASK ABOUT A WEIGHT-LOSS PROGRAM?

Weight-loss program staff should be able to answer questions about the program's features, safety, costs, and results. Find out if the program you are interested in is based on current research about what works for reaching and maintaining a healthy weight.

A first and very important question to ask of commercial weight-loss programs is, "Has your company published any reports in peer-reviewed, scientific journals about the safety and effectiveness of your program?"

If the response is "yes," ask for a copy of the report or how you could get it. If the answer is "no," the program is harder to evaluate and may not be as favorable a choice as programs that have published such information. If you have questions about the findings, discuss the report with your health-care professional.

What Kind of Education or Training Do Staff Members Have?

These questions are especially important if you are considering a medically supervised program that encourages quick weight loss (three or more pounds a week for several weeks):

- Does a doctor or other certified health professional run or oversee the program?
- Does the program include specialists in nutrition, physical activity, behavior change, and weight loss?
- What type of certifications, education, experience, and training do staff members have? How long, on average, have most of the staff been working with the program?

Does the Program or Product Carry Any Risks?

- Could the program cause health problems or be harmful to me in any way?
- Is there ongoing input and follow-up to ensure my safety while I am in the program?
- Will the program's doctor or staff work with my health-care professional if needed—for example, to address how the program may affect an ongoing medical issue?

How Much Does the Program Cost?

- What is the total cost of the program, from beginning to end?

- Are there costs that are not included in that total, such as membership fees or fees for:
  - weekly visits
  - food, meal replacements, supplements, or other products
  - medical tests
  - counseling sessions
  - follow-up to maintain the weight I have lost

What Results Do People in the Program Typically Achieve?

- How much weight does the average person lose?
- How long does the average person keep the weight off?
- Do you have written information on these and other program results?
- Are the results of the program published in a peer-reviewed scientific journal?

What If You Need More Help in Losing Weight?

If a weight-loss program is not enough to help you reach a healthy weight, ask your health-care professional about other types of weight-loss treatments. Prescription medicines to treat overweight and obesity, combined with healthy lifestyle changes, may help some people reach a healthy weight. For some people who have extreme obesity, bariatric surgery may be an option.[5]

---

[5] "Choosing a Safe and Successful Weight-Loss Program," National Institute of Diabetes and Digestive and Kidney Diseases (NIDDK), July 2017. Available online. URL: www.niddk.nih.gov/health-information/weight-management/choosing-a-safe-successful-weight-loss-program. Accessed July 20, 2023.

Chapter 38 | Nutrition Tips for Men

Chapter Contents

Section 38.1 | Healthy Eating for Men

Eating healthy means following a healthy eating pattern that includes a variety of nutritious foods and drinks. It also means getting the number of calories that is right for you (not eating too much or too little).

CHOOSE A MIX OF HEALTHY FOODS

There are lots of healthy choices in each food group! Choose a variety of foods you enjoy, including the following:
- whole fruits—such as apples, berries, oranges, mango, and bananas
- veggies—such as broccoli, sweet potatoes, beets, okra, spinach, peppers, and jicama
- whole grains—such as brown rice, millet, oatmeal, bulgur, and whole-wheat bread
- proteins—such as lean meats and chicken, eggs, seafood, beans and lentils, nuts and seeds, and tofu
- low-fat or fat-free dairy—such as milk, yogurt, cheese, lactose-free dairy, and fortified soy beverages (soy milk) or soy yogurt
- oils—such as vegetable oil, olive oil, and oils in foods, such as seafood, avocado, and nuts

LIMIT CERTAIN NUTRIENTS AND INGREDIENTS
Sodium (Salt)
Sodium is found in table salt—but most of the sodium we eat comes from packaged food or food that is prepared in restaurants.

Added Sugars
Added sugars include syrups and sweeteners that manufacturers add to products, such as sodas, yogurt, and cereals—as well as things you add, such as sugar in your coffee.

Saturated Fat

Saturated fat comes from animal products, such as cheese, fatty meats and poultry, whole milk, and butter and many sweets and snack foods. Some plant products, such as palm and coconut oils, also have saturated fat.

WHAT ABOUT ALCOHOL?

Alcohol includes beer, wine, and liquor. If you choose to drink, drink in moderation—two drinks or less in a day for men. And remember that drinking less is always better for your health than drinking more.

HEALTH BENEFITS
A Healthy Eating Routine Can Help Keep You Healthy

Eating healthy is good for your overall health—and there are many ways to do it.

Making smart food choices can also help you manage your weight and lower your risk for certain chronic (long-term) diseases.

When you eat healthy, you can reduce your risk for:

- overweight and obesity
- heart disease
- type 2 diabetes
- high blood pressure
- some types of cancer

MAKE SMALL CHANGES

Making small changes to your eating habits can make a big difference in your health over time.

Make Healthy Swaps

Try making one or two small changes this week. The following are a few examples:

- Drink sparkling water instead of regular soda.
- Try plain, low-fat yogurt with fruit instead of full-fat yogurt with added sugars.

- Choose low-sodium black beans instead of regular canned black beans.
- Cook with olive oil instead of butter.

SHOP SMART
Shop Smart at the Grocery Store
The next time you go food shopping, do the following:
- Make a shopping list ahead of time—only buy what is on your list.
- Do not shop while you are hungry—eat something before you go to the store.

Use the following tips to make healthy choices:
- Try a variety of vegetables and fruits in different colors.
- Choose fat-free or low-fat dairy—or soy milk and soy yogurt with added calcium, vitamin A, and vitamin D.
- Replace old favorites with options that are lower in calories, sodium, added sugars, and saturated fat.
- Choose foods with whole grains—such as 100 percent whole-wheat or whole-grain bread, cereal, and pasta.
- Buy lean cuts of meat and poultry and eat a variety of foods with protein—such as fish, shellfish, beans, and nuts.
- Save money by getting fruits and vegetables in season or on sale

CHECK THE LABEL
Read the Nutrition Facts Label
Understanding the Nutrition Facts label on food packages can help you make healthy choices (see Figure 38.1).

First, look at the serving size and the number of servings per package—there may be more than one serving!

Then check out the calories. Calories tell you how much energy is in one serving of food.

To stay at a healthy weight, you need to balance the calories you eat and drink with the calories you use.

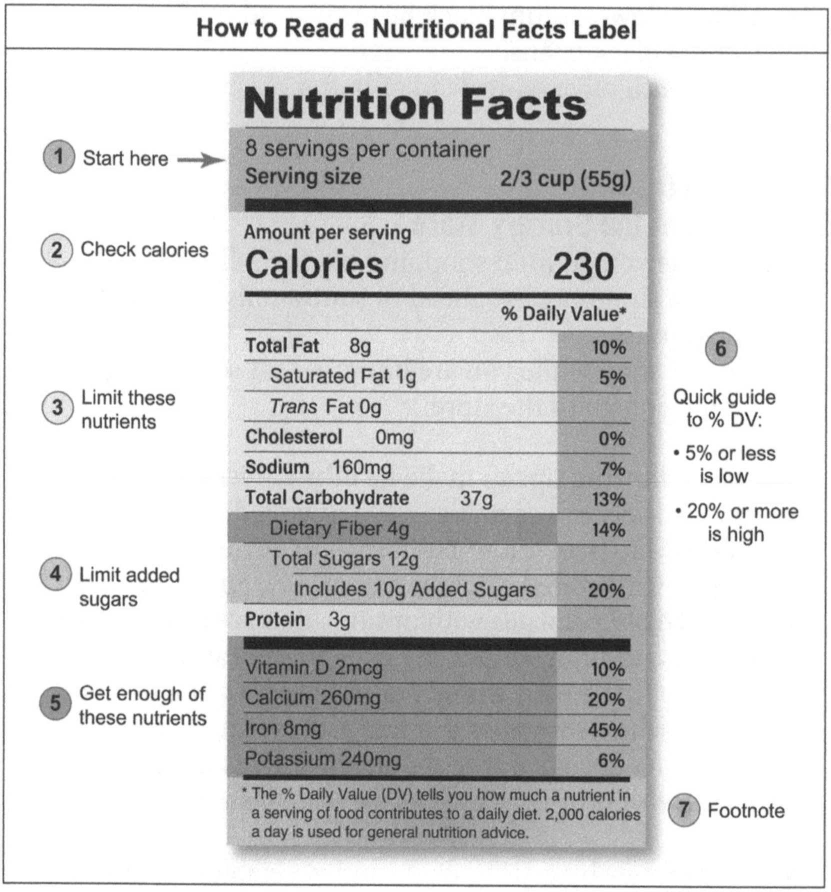

How to Read a Nutritional Facts Label

Nutrition Facts

1) Start here →

8 servings per container
Serving size   2/3 cup (55g)

2) Check calories

Amount per serving
Calories   **230**

% Daily Value*

Total Fat 8g	10%
Saturated Fat 1g	5%
Trans Fat 0g	
Cholesterol 0mg	0%
Sodium 160mg	7%
Total Carbohydrate 37g	13%
Dietary Fiber 4g	14%
Total Sugars 12g	
Includes 10g Added Sugars	20%
Protein 3g	
Vitamin D 2mcg	10%
Calcium 260mg	20%
Iron 8mg	45%
Potassium 240mg	6%

3) Limit these nutrients

4) Limit added sugars

5) Get enough of these nutrients

6) Quick guide to % DV:
• 5% or less is low
• 20% or more is high

* The % Daily Value (DV) tells you how much a nutrient in a serving of food contributes to a daily diet. 2,000 calories a day is used for general nutrition advice.

7) Footnote

© Infobase

Figure 38.1. Nutrition Facts Label

Infobase

Next, look at the percent daily value (% DV) column. The DV shows you if food is higher or lower in certain nutrients. Look for foods that are:

- low in added sugars, sodium, and saturated fat (5% DV or less)
- high in fiber, calcium, potassium, iron, and vitamin D (20% DV or more)

You can also use the DV to compare the amount of calories and nutrients in different foods. Just be sure to check and see if the serving size is the same.

HEALTHY FAMILIES
Be a Healthy Family

Parents and caregivers are important role models for healthy eating. You can teach kids how to choose and prepare healthy snacks and meals.

- Make healthy choices at the grocery store—take your child with you to the store and explain the choices you make.
- Turn cooking into a fun activity for the whole family— try out kid-friendly recipes together.

If you have a family member who has a hard time eating healthy, use these tips to start a conversation about how you can help.

EATING OUT
Eat Healthy Away from Home

You can make smart food choices wherever you are—at work, in your favorite restaurant, or out running errands. Try these tips for eating healthy even when you are away from home:

- Pack healthy snacks, such as fruit, unsalted nuts, or low-fat string cheese sticks.
- Look for calorie information on restaurant menus.
- Choose dishes that are steamed, baked, or grilled instead of fried.
- Ask to have no salt added to your meal.

SEE YOUR DOCTOR
If You Are Worried about Your Eating Habits, Talk to a Doctor

If you need help making healthier food choices, ask your doctor for help. Your doctor may refer you to a registered dietitian. A registered dietitian is a health professional who helps people with healthy eating.

WHAT ABOUT THE COST?

Under the Affordable Care Act (ACA), insurance plans must cover diet counseling for people with risk factors for heart disease, such as high blood pressure (HBP). Depending on your insurance plan, you may be able to get diet counseling at no cost to you. Check with your insurance company to find out more.

Medicare may also cover diet counseling at no cost. Use the tool available at www.medicare.gov/coverage to see what Medicare covers.

If you do not have insurance, you may still be able to get free or low-cost help. Find a health center near you and ask about diet counseling.

MANAGE YOUR HIGH BLOOD PRESSURE OR DIABETES

If you or a loved one has HBP, type 2 diabetes, or heart disease, talk with your doctor or a registered dietitian about how to stay healthy. If you need to follow a special diet, check out the following websites:

- DASH eating plan—www.nhlbi.nih.gov/health/ health-topics/topics/dash
- Living with Diabetes: Eat Well!—www.cdc.gov/ diabetes/managing/eat-well.html[1]

Section 38.2 | Nutrition Tips for Building Muscle Mass

Did you know you have more than 600 muscles in your body? These muscles help you move, lift things, pump blood through your body, and even help you breathe.

When you think about your muscles, you probably think most about the ones you can control. These are your voluntary muscles,

---

[1] Office of Disease Prevention and Health Promotion (ODPHP), "Eat Healthy," U.S. Department of Health and Human Services (HHS), July 14, 2022. Available online. URL: https://health.gov/myhealthfinder/health-conditions/ diabetes/eat-healthy. Accessed June 23, 2023.

which means you can control their movements. They are also called "skeletal muscles" because they attach to your bones and work together with your bones to help you walk, run, play an instrument, or cook a meal. The muscles of your mouth and throat even help you talk.

Keeping your muscles healthy will help you be able to walk, run, jump, lift things, play sports, and do all the other things you love to do. Exercising, getting enough rest, and eating a balanced diet will help keep your muscles healthy for life.

WHY HEALTHY MUSCLES MATTER TO YOU

Healthy muscles let you move freely and keep your body strong. They help you enjoy playing sports, dancing, walking the dog, swimming, and other fun activities. And they help you do those other (not so fun) things that you have to do, such as making the bed, vacuuming the carpet, or mowing the lawn.

Strong muscles also help keep your joints in good shape. If the muscles around your knee, for example, get weak, you may be more likely to injure that knee. Strong muscles also help you keep your balance, so you are less likely to slip or fall.

And remember—the activities that make your skeletal muscles strong will also help keep your heart muscle strong!

DIFFERENT KINDS OF MUSCLES HAVE DIFFERENT JOBS

- **Skeletal muscles**. These muscles are connected to your bones by tough cords of tissue called "tendons." As the muscle contracts, it pulls on the tendon, which moves the bone. Bones are connected to other bones by ligaments, which are like tendons and help hold your skeleton together.
- **Smooth muscles**. These muscles are also called "involuntary muscles" since you have no control over them. Smooth muscles work in your digestive system to move food along and push waste out of your body. They also help keep your eyes focused without you having to think about it.

- **Cardiac muscle**. Did you know your heart is also a muscle? It is a specialized type of involuntary muscle. It pumps blood through your body, changing its speed to keep up with the demands you put on it. It pumps more slowly when you are sitting or lying down and faster when you are running or playing sports, and your skeletal muscles need more blood to help them do their work.

WHAT CAN GO WRONG?
Injuries

Almost everyone has had sore muscles after exercising or working too much. Some soreness can be a normal part of healthy exercise. But, in other cases, muscles can become strained. Muscle strain (streyn) can be mild (the muscle has just been stretched too much) to severe (the muscle actually tears). Maybe you lifted something that was too heavy, and the muscles in your arms were stretched too far. Lifting heavy things in the wrong way can also strain the muscles in your back. This can be very painful and can even cause an injury that will last a long time and make it hard to do everyday things.

Contact sports, such as soccer, football, hockey, and wrestling, can often cause strains. Sports in which you grip something (such as gymnastics or tennis) can lead to strains in your hand or forearm.

The tendons that connect the muscles to the bones can also be strained if they are pulled or stretched too much. If ligaments (remember, they connect bones to bones) are stretched or pulled too much, the injury is called a "sprain (spreyn)." Most people are familiar with the pain of a sprained ankle.

HOW COULD YOU KEEP YOUR MUSCLES MORE HEALTHY?

Muscles that are not used will get smaller and weaker. This is known as "atrophy."

Eat a Healthy Diet

You really do not need a special diet to keep your muscles in good health. Eating a balanced diet will help manage your weight and provide a variety of nutrients for your muscles and overall health. A balanced diet:

- emphasizes fruits, vegetables, whole grains, and fat-free or low-fat dairy products such as milk, cheese, and yogurt
- includes protein from lean meats, poultry, seafood, beans, eggs, and nuts
- is low in solid fats, saturated fats, cholesterol, salt (sodium), added sugars, and refined grains
- is as low as possible in trans fats
- balances calories taken in through food with calories burned in physical activity to help maintain a healthy weight

As you grow and become an adult, iron is an important nutrient. Not getting enough iron can cause anemia, which can make you feel weak and tired because your muscles do not get enough oxygen. This can also keep you from getting enough activity to keep your muscles healthy. You can get iron from foods such as lean beef, chicken, and turkey; beans and peas; spinach; and iron-enriched breads and cereals. You can also get iron from dietary supplements, but it is always good to check with a doctor first.

Some people think that supplements will make their muscles bigger and stronger. However, supplements such as creatine can cause serious side effects, and protein and amino acid supplements are no better than getting protein from your food. Using steroids to increase your muscles is illegal (unless a doctor has prescribed them for a medical problem) and can have dangerous side effects.

No muscle-building supplement can take the place of good nutrition and proper training.

Start Now

Keeping your muscles healthy will help you have more fun and enjoy the things you do. Healthy muscles will help you look your best and feel full of energy. Start good habits now, while you are young, and you will have a better chance of keeping your muscles healthy for the rest of your life.[2]

[2] "Healthy Muscles Matter," National Institute of Arthritis and Musculoskeletal and Skin Diseases (NIAMS), May 2023. Available online. URL: www.niams.nih.gov/health-topics/kids/healthy-muscles. Accessed June 23, 2023.

Chapter 39 | **Physical Activity: Key to a Healthy Life**

Chapter Contents

Section 39.1 | Physical Activity Guidelines for Adults

Physical activity is anything that gets your body moving. Each week adults need 150 minutes of moderate-intensity physical activity and two days of muscle-strengthening activity, according to the current Physical Activity Guidelines for Americans (health.gov/our-work/nutrition-physical-activity/physical-activity-guidelines/current-guidelines).

MOVE MORE AND SIT LESS
Adults should move more and sit less throughout the day. Some physical activity is better than none. Adults who sit less and do any amount of moderate-to-vigorous intensity physical activity gain some health benefits.

RECOMMENDED LEVELS FOR HEALTH BENEFITS
Adults should follow the exercises as specified in the following options.

Example 1
- moderate-intensity aerobic activity (such as brisk walking) for 150 minutes every week (e.g., 30 minutes a day, 5 days a week)
- muscle-strengthening activities on two or more days a week that work all major muscle groups (legs, hips, back, abdomen, chest, shoulders, and arms)

Example 2
- vigorous-intensity aerobic activity (such as jogging or running) for 75 minutes (1 hour and 15 minutes) every week
- muscle-strengthening activities on two or more days a week that work all major muscle groups (legs, hips, back, abdomen, chest, shoulders, and arms)

Example 3
- an equivalent mix of moderate- and vigorous-intensity aerobic activity on two or more days a week

- muscle-strengthening activities on two or more days a week that work all major muscle groups (legs, hips, back, abdomen, chest, shoulders, and arms)

PHYSICAL ACTIVITY FOR GREATER HEALTH BENEFITS

If you go beyond 150 minutes a week of moderate-intensity activity, 75 minutes a week of vigorous-intensity activity, or an equivalent combination, you will gain even more health benefits.

Aerobic Activity

Aerobic activity or "cardio" gets you breathing harder and your heart beating faster. It ranges from pushing a lawn mower to taking a dance class to walking or biking to the store—these types of activities and more count. As long as you are doing aerobic physical activities at a moderate or vigorous intensity, they count toward meeting the aerobic guideline.

Intensity is how hard your body is working during a physical activity.

Moderate-intensity aerobic physical activity means you are working hard enough to raise your heart rate and break a sweat. One way to tell if it is a moderate-intensity aerobic activity is that you will be able to talk but will not be able to sing the words to your favorite song.

Here are some examples of activities that require moderate effort:

- walking fast
- doing water aerobics
- riding a bike on level ground or with few hills
- playing doubles tennis
- pushing a lawn mower

Vigorous-intensity aerobic activity means you are breathing hard and fast, and your heart rate has gone up quite a bit. Here are some examples of activities that require vigorous effort:

- jogging or running
- swimming laps

- riding a bike fast or on hills
- playing singles tennis
- playing basketball

If you are doing moderate-intensity physical activity, such as walking or hiking, you can talk but cannot sing during the activity.

Building Up over Time

If you want to do more vigorous-level activities, slowly replace those that take moderate effort, such as brisk walking, with more vigorous activities, such as jogging.

You can do moderate- or vigorous-intensity aerobic activity or a mix of the two, each week. A rule of thumb is that one minute of vigorous-intensity activity is about the same as two minutes of moderate-intensity activity.

Some people like to do vigorous activity because it gives them about the same health benefits in half the time. If you have not been very active lately, however, increase your physical activity level slowly. If you have a history of a chronic disease, consider telling your doctor you are planning to increase your physical activity, including moving to more vigorous activity. You need to feel comfortable doing moderate-intensity activities before you move on to more vigorous ones.

MUSCLE-STRENGTHENING ACTIVITIES: WHAT COUNTS?

Physical activities to strengthen your muscles are recommended at least two days a week. Activities should work all the major muscle groups of your body—legs, hips, back, chest, abdomen, shoulders, and arms. Muscle-strengthening activities should be done in addition to your aerobic activity.

To gain health benefits, you need to do muscle-strengthening activities to the point where it is hard for you to do another repetition without help. A repetition is one complete movement of an activity, such as lifting a weight or doing a sit-up. Try to do 8–12 repetitions per activity, which counts as one set. Try to do at least one set of muscle-strengthening activities. To gain even more benefits, do two or three sets.

You can do activities that strengthen your muscles on the same or different days that you do aerobic activity—whatever works best for you.

There are many ways you can strengthen your muscles, whether it is at home or the gym. You may want to try the following:

- lifting weights
- working with resistance bands
- doing exercises that use your body weight for resistance (e.g., push-ups, sit-ups)
- heavy gardening (e.g., digging, shoveling)
- some forms of yoga[1]

Section 39.2 | Benefits of Regular Physical Activity

We have all heard it many times before: Regular exercise is good for you, and it can help you lose weight. But, if you are like many Americans, you are busy; you have a sedentary job, and you have not yet changed your exercise habits. The good news is that it is never too late to start. You can start slowly and find ways to fit more physical activity into your life. To get the most benefit, you should try to get the recommended amount of exercise for your age. If you can do it, the payoff is that you will feel better, help prevent or control many diseases, and likely even live longer.

HOW CAN YOU MAKE EXERCISE A PART OF YOUR REGULAR ROUTINE?

- **Make everyday activities more active.** Even small changes can help. You can take the stairs instead of the elevator. Walk down the hall to a coworker's office instead of sending an email. Wash the car yourself. Park further away from your destination.

---

[1] "How Much Physical Activity Do Adults Need?" Centers for Disease Control and Prevention (CDC), June 2, 2022. Available online. URL: www.cdc.gov/physicalactivity/basics/adults/index.htm. Accessed June 23, 2023.

- **Be active with friends and family**. Having a workout partner may make you more likely to enjoy exercise. You can also plan social activities that involve exercise. You may also consider joining an exercise group or class, such as a dance class, hiking club, or volleyball team.
- **Keep track of your progress**. Keeping a log of your activity or using a fitness tracker may help you set goals and stay motivated.
- **Make exercise more fun**. Try listening to music or watching television while you exercise. Also, mix things up a little bit; if you stick with just one type of exercise, you might get bored. Try doing a combination of activities.
- **Find activities that you can do even when the weather is bad**. You can walk in a mall, climb stairs, or work out in a gym even if the weather stops you from exercising outside.

WHAT ARE THE HEALTH BENEFITS OF EXERCISE?

Regular exercise and physical activity may do the following:
- **Help you control your weight**. Along with diet, exercise plays an important role in controlling your weight and preventing obesity. To maintain your weight, the calories you eat and drink must equal the energy you burn. To lose weight, you must use more calories than you eat and drink.
- **Reduce your risk of heart diseases**. Exercise strengthens your heart and improves your circulation. The increased blood flow raises the oxygen levels in your body. This helps lower your risk of heart diseases, such as high cholesterol, coronary artery disease (CAD), and heart attack. Regular exercise can also lower your blood pressure and triglyceride levels.
- **Help your body manage blood sugar and insulin levels**. Exercise can lower your blood sugar level and help your insulin work better. This can cut down your risk for metabolic syndrome and type 2 diabetes. And,

if you already have one of those diseases, exercise can help you manage it.

- **Help you quit smoking**. Exercise may make it easier to quit smoking by reducing your cravings and withdrawal symptoms. It can also help limit the weight you might gain when you stop smoking.
- **Improve your mental health and mood**. During exercise, your body releases chemicals that can improve your mood and make you feel more relaxed. This can help you deal with stress and reduce your risk of depression.
- **Help keep your thinking, learning, and judgment skills sharp as you age**. Exercise stimulates your body to release proteins and other chemicals that improve the structure and function of your brain.
- **Strengthen your bones and muscles**. Regular exercise can help kids and teens build strong bones. Later in life, it can also slow the loss of bone density that comes with age. Doing muscle-strengthening activities can help you increase or maintain your muscle mass and strength.
- **Reduce your risk of some cancers**. This includes colon, breast, uterine, and lung cancer.
- **Reduce your risk of falls**. For older adults, research shows that doing balance and muscle-strengthening activities in addition to moderate-intensity aerobic activity can help reduce your risk of falling.
- **Improve your sleep**. Exercise can help you fall asleep faster and stay asleep longer.
- **Improve your sexual health**. Regular exercise may lower the risk of erectile dysfunction (ED) in men. For those who already have ED, exercise may help improve their sexual function.
- **Increase your chances of living longer**. Studies show that physical activity can reduce your risk of dying early from the leading causes of death, such as heart disease and some cancers.[2]

---

[2] MedlinePlus, "Benefits of Exercise," National Institutes of Health (NIH), August 30, 2017. Available online. URL: https://medlineplus.gov/benefitsofexercise.html. Accessed July 20, 2023.

Chapter 40 | Vaccinations for Men

Chapter Contents

Section 40.1 | Recommended Adult Vaccinations

Every year, thousands of adults in the United States get sick and are hospitalized from vaccine-preventable diseases. Getting vaccinated will help you stay healthy, so you will miss less work and also have more time for your family and friends.

Did you know that when you get vaccinated, you also help protect your family and your community? Vaccines help keep diseases from spreading to people who may not be able to get certain vaccines, such as newborn babies.

ADULTS BETWEEN THE AGES OF 19 AND 26

Young adults need vaccines, too. Vaccines protect young adults from getting serious and even deadly diseases. They may be especially important if you are living in close quarters with others—such as in college dorms—and sharing bedrooms, bathrooms, and food. This can make you more likely to come into contact with dangerous germs.

By getting vaccinated, you can help keep yourself, your family, and your community healthy.

Which Vaccines Are Recommended for Adults between the Ages of 19 and 26?

It is important for young adults to get vaccines that protect against diseases such as the flu and whooping cough. You also need to be up-to-date on meningococcal and human papillomavirus (HPV) vaccines.

You may also need other vaccines, especially when you are planning to travel outside the United States.

Make Sure Your Childhood Vaccines Are Up-to-Date

In addition to getting the vaccinations you need now as a young adult, it is important to make sure you have had all of your childhood vaccinations.

It is also a good idea to ask your doctor about any childhood shots that you may have missed or new vaccines that are now available.

ADULTS BETWEEN THE AGES OF 27 AND 64

Did you know that it is just as important for you to stay on top of your vaccinations now as it was when you were a child?

You need a flu shot every year, and you may need additional doses of some vaccines to help you stay protected from diseases. As you age or your lifestyle or health conditions change, you may need protection from different diseases.

Getting vaccinated can help keep you, your family, and your community healthy.

ADULTS AGED 65 AND OLDER

Vaccines are especially important for older adults. As you get older, your immune system weakens, and it can be more difficult to fight off infections. You are more likely to get diseases such as the flu, pneumonia, and shingles, and you are more likely to have complications that can lead to long-term illness, hospitalization, and even death.

If you have an ongoing health condition, such as diabetes or heart disease, getting vaccinated is especially important. Vaccines can protect you from serious diseases (and related complications), so you can stay healthy as you age.

Does Medicare Cover Vaccines for Older Adults?

- **Medicare Part B**. This covers vaccines that protect against the flu and pneumococcal disease—and the hepatitis B vaccine if you are at increased risk for hepatitis B. It also covers vaccines that you might need after an injury (such as the tetanus vaccine) or coming into contact with a disease (such as the rabies vaccine).
- **Medicare Part D plans**. These plans generally cover more vaccines than Part B. But, depending on your Medicare

Part D plan, you may have out-of-pocket costs for these vaccines. Contact Medicare to find out what is covered.

YOU HAVE GOTTEN ALL YOUR CHILDHOOD VACCINES. WHY DO YOU NEED MORE?

Adults need vaccines for several reasons. The following are a few examples:

- Some vaccines are recommended only for adults who are more at risk for certain diseases, such as shingles.
- Protection from childhood vaccines wears off over time, so you need additional doses of certain vaccines to stay protected.
- You may not have gotten some of the newer vaccines that are now available.
- Some viruses, such as the virus that causes the flu, can change over time.
- You may be at an increased risk for diseases based on travel plans, your job, or health conditions.

HOW DO YOU KNOW WHICH VACCINATIONS YOU HAVE HAD AND WHICH ONES YOU NEED?

To find out which vaccinations you have had, you will need to find your vaccination record. Your vaccination record is the history of all the vaccines you have had as a child and as an adult. To find your vaccination record, do the following:

- Ask your parents or caregivers if they have your vaccination record.
- Contact current or previous doctors and ask for your record.
- Contact your state health department. Some states have registries (immunization information systems (IISs)) that can provide information about your vaccination records.

If you cannot find your record, ask your doctor if you should get some vaccinations again.[1]

---

[1] Vaccines.gov, "Vaccines for Adults," U.S. Department of Health and Human Services (HHS), April 29, 2021. Available online. URL: www.hhs.gov/immunization/who-and-when/adults/index.html. Accessed July 21, 2023.

Section 40.2 | Human Papillomavirus Vaccination for Young Men

WHAT IS HUMAN PAPILLOMAVIRUS?
Human papillomavirus (HPV) is a group of more than 150 viruses. Many people who get HPV have no symptoms. Some people who get HPV develop warts in their genital area.

Some HPV infections do not go away and can cause cancer, including the following:
- cancer of the penis (penile cancer)
- cancer of the anus (anal cancer) or rectum (rectal cancer)
- cancer of the throat (oropharyngeal cancer), including the base of the tongue and tonsils

HPV spreads through intimate skin-to-skin contact. Most of the time, it spreads when a person who has an HPV infection has vaginal, oral, or anal sex. And, since HPV may not cause symptoms, people can have it—and spread it to others—without knowing.

WHY IS THE HUMAN PAPILLOMAVIRUS VACCINE IMPORTANT?
Human papillomavirus infections are so common that nearly all men get at least one type of HPV at some point in their lives—and the complications can be serious. Many of these cancers do not cause symptoms until they have gotten serious and are hard to treat.

Getting vaccinated against HPV can protect your child from HPV infections that cause cancer.

WHO NEEDS TO GET THE HUMAN PAPILLOMAVIRUS VACCINE?
Everyone needs to get the HPV vaccine—doctors recommend that boys and girls get the HPV vaccine at the age of 11 or 12 to take advantage of the best immune response. The HPV vaccine can be routinely given as early as age 9–26, and some adults up to age 45 may get the vaccine after speaking with their health-care provider.

Preteens and Teens Aged 9–14

Preteens and teens need two doses of the HPV vaccine as part of their routine vaccine schedule. They get the second dose about 6–12 months after the first dose. Preteens usually get the HPV vaccine at age 11 or 12 though vaccination can start as early as age 9.

Teens and Young Adults Aged 15–26

If you did not get the HPV vaccine as a preteen, you can still get it. Teens and young adults need three doses of the HPV vaccine. They need to get the second dose one to two months after the first dose—and the third dose six months after the first dose.

Adults Aged 27–45

Some adults older than age 26 may need to get the HPV vaccine, but it is not recommended for everyone. Talk to your doctor about the risk of new HPV infections and the possible benefits of vaccination.

WHO SHOULD NOT GET THE HUMAN PAPILLOMAVIRUS VACCINE?

You should not get the HPV vaccine if you have had a life-threatening allergic reaction to the HPV vaccine or any ingredient in the vaccine.

WHAT ARE THE SIDE EFFECTS OF THE HUMAN PAPILLOMAVIRUS VACCINE?

Side effects are usually mild and go away in a few days. They may include the following:
- pain, redness, and swelling where the shot was given
- fever
- headache

It is very unlikely that the HPV vaccine could cause a serious reaction. Keep in mind that getting the HPV vaccine is much safer than getting cancer caused by an HPV infection.[2]

[2] Vaccines.gov, "HPV (Human Papillomavirus)," U.S. Department of Health and Human Services (HHS), April 29, 2021. Available online. URL: www.hhs.gov/immunization/diseases/hpv/index.html. Accessed July 21, 2023.

Section 40.3 | Seasonal Influenza Vaccination

Every year, millions of people get the flu. The good news is that the seasonal flu vaccine can lower the risk of getting the flu by about half. Getting the yearly flu vaccine is the best way to protect yourself from the flu.

WHAT IS THE FLU?

The flu is caused by a virus. Common symptoms of the flu include the following:

- fever and chills
- cough
- sore throat
- runny or stuffy nose
- muscle or body aches
- headache
- fatigue

Some people with the flu may throw up or have diarrhea (watery poop)—this is more common in children than adults. It is also important to know that not everyone with the flu will have a fever.

The flu is worse than the common cold. It is a common cause of problems such as sinus or ear infections. It can also cause serious complications such as:

- pneumonia (lung infection)
- worsening of long-term health problems, such as asthma or heart failure
- inflammation of the brain, heart, or muscles
- sepsis, a life-threatening inflammatory condition
- multi-organ failure

The flu is contagious, meaning it can spread from person to person. The flu can spread when:

- someone with the flu coughs, sneezes, or talks—and droplets from their mouth or nose get into the mouths or noses of people nearby

- someone touches a surface that has flu virus on it and then touches their mouth, nose, or eyes

People can spread the flu before they know they are sick—and while they have the flu.

WHO NEEDS TO GET THE FLU VACCINE?

Everyone aged six months and older needs to get the flu vaccine every year. It is part of the routine vaccine schedules for children, teens, and adults.

It is important to get the flu vaccine every year. That is important for two reasons. First, immunity (protection) decreases with time. Additionally, the flu viruses are constantly changing—so the vaccine is often updated to give the best protection.

People at Increased Risk for Complications from the Flu

It is especially important for people who are at high risk of developing complications from the flu to get the vaccine every year. People at high risk for complications from the flu include the following:

- adults aged 65 and older
- children younger than six years—and especially children younger than two years
- people with long-term health conditions, such as asthma, diabetes, or cancer
- people in long-term care or nursing homes

Health-Care Professionals and Caregivers

It is also very important for people who spend a lot of time with people at high risk for complications from the flu to get the vaccine—for example, health-care professionals and caregivers.

Talk with your doctor about how to protect your family from the flu.

WHO SHOULD NOT GET THE FLU VACCINE?

Children younger than six months should not get the flu vaccine.

Be sure to tell your doctor before getting vaccinated if you:
- have had a life-threatening allergic reaction to a dose of the flu vaccine or any ingredient in the vaccine (such as eggs or gelatin)
- have had Guillain-Barré syndrome (an immune system disorder)

If you are sick, you may need to wait until you are feeling better to get the flu vaccine.

WHAT ARE THE SIDE EFFECTS OF THE FLU VACCINE?

Side effects are usually mild and go away in a few days. These side effects are not the flu—the flu vaccine cannot cause the flu.

Side effects from the flu vaccine may include the following:
- pain, swelling, or redness where the shot was given
- headache
- muscle aches
- fever
- upset stomach

Serious side effects from the flu vaccine are very rare.

Like any medicine, there is a very small chance that the flu vaccine could cause a serious reaction. Keep in mind that getting the flu vaccine is much safer than getting the flu.[3]

---

[3] Vaccines.gov, "Flu (Influenza)," U.S. Department of Health and Human Services (HHS), May 6, 2022. Available online. URL: www.hhs.gov/immunization/diseases/flu/index.html. Accessed July 21, 2023.

Part 6 | **Additional Help and Information**

Chapter 41 | **Glossary of Terms Related to Men's Health**

abstinence: Not having sexual intercourse.

active surveillance: Closely watching a cancer patient's condition but not giving treatment unless there are changes in test results.

addiction: A chronic, relapsing disease, characterized by compulsive drug seeking and use accompanied by neurochemical and molecular changes in the brain.

adjuvant therapy: Treatment given after the main treatment to help cure a disease.

allergy: An abnormally high sensitivity to certain substances, such as pollens or foods.

alopecia: The lack or loss of hair from areas of the body where hair is usually found.

anemia: A condition in which the number of red blood cells (RBCs) is less than normal, resulting in less oxygen carried to the body's cells.

aneurysm: A weak or thin spot on an artery wall that has stretched or ballooned out from the wall and filled with blood or damage to an artery leading to pooling of blood between the layers of the blood vessel walls.

antiandrogen: A substance that prevents cells from making or using androgens (hormones that play a role in the formation of male sex characteristics).

antibiotic: A drug that can destroy or prevent the growth of bacteria.

This glossary contains terms excerpted from documents produced by several sources deemed reliable.

antiretroviral therapy (ART): The recommended treatment for human immunodeficiency virus (HIV) infection.

artery: Any of the thick-walled blood vessels that carry oxygenated blood away from the heart to other parts of the body.

atherosclerosis: A blood vessel disease characterized by deposits of lipid material on the inside of the walls of large to medium-sized arteries, which make the artery walls thick, hard, brittle, and prone to breaking.

basal cell: A small, round cell found in the lower part (or base) of the epidermis, the outer layer of the skin.

biopsy: To remove cells or tissues from the body for testing and examination under a microscope.

calories: The energy provided by food/nutrients.

carcinoma: Cancer that begins in the skin or in tissues that line or cover internal organs.

chlamydia: A common sexually transmitted disease (STD) caused by the bacterium *Chlamydia trachomatis*.

cholesterol: A waxy substance, produced naturally by the liver and also found in foods, that circulates in the blood and helps maintain tissues and cell membranes.

cocaine: A highly addictive stimulant drug derived from the coca plant that produces profound feelings of pleasure.

condom: A thin rubber sheath worn on a man's penis during sexual intercourse to block semen from coming in contact with the inside of the vagina.

depression: A disorder marked by sadness, inactivity, difficulty with thinking and concentration, significant increase or decrease in appetite and time spent sleeping, feelings of dejection and hopelessness, and, sometimes, suicidal thoughts or an attempt to commit suicide.

diabetes: A condition characterized by high blood glucose, resulting from the body's inability to use blood glucose for energy.

dialysis: The artificial process of filtering waste products and excess fluids from the blood in cases of kidney failure.

diuretic: A chemical that stimulates the production of urine.

dopamine: A neurotransmitter present in regions of the brain that regulate movement, emotion, motivation, and the feeling of pleasure.

edema: The swelling of a cell that results from the influx of large amounts of water or fluid into the cell.

emphysema: A disease that affects the tiny air sacs in the lungs.

gene: The basic unit of heredity. Genes play a role in how high a person's risk is for certain diseases.

genital warts: A sexually transmitted disease (STD) caused by the human papillomavirus.

germ cell tumor: A type of tumor that begins in the cells that give rise to sperm or eggs.

hormone: A substance that stimulates the function of a gland.

human immunodeficiency virus (HIV): The virus that causes acquired immunodeficiency syndrome (AIDS), which is the most advanced stage of HIV infection.

human papillomavirus (HPV): The virus that causes HPV infection, the most common sexually transmitted infection (STI).

hypertension: Characterized by persistently high arterial blood pressure defined as a measurement greater than or equal to 140 mm/Hg systolic pressure over 90 mm/Hg diastolic pressure.

imaging: In medicine, a process that makes pictures of areas inside the body.

immune system: The complex group of organs and cells that defends the body against infections and other diseases.

incontinence: The inability to control urination.

injection drug use: A method of illicit drug use. The drugs are injected directly into the body into a vein, into a muscle, or under the skin with a needle and syringe.

invasive cancer: Cancer that has spread beyond the layer of tissue in which it developed and is growing into surrounding, healthy tissues.

jaundice: A condition in which the skin and the whites of the eyes become yellow, urine darkens, and the color of stool becomes lighter than normal.

lipoprotein: Small globules of cholesterol covered by a layer of protein, produced by the liver.

lobe: A portion of an organ, such as the liver, lung, breast, thyroid, or brain.

lupus: A chronic inflammatory disease that occurs when the body's immune system attacks its own tissues and organs.

lymph nodes: Small glands that help the body fight infection and disease. They filter a fluid called "lymph" and contain white blood cells (WBCs).

magnetic resonance imaging (MRI): A type of imaging involving the use of magnetic fields to detect subtle changes in the water content of tissues.

medical test: Tests designed to rule out or avoid disease.

melanoma: A form of skin cancer that begins in melanocytes (cells that produce the pigment melanin).

metabolism: It refers to all of the processes in the body that make and use energy, such as digesting food and nutrients and removing waste through urine and feces.

mutation: Any change in the deoxyribonucleic acid (DNA) of a cell. Mutations may be caused by mistakes during cell division, or they may be caused by exposure to DNA-damaging agents in the environment.

neoplasm: An abnormal mass of tissue that results when cells divide more than they should or do not die when they should.

nonseminoma: A group of testicular cancers that begin in the germ cells (cells that give rise to sperm).

obstruction: A clog or blockage that prevents liquid from flowing easily.

oncologist: A doctor who specializes in treating cancer. Some oncologists specialize in a particular type of cancer treatment.

opioid: A natural or synthetic psychoactive chemical that binds to opioid receptors in the brain and body.

opportunistic infection: An infection that occurs more frequently or is more severe in people with weakened immune systems, such as people with HIV or people receiving chemotherapy, than in people with healthy immune systems.

outpatient surgery: A procedure in which the patient is not required to stay overnight in a hospital.

pancreas: A large gland that helps digest food and also makes some important hormones.

positron emission tomography (PET) scan: In a PET scan, the patient is given radioactive glucose (sugar) through a vein. A scanner then tracks the glucose in the body.

plaque: Fatty cholesterol deposits found along the inside of artery walls that lead to atherosclerosis and stenosis of the arteries.

Glossary of Terms Related to Men's Health

prognosis: A prediction of the probable outcome of a disease.

pubic lice: Also called "crab lice" or "crabs," pubic lice are parasitic insects found primarily in the pubic or genital area of humans.

radiation: The emission of energy in waves or particles. Often used to treat cancer cells.

recurrence: When cancer comes back after a period when no cancer could be found.

relapse: Return of the manifestations of a disease after an interval of improvement.

resection: Surgery to remove tissue, an organ, or part of an organ.

scabies: An infestation of the skin by the human itch mite (*Sarcoptes scabiei* var. *hominis*). The most common symptoms of scabies are intense itching and a pimple-like skin rash.

scrotum: The sac of skin that contains the testes.

semen: The fluid, containing sperm, which comes out of the penis during sexual excitement.

serotonin: A neurotransmitter used in widespread parts of the brain, which is involved in sleep, movement, and emotions.

sexually transmitted disease (STD): An infectious disease that spreads from person to person during sexual contact.

spermicide: A topical preparation or substance used during sexual intercourse to kill sperm.

stage: How much cancer is in the body and how far it has spread.

stroke: A stroke occurs when blood flow to your brain stops due to a blocked or ruptured blood vessel.

subarachnoid hemorrhage: Bleeding within the meninges, or outer membranes, of the brain into the clear fluid that surrounds the brain.

testes: The male reproductive glands where sperm are produced.

transmission: The spread of disease from one person to another.

trichomoniasis: A sexually transmitted disease (STD) caused by a parasite.

triglycerides: A type of fat in your blood. Triglycerides can contribute to the hardening and narrowing of your arteries if levels are too high.

ulcer: An open lesion on the surface of the skin or a mucosal surface, caused by superficial loss of tissue, usually with inflammation.

ultrasound: A type of test in which sound waves too high to hear are aimed at a structure to produce an image of it.

urinalysis: A test of a urine sample that can reveal many problems of the urinary tract and other body systems.

urinary tract: The path that urine takes as it leaves the body. It includes the kidneys, ureters, bladder, and urethra.

vaccine: A substance meant to help the immune system respond to and resist disease.

virus: A microscopic infectious agent that requires a living host cell in order to replicate.

x-ray: A type of high-energy radiation. In low doses, x-rays are used to diagnose diseases by making pictures of the inside of the body.

yoga: A mind and body practice with origins in ancient Indian philosophy. The various styles of yoga typically combine physical postures, breathing techniques, and meditation or relaxation.

Chapter 42 | Directory of Resources That Provide Information about Men's Health

GENERAL

Eunice Kennedy Shriver National Institute of Child Health and Human Development (NICHD)
P.O. Box 3006
Rockville, MD 20847
Toll-Free: 800-370-2943
Toll-Free Fax: 866-760-5947
Website: www.nichd.nih.gov
Email:
NICHDInformationResource
Center@mail.nih.gov

Mayo Clinic
200 First St., S.W.
Rochester, MN 55905
Phone: 507-284-2511
Toll-Free: 844-217-9591
Website: www.mayoclinic.org

National Human Genome Research Institute (NHGRI)
9000 Rockville Pike, Bldg. 31,
Rm. 4B09
31 Center Dr., MSC 2152
Bethesda, MD 20892-2152
Phone: 301-402-0911
Fax: 301-402-2218
Website: www.genome.gov

National Institute of Diabetes and Digestive and Kidney Diseases (NIDDK)
9000 Rockville Pike
Bethesda, MD 20892
Toll-Free: 800-860-8747
Website: www.niddk.nih.gov
Email: healthinfo@niddk.nih.gov

Resources in this chapter were compiled from several sources deemed reliable; all contact information was verified and updated in September 2023.

Occupational Safety and Health Administration (OSHA)
200 Constitution Ave., N.W.
Rm. N3626
Washington, DC 20210
Toll-Free: 800-321-6742 (OSHA)
Website: www.osha.gov

United Network for Organ Sharing (UNOS)
700 N. Fourth St.
Richmond, VA 23219
Phone: 804-782-4800
Toll-Free: 800-292-9548
Website: www.unos.org
Email: patientservices@unos.org

U.S. Department of Health and Human Services (HHS)
200 Independence Ave., S.W.
Hubert H. Humphrey Bldg.
Washington, DC 20201
Toll-Free: 877-696-6775
Website: www.hhs.gov

U.S. Food and Drug Administration (FDA)
10903 New Hampshire Ave.
Silver Spring, MD 20993-0002
Toll-Free: 888-463-6332
(888-INFO-FDA)
Website: www.fda.gov

CANCER

Abramson Cancer Center
3400 Spruce St.
Philadelphia, PA 19104
Phone: 215-662-4000
Toll-Free: 800-789-7366
Website: www.pennmedicine.org/cancer

American Association for Cancer Research (AACR)
615 Chestnut St.
17th Fl.
Philadelphia, PA 19106-4404
Phone: 215-440-9300
Website: www.aacr.org
Email: aacr@aacr.org

American Cancer Society (ACS)
3380 Chastain Meadows Pkwy., N.W., Ste. 200
Kennesaw, GA 30144
Toll-Free: 800-227-2345
Website: www.cancer.org

American Institute for Cancer Research (AICR)
P.O. Box 97167
Washington, DC 20090
Toll-Free: 800-843-8114
Fax: 202-328-7226
Website: www.aicr.org
Email: communications@aicr.org

Association of Community Cancer Centers (ACCC)
1801 Research Blvd., Ste. 400
Rockville, MD 20850
Phone: 301-984-9496
Fax: 301-770-1949
Website: www.accc-cancer.org

Cancer Care
275 Seventh Ave.
22nd Fl.
New York, NY 10001
Phone: 212-712-8400
Toll-Free: 800-813-4673
Fax: 212-712-8495
Website: www.cancercare.org
Email: info@cancercare.org

Montefiore Einstein Cancer Center
1300 Morris Park Ave.
Chanin Bldg.
Bronx, NY 10461
Phone: 718-430-2302
Toll-Free: 833-632-2623
Website: cancer.montefioreeinstein.org
Email: mecc@einsteinmed.edu

DRUG ABUSE

Florida Alcohol and Drug Abuse Association (FADAA)
316 E. Park Ave.
Tallahassee, FL 32301
Phone: 850-878-2196
Website: www.fadaa.org
Email: fadaa@fadaa.org

National Council on Alcoholism and Drug Dependence, Inc. (NCADD)
28 E. Ostend St., Ste. 303
Baltimore, MD 21230
Website: www.ncadd.us
Email: adminl@ncadd.us

National Institute on Drug Abuse (NIDA)
3WFN MSC 6024
16071 Industrial Dr., Dock 11
Gaithersburg, MD 20892
Phone: 301-443-6441
Website: nida.nih.gov

Substance Abuse and Mental Health Services Administration (SAMHSA)
5600 Fishers Ln.
Rockville, MD 20857
Toll-Free: 877-SAMHSA-7
(877-726-4727)
Toll-Free TTY: 800-487-4889
Website: www.samhsa.gov
Email: SAMHSAInfo@samhsa.hhs.gov

EATING DISORDERS

The Academy for Eating Disorders (AED)
11130 Sunrise Valley Dr., Ste. 350
Reston, VA 20191
Phone: 703-234-4079
Website: www.aedweb.org
Email: info@aedweb.org

Alaska Eating Disorders Alliance (AKEDA)
440 Oceanview Dr.
Anchorage, AK 99515
Phone: 907-308-8400
Website: www.
akeatingdisordersalliance.org
Email: info.
akeatingdisordersalliance@gmail.
com

Center for Eating Disorders (CED)
1100 N. Main St.
Ann Arbor, MI 48104
Phone: 734-668-8585
Fax: 734-668-2645
Website: www.center4ed.org
Email: info@center4ed.org

The Eating Disorders Information Network
4780 Ashford Dunwoody Rd.
Ste. 375
Atlanta, GA 30338
Website: www.myedin.org
Email: inquiries@myedin.org

National Alliance for Eating Disorders
4400 N. Congress Ave., Ste. 100
West Palm Beach, FL 33407
Toll-Free: 866-662-1235
Website: www.
allianceforeatingdisorders.com/
contact
Email: info@
allianceforeatingdisorders.com

National Eating Disorders Association (NEDA)
333 Mamaroneck Ave., Ste. 214
White Plains, NY 10605
Phone: 212-575-6200
Toll-Free: 800-931-2237
Website: www.
nationaleatingdisorders.org
Email: info@
nationaleatingdisorders.org

HEART DISEASE

American Association of Cardiovascular and Pulmonary Rehabilitation (AACVPR)
330 N. Wabash Ave., Ste. 2000
Chicago, IL 60611
Phone: 312-321-5146
Fax: 312-673-6924
Website: www.aacvpr.org
Email: aacvpr@aacvpr.org

American Heart Association (AHA)
7272 Greenville Ave.
Dallas, TX 75231
Phone: 214-570-5943
Toll-Free: 800-AHA-USA-1
(800-242-8721)
Website: www.heart.org

Cardiovascular Research Foundation (CRF)
1700 Bdwy.
9th Fl.
New York, NY 10019
Phone: 646-434-4500
Website: www.crf.org
Email: info@crf.org

Heart Rhythm Society (HRS)
1325 G St., N.W., Ste. 500
Washington, DC 20005
Phone: 202-464-3400
Fax: 202-464-3401
Website: www.hrsonline.org
Email: info@HRSonline.org

National Heart, Lung, and Blood Institute (NHLBI)
Bldg. 31
Bethesda, MD 20892
Toll-Free: 877-NHLBI4U
(877-645-2448)
Website: www.nhlbi.nih.gov
Email: nhlbiinfo@nhlbi.nih.gov

LIVER DISEASE

American Association for the Study of Liver Diseases (AASLD)
1001 N. Fairfax St.
4th Fl.
Alexandria, VA 22314
Phone: 703-299-9766
Fax: 703-299-9622
Website: www.aasld.org
Email: aasld@aasld.org

American Liver Foundation (ALF)
P.O. Box 299
West Orange, NJ 07052
Phone: 212-668-1000
Toll-Free: 800-465-4837
Website: www.liverfoundation.org
Email: info@liverfoundation.org

Children's Liver Association for Support Services (CLASS)
P.O. Box 186
Monaca, PA 15061
Phone: 724-581-5527
Website: www.classkids.org
Email: classkidscares@gmail.com

MENTAL HEALTH ISSUES

Center for Mental Health Services (CMHS)
5600 Fishers Ln.
Rockville, MD 20857
Phone: 240-276-1310
Website: www.samhsa.
gov/about-us/who-we-are/
offices-centers/cmhs

Depression and Bipolar Support Alliance (DBSA)
55 E. Jackson Blvd., Ste. 490
Chicago, IL 60604
Toll-Free: 800-826-3632
Fax: 312-642-7243
Website: www.dbsalliance.org
Email: info@dbsalliance.org

Mental Health America (MHA)
500 Montgomery St., Ste. 820
Alexandria, VA 22314
Phone: 703-684-7722
Toll-Free: 800-969-6642
Fax: 703-684-5968
Website: www.
mentalhealthamerica.net
Email: info@mhanational.org

MentalHealth.gov
200 Independence Ave., S.W.
Washington, DC 20201
Website: www.samhsa.gov/
mental-health

National Institute of Mental Health (NIMH)
6001 Executive Blvd.
Rm. 6200, MSC 9663
Bethesda, MD 20892-9663
Toll-Free: 866-615-6464
Toll-Free TTY: 866-415-8051
Website: www.nimh.nih.gov
Email: nimhinfo@nih.gov

National Association of State Mental Health Program Directors (NASMHPD)
675 N. Washington St., Ste. 470
Alexandria, VA 22314
Phone: 703-739-9333
Website: www.nasmhpd.org

World Federation for Mental Health (WFMH)
Website: www.wfmh.global

PROSTATE AND UROLOGICAL DISORDERS

The American Urological Association Foundation
1000 Corporate Blvd.
Linthicum, MD 21090
Phone: 410-689-3700
Toll-Free: 800-828-7866
Fax: 410-689-3998
Website: www.urologyhealth.org
Email: info@
UrologyCareFoundation.org

Prostatitis Foundation (PF)
1063 30th St.
Smithshire, IL 61478
Website: www.prostatitis.org
Email: info@prostatitis.org

SEXUALLY TRANSMITTED DISEASES

AIDS Healthcare Foundation (AHF)
6255 Sunset Blvd.
21st Fl.
Los Angeles, CA 90028
Phone: 323-860-5200
Website: www.aidshealth.org

Gay Men's Health Crisis (GMHC)
307 W. 38th St.
4th Fl.
New York, NY 10018
Phone: 212-367-1000
Website: www.gmhc.org
Email: info@gmhc.org

Sexuality Information and Education Council of the United States (SIECUS)
1012 14th St., N.W., Ste. 1108
Washington, DC 20005
Phone: 202-265-2405
Website: www.siecus.org
Email: info@siecus.org

SUICIDE

American Association of Suicidology (AAS)
448 Walton Ave.
Unit 790
Hummelstown, PA 17036
Toll-Free: 888-9 PREVENT
(888-977-3836)
Website: suicidology.org
Email: info@suicidology.org

American Foundation for Suicide Prevention (AFSP)
199 Water St.
11th Fl.
New York, NY 10038
Phone: 212-363-3500
Toll-Free: 888-333-AFSP
(888-333-2377)
Fax: 212-408-9684
Website: afsp.org
Email: info@afsp.org

Suicide Awareness Voices of Education (SAVE)
7900 Xerxes Ave., S., Ste. 810
Bloomington, MN 55431
Phone: 952-946-7998
Website: save.org
Email: save@save.org

Suicide Prevention Resource Center (SPRC)
1000 N.E. 13th St., Ste. 5900
Nicholson Twr.
Oklahoma City, OK 73104
Toll-Free: 877-GET-SPRC
(877-438-7772)
Website: www.sprc.org
Email: info@sprc.org

Yellow Ribbon Suicide Prevention
7300 Lowell Blvd., Ste. 35
Westminster, CO 80030
Phone: 303-429-3530
Toll-Free: 800-273-8255
Website: www.yellowribbon.org
Email: ask4help@yellowribbon.org

INDEX

INDEX

Page numbers followed by "n" refer to citation information; by "t" indicate tables; and by "f" indicate figures.

Index

Index

Index

Index

Index

diuretics
bulimia nervosa 588
heart failure 110
kidney stones 171
DMD *see* Duchenne muscular
dystrophy
dopamine
Lesch-Nyhan syndrome
(LNS) 238
Parkinson disease (PD) 196
DRE *see* digital rectal exam
drowning, falls overboard 539
drowsy driving, overview 522–524
drug-impaired driving,
overview 524–526
drugs
depression 325
erectile dysfunction (ED) 395
heart failure 105
hepatitis B 436
Lesch-Nyhan syndrome (LNS) 240
lung cancer 284
motor vehicle accidents 525
overview 36–40
painkiller abuse 29
Parkinson disease (PD) 200
pneumonia 141
sexual health issues 466
sleep disorders 605
dry eye
sleep apnea 266
vision disorders 32
dry skin
chronic kidney disease (CKD) 182
type 1 diabetes 96
dual-energy x-ray absorptiometry
(DXA)
body mass index (BMI) 621
osteoporosis 243
Duchenne muscular dystrophy
(DMD), muscular
dystrophy (MD) 226

ductal carcinoma in situ (DCIS),
breast cancer 273
Dupuytren disease, Peyronie
disease 379
DXA *see* dual-energy x-ray
absorptiometry
dyslipidemia
diabetes screening 57
obesity 625
dysthymia, depression 322

E

eating disorders
depression 23
overview 585–589
The Eating Disorders Information
Network, contact information 688
echocardiography, heart failure 107
ecstasy
priapism 375
tobacco smoking 38
eczema
balanitis 367
phimosis 386
ED *see* erectile dysfunction
edema
chronic kidney disease (CKD) 182
cirrhosis 159
Effective Health Care Program
publications
pancreatic
adenocarcinoma 290n, 294n
ejaculation
benign prostatic hyperplasia
(BPH) 473
orchitis 411
prostate cancer 303
prostatitis 483
sexual health 353
withdrawal 494
workplace exposures 504t

EKG *see* electrocardiogram

electrical burns, fire-related injuries 546

electrocardiogram (EKG), heart failure 108

electromyography (EMG), muscular dystrophy (MD) 232

emergency medical services (EMS), heart attack 120

EMG *see* electromyography

emotional distress
  mental health 321
  Peyronie disease 380

EMS *see* emergency medical services

endoscopic ultrasound-guided fine-needle aspiration (EUS-FNA), pancreatic cancer 292

EPA *see* U.S. Environmental Protection Agency

epididymis
  depicted 496
  overview 405–410
  reproductive hazards 504t
  spermatocele 420
  testicular cancer 309
  testicular self-examination (TSE) 84
  vasectomy 495

epididymitis
  overview 405–410
  spermatocele 420

epididymo-orchitis *see* epididymitis

epigastric pain, pancreatic cancer 291

erectile dysfunction (ED)
  male infertility 361
  overview 391–401
  perineal injury 255
  physical activity 666
  priapism 375
  prostate cancer screening 89, 306
  sexual and reproductive health 34
  sexual health issues 466

smoking 577
  workplace exposures 504

erection
  cancer 577
  described 353
  erectile dysfunction (ED) 398
  penile cancer 295
  perineal injury 253
  phimosis 386
  priapism 374
  sexual health issues 466
  vasectomy 499

erythromycin, balanitis 368

erythroplasia of Queyrat *see* penile intraepithelial neoplasia (PEIN)

erythropoietin, anabolic steroids 580

esketamine, depression 326

estrogen
  autoimmune disorders 22
  benign prostatic hyperplasia (BPH) 473
  biological factors 14
  breast cancer 274
  breast self-examination 71
  gynecomastia 461
  infertility 501
  osteoporosis 242
  stimulants 37

Eunice Kennedy Shriver National Institute of Child Health and Human Development (NICHD)
  contact information 685
  publications
    fragile X syndrome (FXS) 209n
    Klinefelter syndrome (KS) 225n
    men's reproductive health 361n
    sexually transmitted diseases (STDs) 426n
    vasectomy 499n

EUS-FNA *see* endoscopic ultrasound-guided fine-needle aspiration

Index

Index

hepatitis, *continued*
  sexually transmitted diseases
    (STDs)/sexually transmitted
    infections (STIs) 423
hernia
  hydrocele 417
  male infertility 360
heroin
  gynecomastia 462
  opioids 569
  painkiller abuse 28
  tobacco smoking 38
herpes simplex viruses (HSV), sexually
  transmitted diseases (STDs)/
  sexually transmitted infections
  (STIs) 423
HFpEF *see* heart failure with preserved
  ejection fraction
HFrEF *see* heart failure with reduced
  ejection fraction
hHG *see* human growth hormone
Hib *see* Haemophilus influenzae type b
high blood pressure (HBP) *see*
  hypertension
high-density lipoprotein (HDL)
  cholesterol levels 600
  cholesterol screening 62
highly active antiretroviral therapy
  (HAART), sexually transmitted
  diseases (STDs)/sexually
  transmitted infections (STIs) 426
HIV *see* human immunodeficiency
  virus
HIVinfo
  publication
    HIV and AIDS 443n
HPV *see* human papillomavirus
HSV *see* herpes simplex viruses
human growth hormone (hHG),
  anabolic steroids 580
human immunodeficiency virus (HIV)
  condoms 491

epididymitis 409
genital herpes 430
heart failure 105
hepatitis B 437
human papillomavirus (HPV) 443
kidney stones 171
male reproductive health 359
pneumonia 141
safer sex 509
screening tests for men 52
sexual assault 560
sexually transmitted diseases
  (STDs)/sexually transmitted
  infections (STIs) 423
syphilis 454
trichomoniasis (trich) 459
withdrawal 494
human papillomavirus (HPV)
  adult vaccines 669
  condoms 491
  male reproductive health 359
  oral cancer 73
  overview 443–446
  penile cancer 297
  penile intraepithelial neoplasia
    (PEIN) 370
  sexually transmitted diseases
    (STDs)/sexually transmitted
    infections (STIs) 423
  vaccination for young men 672
hydrocele
  epididymitis 406
  overview 416–418
hydrocelectomy, hydrocele
  treatment 417
hypercalciuria, kidney stones 170
hyperparathyroidism, kidney
  stones 171
hypertension
  cirrhosis 158
  COVID-19 42
  diabetes screenings 57

Index

Index

Index

Index

Index

Index

Index

Index

urinary incontinence (UI)
    benign prostatic hyperplasia
        (BPH) 473
    kidney stones 176
    overview 186–189
    perineal trauma 255
    prostate cancer 89, 306
urinary tract infections (UTIs)
    benign prostatic hyperplasia
        (BPH) 474
    bladder cancer 289
    circumcision 366
    cirrhosis 159
    lupus 25
    orchitis 411
    phimosis 386
    prostatitis 480
    urinary incontinence (UI) 186
urine albumin-to-creatinine ratio
    (UACR), chronic kidney disease
    (CKD) 184
urodynamic tests
    benign prostatic hyperplasia
        (BPH) 477
    prostatitis 484
USPSTF see U.S. Preventive Services
    Task Force
UTIs see urinary tract infections
UV rays see ultraviolet rays

V

vaccines
    chronic obstructive pulmonary
        disease (COPD) 131
    COVID-19 intervention
        strategies 48
    healthy lifestyle choices 669
    human papillomavirus (HPV) 443
Vaccines.gov
    publications
        human papillomavirus
            (HPV) 673n

influenza (flu) 676n
    vaccines 671n
vagus nerve stimulation (VNS),
    depression treatment 328
vaped nicotine, tobacco use 568
varicocele
    male infertility 360, 500
    overview 413–415
vas deferens
    depicted 471
    male contraception 358
    testicular cancer 309
    vasectomy 495
vasectomy
    epididymitis 408
    overview 495–499
    reproductive health 358
verapamil, Peyronie disease 383
very-low-density lipoprotein (VLDL),
    lipoprotein panel 600
viagra, erectile dysfunction (ED) 398
viral load, antiretroviral therapy
    (ART) 443
vitamin D supplement, fall
    prevention 538
VLDL see very-low-density lipoprotein
VNS see vagus nerve stimulation

W

WBCs see white blood cells
wheezing
    chronic obstructive pulmonary
        disease (COPD) 130
    lung cancer 280
white blood cells (WBCs)
    epididymitis 407
    Peyronie disease 383
    X-linked agammaglobulinemia
        (XLA) 236
withdrawal
    depression 326

Index